INFECTION CONTROL IN THE ICU ENVIRONMENT

PERSPECTIVES ON CRITICAL CARE INFECTIOUS DISEASES

Jordi Rello, M.D., Series Editor

1. N. Singh and J.M. Aguado (eds.): Infectious Complications in Transplant Recipients. 2000. ISBN 0-7923-7972-1
2. P.O. Eichacker and J. Pugin (eds.): Evolving Concepts in Sepsis and Septic Shock. 2001. ISBN 0-7923-7235-2
3. J. Rello and K. Leeper (eds.): Severe Community Acquired Pneumonia. 2001. ISBN 0-7923-7338-3
4. R.G. Wunderink and J. Rello (eds.): Ventilator Associated Pneumonia. 2001. ISBN 0-7923-7444-4
5. R.A. Weinstein and M. Bonten (eds.): Infection Control in the ICU Environment. 2002. ISBN 0-7923-7415-0

INFECTION CONTROL IN THE ICU ENVIRONMENT

Edited by
ROBERT A. WEINSTEIN
Cook County Hospital and Rush Medical College
1835 W. Harrison St.
Room 129, Durand Bldg.
Chicago, Illinois, USA 60612

MARC J.M. BONTEN
Department of Internal Medicine
Division of Infectious Diseases and Aids
University Medical Center Utrecht
Heidelberglaan 100
Utrecht
The Netherlands

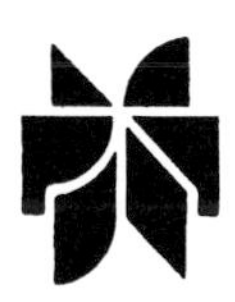

KLUWER ACADEMIC PUBLISHERS
BOSTON / DORDRECHT / LONDON

Distributors for North, Central and South America:
Kluwer Academic Publishers
101 Philip Drive
Assinippi Park
Norwell, Massachusetts 02061 USA
Telephone (781) 871-6600
Fax (781) 681-9045
E-Mail <kluwer@wkap.com>

Distributors for all other countries:
Kluwer Academic Publishers Group
Distribution Centre
Post Office Box 322
3300 AH Dordrecht, THE NETHERLANDS
Telephone 31 78 6392 392
Fax 31 78 6392 254
E-Mail <services@wkap.nl>

Electronic Services <http://www.wkap.nl>

Library of Congress Cataloging-in-Publication Data

Infection control in the ICU environment / edited by Robert A. Weinstein, Marc J.M. Bonten.
p. ; cm. -- (Perspectives on critical care infectious diseases ; 5)
Includes bibliographical references and index.
ISBN 0-7923-7415-0 (hardback : alk. paper)
1. Intensive care units. 2. Nosocomial infections--Prevention. 3. Critical care medicine. I. Weinstein, Robert A. (Robert Alan), 1946- II. Bonten, Marc J. M. III. Series.
[DNLM: 1. Infection Control--methods. 2. Cross Infection--prevention & control. 3. Intensive Care Units. WX 167 I4237 2002]
RA975.5.I56 I565 2002
614.4'4--dc21

2001038474

Printed on acid-free paper.

Printed in the United States of America

CONTENTS

PERSPECTIVES ON CRITICAL CARE INFECTIOUS DISEASES

An Introduction to the Series

Different models of intensive care medicine have been developed worldwide, involving surgeons, anesthetists, internists and critical care physicians. All intensive care departments of hospitals have in common, the highest incidence of antibiotic consumption, the highest incidence of nosocomial infections and community-acquired infections with high degrees of severity. Intensive care areas of hospitals have the largest number of infection outbreaks and require differentiated strategies of prevention.

The specific characteristics of the involved population require differentiated approaches in diagnosis and therapy from those required in classical infectious problems. The specific pharmacodynamic conditions of patients requiring mechanical ventilation or continuous renal replacement, require participation of experts in pharmacology.

The specific objective of this Series is to update therapeutic implications and discuss controversial topics in specific infectious problems involving critically ill patients. Each topic will be discussed by two authors representing the different management perspectives for these controversial and evolving topics. The Guest Editors, one from North America and one from Europe, have invited contributors to present the most recent findings and the specific infectious disease problems and management techniques for critically ill patients, from their perspective.

Jordi Rello, M.D.
Series Editor

PREFACE

Infections are serious and common complications of the treatment of critically ill patients. Intensive Care Unit (ICU) patients become more prone to develop infections as their severity of illness, the complexity of underlying diseases, and the numbers of interventions that breach their host defenses increase. To further complicate care, resistance of ICU pathogens to the newest antimicrobial therapy is emerging, despite current prevention efforts. In such an environment, heightened infection control is of key importance. *Infection Control in the ICU Environment* provides an overarching review that details the most current and high profile infection control problems in ICUs. Authors include noted scientists, intensivisits, and epidemiologists from the United States and Europe and infection control experts from the U.S. Centers for Disease Control and Prevention. The latest problem pathogens in ICUs, particularly Acinetobacter, methicillin-resistant *Staphylococcus aureus*, and vancomycin-resistant Enterococci, are examined in detail. Cutting edge information regarding the potential for prophylactic and/or pre-emptive therapy of fungal infections in ICUs is reviewed. The latest innovations in vascular catheter care and prevention of bloodstream infections are discussed. An up-to-date review of ventilator-associated pneumonia and its prevention is provided. Dissecting fact from fiction and value from ritual in ICU procedures is thoughtfully explored. Finally, the newest innovations in use of mathematical modeling to understand the epidemiology and control of infections in ICUs are presented. The issues discussed in this book are timely, are of global importance, and will remain on our agenda well into the next decade(s).

Marc Bonten, M.D., Ph.D.
Robert A. Weinstein, M.D.

INFECTION CONTROL IN THE ICU ENVIRONMENT

1. SCOPE AND MAGNITUDE OF NOSOCOMIAL ICU INFECTIONS

JUAN ALONSO-ECHANOVE, MD AND
ROBERT P. GAYNES, MD

Centers for Disease Control and Prevention, Atlanta, GA, 30333 USA

INTRODUCTION

Intensive care units (ICUs) are a primary component of modern medicine and are currently in more than 95% of acute-care hospitals in the United States. Although ICUs account for only 5% of hospital beds, they represent 8% to 15% of hospital admissions. Moreover, current health care trends indicate that although the number of beds in U. S. hospitals is decreasing, the number of intensive care beds is increasing. More than one third of patients hospitalized in ICUs develop unexpected complications. In particular, these patients are at high risk of developing nosocomial infections. This is a result of the patients' severity of illness and exposure to life-saving invasive devices and procedures. Numerous studies have reported high rates of infection in ICU patients accounting for >20% of nosocomial infections, with increased morbidity and financial cost and a mortality exceeding 40% (1–7).

The epidemiology of nosocomial infections in ICUs has been extensively studied. Major sites of infection, associated pathogens, and rates vary considerably within hospitals by type of ICU, reflecting differences in the hosts' underlying conditions, types and frequency of invasive devices, patterns of antibiotic use and the selection pressure, and the unique ICU environments (8–11). These observations suggest that each type of ICU may require different control measures. In this chapter, we will provide an overview of predisposing factors for ICU infections, current rates of infection and the distribution by infection site and pathogens in U. S. hospitals.

R.A. Weinstein and M.J.M. Bonten (eds.). INFECTION CONTROL IN THE ICU ENVIRONMENT.

THE ICU ENVIRONMENT AND PREDISPOSING FACTORS FOR NOSOCOMIAL ICU INFECTIONS

ICU-acquired infections are the result of a complex interaction of several factors, including host defense mechanisms and underlying conditions, medical devices, infectious agents and antimicrobial resistance, sources of colonization, and cross-infection.

Natural host defense mechanisms in ICU patients are frequently impaired by underlying diseases or as a result of medical or surgical interventions. The normal skin barriers are broken by vascular cannulas, chemical barriers in the stomach are neutralized by acid-reducing medications, and cleaning mechanisms of hollow organs are disrupted by several types of tubes and catheters. In addition, patients at the extremes of age or with certain underlying diseases may have impaired immune response to infectious agents. Finally, malnutrition occurs in 10% to 50% of ICU patients, as a result of both suspending food intake and having conditions that increase the metabolic demands, e.g., injuries, fever, tachycardia, and perfusion deficits (12). Although its clinical significance is not well established, poor nutritional status may increase a patient's risk of acquiring nosocomial infections (13–15).

The importance of medical devices as risk factors for infections has been demonstrated repeatedly. Pneumonia and bloodstream and urinary tract infections, the three most common ICU-related infections, are almost always associated with the use of an invasive device. Therefore, presence of ventilators, central lines, and urinary catheters and the duration of use of such devices are the two most important risk factors for device-associated infections (16,17). These findings emphasize the importance of monitoring device use and assessing such use as a risk factor when examining an ICU's nosocomial infection experience.

Increasing rates of nosocomial infections have been observed among patients with more severe illnesses. In order to estimate the risk of acquiring nosocomial infections, several severity-of-illness score systems have been proposed. Unfortunately, since most were developed to predict mortality, these indices are inconsistent predictors of nosocomial infections in ICUs; when controlling for device utilization, none of them has proved useful when assessing the site-specific risk of acquiring device-associated infections (18).

Colonization with organisms and cross-transmission between patients via a "contaminated carrier" play a critical role in the pathogenesis of ICU-related nosocomial infections. Host colonization precedes infection with the same organism in >50% of ICU-acquired infections (19–23). Factors associated with microorganism colonization are similar to those associated with development of infection, including length of stay, invasive devices, antibiotic therapy, elimination of the patient's normal flora, and disruption of normal mechanical defense mechanisms. Several factors unique to ICUs contribute to cross-transmission of organisms. Among these, the large number and wide variety of health care workers and the urgent nature of critical care may alter the level of compliance with hand-washing and isolation practices. Also, the degree of asepsis used in maintaining invasive devices and specific agents used for hand-washing may facilitate cross-transmission of pathogens (24,25).

SITE DISTRIBUTION OF NOSOCOMIAL ICU INFECTIONS

Urinary tract infection (UTI), pneumonia, and primary bloodstream infection (BSI) are the three sites of adult and pediatric ICU-related nosocomial infections and constitute 64% to 77% of reported infections. Surgical site infection (SSI) account for 12% of nosocomial infections in surgical ICUs (SICUs) and 8% in medical-surgical ICUs (MS-ICUs), and are less common in medical (MICUs) and coronary care units (CCUs) (<4%). The distribution of major sites of infection varies by type of ICU (Figure 1). In addition, within pediatric ICUs (PICUs) and neonatal ICUs (NICUs), major sites of infection vary by age group and birth weight (Table 1).

Data for Figure 1 and Table 1 come from 112 MICUs, 102 CCUs, 205 MS-ICUs, and 142 SICUs from hospitals participating in the Centers for Disease Control and Prevention's (CDC's) National Nosocomial Infections Surveillance (NNIS) System; from 1992 through 1997, these ICU groups reported over 14,000, 6,000, 29,000, and 26,000 infections respectively (26–28). Among MICUs and CCUs, UTI was the most frequent nosocomial infection (31% and 35%, respectively) followed by pneumonia (27% and 24%) and primary BSI (19% and 17%). In SICUs and MS-ICUs, pneumonia was the most frequent site of infection (33% and 32%) followed by UTI (20% and 23%) and BSI (16% and 14%). Among the over 6000 nosocomial infections reported by 61 PICUs during the same study period, primary BSI was the most frequent (21% to 34%), followed by pneumonia (18% to 26%) and UTI (12% to 22%) (29). This may reflect lower rates of urinary catheter use in PICUs. Finally, among the more than 13,000 nosocomial infections reported by 99 NICUs from 1986 through 1994, primary BSI (32% to 49%) and pneumonia (12% to 18%) were also the first and second most frequent infections respectively, with eye, ear, nose and throat (EENT) infections third (8% to 21%) (30). Most nosocomial UTIs (77% to 95%), pneumonias (82 to 99%), and primary BSIs (82 to 91%) were strongly associated with the use of urinary catheters, ventilators, and central lines, respectively. This association was observed consistently across different types of units, age groups, and birth weight categories.

The distribution of specific sites of nosocomial infection also varied by type of ICU, age, and birth weight. Within MS-ICUs, the distribution was very similar among surgical and medical patients except for SSIs. Among primary BSIs, laboratory-confirmed bloodstream infections consistently constituted the vast majority across different types of ICUs (91% to 93% of all primary BSIs). However, in NICUs clinical sepsis accounted for a substantial proportion of primary BSIs (13% to 20%). Asymptomatic UTIs represented a larger proportion of UTIs in adult ICUs (37% to 44%) than in PICUs (16% to 19%). Endocarditis was quite uncommon in adult ICUs (<2%) but relatively more frequent in PICUs (13% to 45% of all cardiovascular infections). Sinusitis was the most common EENT infection among children >5 years old and adults (>51%) whereas conjuctivitis and other eye infections were the most common in NICUs and children ≤2 months old (>54%). Skin and soft tissue infections were consistently the most common SSI in all types of ICUs and accounted for 50% to 78% of the SSIs.

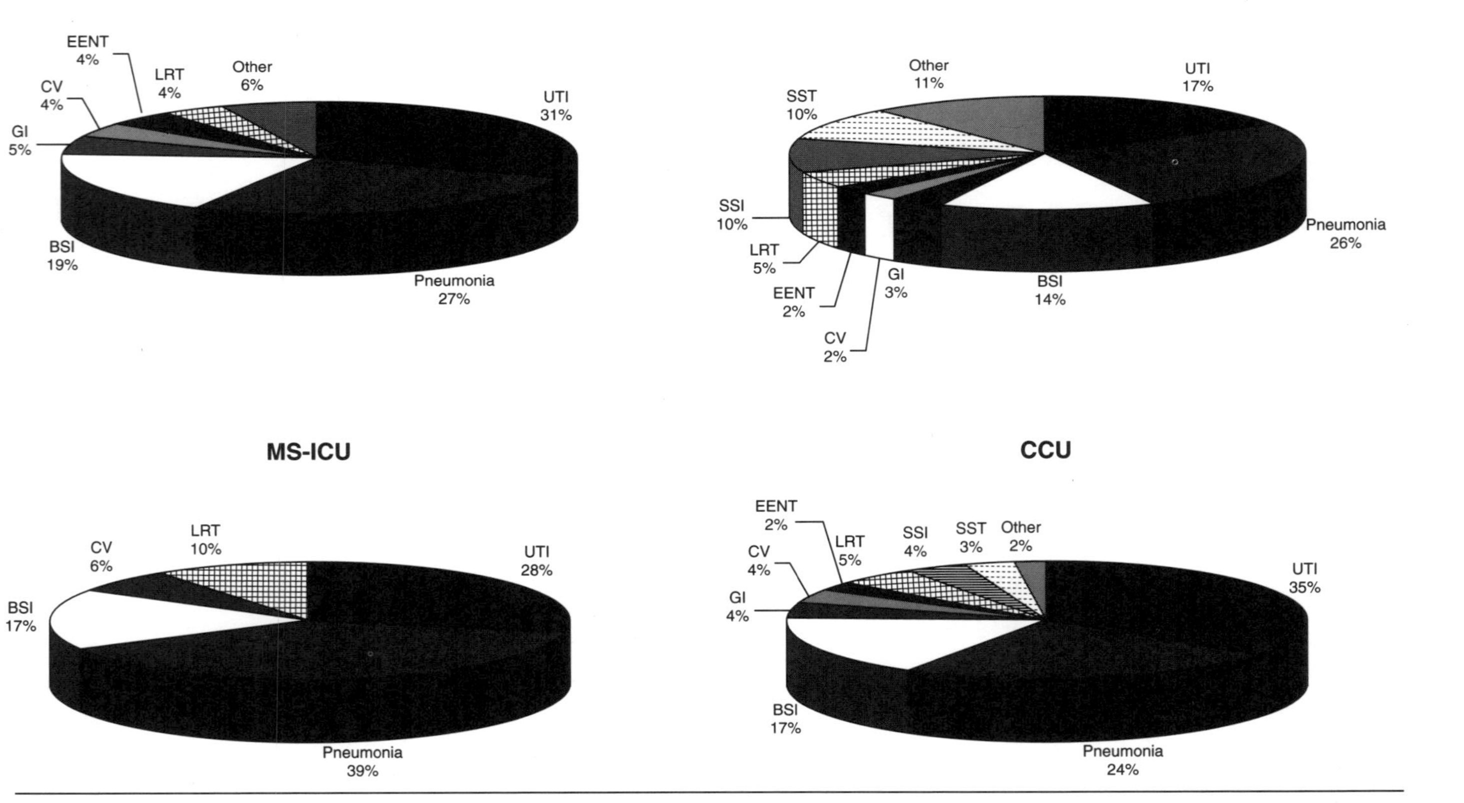

Figure 1. Distribution of ICU-associated nosocomial infections reported to the CDC's National Nosocomial Infection Surveillance System by type of ICU, 1992–1997.

Type of ICU: MICU = Medical ICU; SICU = Surgical ICU; MS-ICU = Medical-Surgical ICU; CCU = Coronary Care Unit.
Major infection site: UTI = Urinary tract infections; BSI = Primary bloodstream infections; GI = Gastrointestinal infections; CV = Cardiovascular infections;

Table 1. Distribution of Percentages of ICU-associated Nosocomial Infections Among Neonatal and Pediatric ICUs Participating in NNIS, by Birth Weight (NICUs), and Age (PICUs)

	NICU[1]				PICU[2]			
Infections	≤1000 g	>1000 g and ≤1500 g	>1500 g and ≤2500 g	>2500 g	≤2 Months	>2 Months and ≤5 Years	>5 Years and ≤12 Years	>12 Years
UTI[3]	—	—	—	—	12	14	17	22
Pneumonia	16	12	13	18	18	20	26	21
BSI[4]	49	45	32	36	34	28	21	25
Gastrointestinal	7	10	11	5	4	5	4	4
Cardiovascular	—	—	—	—	2	2	2	1
EENT[5]	8	14	21	13	5	7	7	7
Lower resp. tract	—	—	—	—	10	13	11	9
SSI[6]	1	1	3	7	10	6	7	6
Skin and soft tissues	6	7	10	9	3	3	3	3
Other	13	11	10	12	2	2	2	2

[1] NICU = Neonatal ICU; [2] PICU = Pediatric IC; [3] UTI = Urinary tract infections; [4] BSI = Primary bloodstream infections; [5] EENT = Ear, Eye, Nose and Throat; [6] SSI = Surgical site infections.

Other authors have reported similar distributions of infections by type of ICU (8). However, pneumonia has been reported as the most frequent major site of infection in medical (37% to 54%) and pediatric (20%–50%) ICUs in several studies (8,31).

These differences most likely reflect differences in patient mix and critical care practices, especially in device utilization.

PATHOGEN DISTRIBUTION OF NOSOCOMIAL ICU INFECTIONS

Based on data reported to the NNIS system by MICUs, SICUs, MS-ICUs, and PICUs from 1992 through 1997, and from NICUs from 1990 through 1995, gram-negative aerobes accounted for the majority of ICU-related nosocomial infections (>50%), followed in frequency by gram-positive aerobes (>30%) and fungi (>10%). *P. aeruginosa*, *S. aureus*, coagulase-negative staphylococci, *Enterococcus* spp. and *Enterobacter* spp. were the five most common pathogens, with each accounting for approximately 10% of the infections. However, the distribution of pathogens differed markedly by infection site and also by type of ICU (Table 2) (26–30).

Urinary tract infections. Nosocomial UTIs are caused predominantly by aerobic gram-negative bacteria in all types of ICUs (40%–56%), followed by fungi, which are almost as frequent as gram-negative bacteria in MICUs (39%) and MS-ICUs (31%). *Escherichia coli*, *Candida albicans*, and *Enterococcus* spp., accounted for almost 50% of all UTIs. *P. aeruginosa* was also a frequent pathogen, accounting for 7% to 13% of UTIs. *Candida* spp. were usually associated with asymptomatic UTIs and also were more commonly reported in catheter-associated UTIs than in non-catheter associated infections (26). This increased frequency of UTIs caused by fungi observed in the last decade may partially reflect more extensive use of broad-spectrum antimicrobial agents.

Nosocomial pneumonia. Nosocomial pneumonias were largely caused by aerobic gram-negative bacteria (40% to 52%) in all types of ICUs except NICUs, where gram-positive cocci were equally reported as a frequent cause of pneumonia. In 7% to 10% of nosocomial pneumonias, no organism was reported. *P. aeruginosa*, *S. aureus* and *Enterobacter* spp. were the three most common causes of nosocomial pneumonia in adult ICUs, accounting for 44% to 50% of all such episodes. In PICUs and NICUs, *H. influenzae* and coagulase-negative staphylococcus respectively were also frequent pneumonia pathogens. *S. aureus* has been reported as a cause of 2% to 48% of nosocomial pneumonias in studies from single institutions (32–34). This range partially reflects variation in the ICU patient population as demonstrated in NNIS hospitals, but also differences in the invasive techniques used for the diagnosis of nosocomial pneumonia. In NNIS hospitals, the microbiology of pneumonia is based predominantly on sputum cultures.

Primary bloodstream infections. There is substantial consistency in the pathogen distribution primary BSIs among different types of ICUs. Gram-positive cocci were the most common pathogens (59% to 75%). Gram-negative organisms

Table 2. Percent Distribution of Selected Pathogens Reported to NNIS for the Three Most Common Sites of Infections, by type of ICU

Infection Site	Pathogens	[1]NICU (N = 99)	[2]PICU (N = 61)	[3]MICU (N = 112)	[4]SICU (N = 142)	[5]MS-ICU (N = 205)	[6]CCU (N = 102)
Bloodstream Infections	Coag-neg staphylococcus	51	38	36	36	39	37
	Enterococcus spp.	6	11	16	15	11	10
	Staphylococcus aureus	7	9	13	11	11	24
	Candida albicans	7	5	6	4	6	3
	Klebsiella pneumoniae	2	4	4	4	2	2
	P. aeruginosa	—	5	3	4	4	2
	Escherichia coli	4	3	3	3	2	3
	Enterobacter	3	6	3	6	4	3
	Group B streptococcus	8	<1	—	0	—	—
Pneumonia	*P. aeruginosa*	12	22	21	17	16	14
	Staphylococcus aureus	17	17	20	17	17	21
	Enterobacter	8	2	9	13	11	9
	Klebsiella pneumoniae	6	5	8	7	7	8
	Acinetobacter	—	3	6	6	3	3
	Candida albicans	—	2	5	4	6	6
	Escherichia coli	6	4	3	5	4	4
	Serratia marcescens	—	4	1	4	4	4
	Group B streptococcus	6	<1	—	0	—	—
	Coag-neg staphylococcus	16	1	1	1	2	2
Urinary Tract Infections	*Candida albicans*	—	14	21	16	15	6
	Enterococci	—	10	14	14	14	14
	Escherichia coli	—	19	14	15	18	28
	P. aeruginosa	—	13	10	13	10	7
	Other fungi	—	2	8	5	16	5
	Klebsiella pneumoniae	—	7	6	6	5	6
	Enterobacter	—	10	5	6	4	4
	Proteus mirabilis	—	—	2	3	—	4

[1]NICU = Neonatal ICU; [2]PICU = Pediatric ICU; [3]MICU = Medical ICU; [4]SICU = Surgical ICU; [5]MS-ICU = Medical-Surgical ICU; [6]CCU = Coronary Care Unit.

were reported in 9% to 22% and fungi in 7% to 15% of nosocomial BSIs. Coagulase-negative staphylococcus was the most common BSI pathogen reported in all types of ICUs (36% to 51%), and was two to seven times more common than either *Enterococcus* spp. (6% to 16%) or *S. aureus* (7% to 24%). The latter two pathogens were reported with similar frequency but *Enterococcus* spp. was more common than *S. aureus* in MICUs and SICUs and *S. aureus* was more common in CCUs. Group B streptococcal infections were reported frequently in NICUs (8% of all nosocomial infections) but most were maternally-acquired infections. Little difference was observed in the distribution of gram-negative species. Finally, fungi, particularly *C. albicans,* were reported in a substantial proportion of nosocomial bloodstream infections.

PATHOGEN DISTRIBUTION AND THE USE OF INVASIVE DEVICES

The pathogen distribution for device-associated infections is different from that of non-device-associated infections (26,28,29) for certain types of ICUs.

Fungi and specifically *C. albicans* were reported significantly more often in catheter-associated UTIs than in non-catheter-associated infections in MICUs, MS-ICUs, and PICUs. Likewise, *P. aeruginosa* was reported more commonly in catheter-associated UTIs in PICUs.

An association with ventilator use was observed with certain gram-negative organisms in MICUs and MS-ICUs. *P. aeruginosa*, *Acinetobacter* spp., and *Enterobacter* spp. were reported more frequently in ventilator-associated pneumonias than in non-ventilator-associated pneumonias in MS-ICUs, and the first two also were reported more frequently in ventilator-associated pneumonias in MICUs. Conversely, *E. coli* was less commonly reported in ventilator-associated pneumonias in both types of ICUs, as were viral pneumonia in PICUs.

Similarly, some pathogens were associated with the use of central lines. In MS-ICUs and PICUs, coagulase-negative staphylococci and *C. albicans* were reported significantly more often in primary BSIs associated with central lines than in non-central line-associated infections. Coagulase-negative staphylococci, but not *C. albicans,* was also reported more frequently in central line-associated BSIs in MICUs. Finally, *S. aureus* was significantly more common in non-central line associated BSI in MS-ICUs.

TEMPORAL CHANGES IN PATHOGEN DISTRIBUTION

Significant changes in pathogen distribution have been observed over the last few years, especially in UTIs and BSIs (Table 3).

From 1986 through 1995, over 600 ICUs reported at least one complete month of data to the NNIS system. Over the last 5 years, there was an increase in the proportion of catheter-associated UTIs caused by fungi, in the proportion of ventilator-associated pneumonias caused by gram-positive cocci and fungi, and in the proportion of central line-associated BSIs caused by gram-positive cocci. For all three sites, the proportion of device-associated nosocomial infections caused by

Table 3. Pathogens Associated with the Three Most Common ICU-acquired Nosocomial Infections, NNIS System, 1986–1995

	1986–1989		1990–1995	
Infection Site and Pathogen	N	%	N	%
Central line-associated [1]*BSI*				
Gram-negative pathogens	2832	57.2	7938	64.0
Gram-positive pathogens	1149	23.2	2420	19.5
Fungal pathogens	608	12.3	1362	11.0
Anaerobic pathogens	68	1.4	85	0.7
Other	289	5.9	611	4.8
Ventilator-associated Pneumonia				
Gram-negative pathogens	7038	72.8	15388	67.1
Gram-positive pathogens	1968	21.2	5580	24.3
Fungal pathogens	468	5.0	1477	6.4
Viral pathogens	37	0.4	87	0.4
Other	64	0.7	391	1.8
Catheter-associated [2]*UTI*				
Gram-negative pathogens	6132	52.2	10033	47.0
Fungal pathogens	2595	22.1	6249	29.3
Gram-positive pathogens	2545	22.0	4270	20.0
Viral pathogens	2	0.0	5	0.0
Other	474	3.7	802	3.7

[1] BSI = Bloodstream infection; [2] UTI = Urinary tract infection.

gram-negative pathogens decreased. Finally, the proportion of central line-associated BSIs caused by fungi and specifically by *C. albicans* also decreased.

When we looked at trends over time in the pathogen distribution of device-associated infections from 1992 through 1997 for specific types of ICUs, we demonstrated significant changes in the distribution of only a few bacteria in MS-ICUs and PICUs (28,29). We observed significant increases in the proportion of patients with device-associated infections caused by specific organisms. Ventilator-associated pneumonias caused by *Enterobacter* spp. increased in PICUs (7% to 13%) and MS-ICUs (9% to 13%). Central line-associated bloodstream infections caused by coagulase-negative staphylococci increased in MS-ICUs (31% to 45%) and those caused by *P. aeruginosa* increased in PICUs (3% to 7%). Finally, SSIs caused by *S. aureus* increased in MS-ICUs (8% to 11%).

COMPARING NOSOCOMIAL INFECTION RATES AMONG ICUS

We have previously demonstrated in the NNIS system that the commonly reported overall patient and patient-day nosocomial infection rates may be misleading because they are strongly correlated with average length of stay and device use (11). Therefore, differences in rates among several units or within the same unit over time may be related to variation in either the length of stay or the frequency or intensity of device use rather than to an increase in the infection risk. However, when we used device-days as the denominator, the resulting site-specific device-associated infection rates were no longer confounded by these factors or other hospital or ICU characteristics, i.e., hospital bed-size, ICU bed-size, or teaching affiliation.

We have also demonstrated that site-specific device-associated infection rates vary by ICU type (11). Therefore, combining data from all of a hospital's ICUs when calculating and comparing ICU infection rates can also be misleading. In the NNIS system, rates of device-associated infections are aggregated from approximately 300 hospitals and reported every 6 months stratified by type of ICU. Significant differences in the median and the distribution of device-specific rates are observed across different types of ICUs. For instance, we reviewed data recently reported from medical and pediatric ICUs from 1992 through 1997 (26,29). In this review, we observed that the rates of ventilator-associated pneumonia and catheter-associated UTIs were lower in adult MICUs than in PICUs (5.9 vs 9.1 and 5.9 vs 9.5 infections/1000 device-days, respectively), but the rate of central line associated BSIs was higher (7.3 vs 3.1 infections/1000 device-days). Therefore, the ventilator-associated pneumonia rate, central line-associated BSI rate, and catheter-associated UTI rate stratified by ICU type are currently the most useful rates for inter- and intra-hospital comparison and for comparison over time.

Even after stratifying by type of ICU, considerable variation is observed in the distribution of device-associated infection rates across participating type-specific ICUs (Table 4).

This suggests that there are differences in the distribution of other intrinsic or extrinsic risk factors, including hospital characteristics, severity of illness, underlying conditions, duration of device use at a patient level, different types of invasive devices, or drugs administered during the ICU stay. In a recent review of MS-ICUs we identified major teaching affiliation as a hospital characteristic that was significantly associated with an increased risk of infection for each of the three most frequent device-specific infection sites (28). As a result, device-associated rates for MS-ICUs are further stratified in "Major teaching" and "All others" categories. Ongoing research within a selected number of ICUs participating in the NNIS system is currently addressing this issue in the Detailed ICU Surveillance Component (DISC) study, a prospective multicenter observational study that will hopefully help us to identify one or several significant risk factors useful for surveillance purpose.

COMMENTS

Nosocomial infections are a major cause of morbidity and mortality in ICU patients. Many factors influence the risk of nosocomial infections in these patients, and considerable progress has been made in the last decade in understanding the epidemiology of this common complication. Particularly, we have learned that the type of ICU is a surrogate for a certain patient-mix and for certain medical practices that are reflected in the different distributions of infections, pathogens, and device-associated rates of infection observed in each type of ICU. We also have learned the importance of the infection site and device use in determining the likely pathogen causing an infection, which in turn may direct empiric therapy. Finally, we have

Table 4. Selected Percentiles for Distribution of Device-associated Infection Rates*, by Type of ICU, NNIS System, January 1992–October 1998

					[4]MS-ICU		
Infection Site	Percentile	[1]PICU (N = 62)	[2]MICU (N = 125)	[3]SICU (N = 146)	Major teaching (N = 83)	All others (N = 148)	[5]CCU (N = 105)
Central-line associated							
[6]BSI	10%	1.7	1.5	1.3	1.7	1.1	0.0
	Median	7.1	5.4	4.9	6.1	3.8	4.1
	90%	12.8	10.2	9.8	9.3	6.9	8.9
Ventilator-associated							
Pneumonia	10%	0.0	1.8	5.4	3.7	3.6	0.1
	Median	4.0	7.4	12.3	11.0	9.6	7.3
	90%	11.4	15.5	25.1	18.8	15.4	16.5
Catheter-associated							
[7]UTI	10%	0.9	1.9	1.1	2.8	1.1	1.2
	Median	4.9	6.8	4.9	7.4	4.3	6.2
	90%	11.1	12.2	9.3	10.8	7.1	13.8

[1] PICU = Pediatric ICU; [2] MICU = Medical ICU; [3] SICU = Surgical ICU; [4] MS-ICU = Medical-Surgical ICU; [5] CCU = Coronary Care Unit; [6] BSI = Bloodstream infection; [7] UTI = Urinary tract infection.
*Rate = Number of device-associated infections/1000 device-days; N = number of reporting ICUs.

learned that device utilization is, to date, the single most important independent risk factor for acquiring any of the three most common nosocomial infections, and that device-associated nosocomial infection rates are currently the most useful rates for inter- and intra-hospital comparison, and comparison over time.

REFERENCE LIST

1. Wenzel R. Epidemiology and control of nosocomial infections in adult intensive care units. Am J Med 1991;91(Supp 3B):179S–184S.
2. Archibald L, Phillips L, Monnet D, et al. Antimicrobial resistance in isolates from impatients and outpatients in the United States: increasing importance of the intensive care unit. Clin Infect Dis 1997;24:211–215.
3. Donowitz LG, Wenzel R, Hoyt JW. High risk of hospital-acquired infections in the ICU patient. Infect Control Hosp Epidemiol 1982;10:355–357.
4. Emori T, Gaynes R. An overview of nosocomial infections, including the role of the microbiology laboratory. Clin Microbiol Rev 1993;428–442.
5. Weinstein JW, Mazon D, Pantelick E, Reagan-Cirincione P, Dembry LM, Hierholzer WJ. A decade of prevalence surveys in a tertiary-care center: trends in nosocomial infection rates, device utilization, and patient acuity. Infect Control Hosp Epidemiol 1999;20(8):543–548.
6. Brown RB, Colodny SM, Drapkin MS, et al. One-day prevalence study of nosocomial infections, antibiotic usage, and selected infection control practices in adult medical/surgical intensive care units in the United States [Abstract]. The Fifth Annual Meeting of the Society for Healthcare Epidemiology, San Diego, CA, April 2–5, 1995. Infect Control Hosp Epidemiol 1995;(supp).
7. Wenzel R, Thompson RL, Landry SM, et al. Hospital-acquired infections in intensive care unit patients: an overview with emphasis on epidemics. Infect Control Hosp Epidemiol 1983;4:371–375.
8. Pittet D, Herwaldt LA, Massanari RM. The Intensive Care Unit. In: Brachman P, Bennett J, editors. Hospital Infections. Boston: Little, Brown and Company, 1992:405–439.
9. Daschner F, Frey P, Wolff G, Baumann P. Nosocomial infections in intensive care wards: a multicenter prospective study. Intensive Care Med 1982;8:5–9.
10. Goldmann DA, Durbin WA, Freeman J. Nosocomial infections in a neonatal intensive care unit. J Infect Dis 1981;144:449–451.
11. Jarvis WR, Edwards JR, Culver D, et al. Nosocomial infection rates in adult and pediatric intensive care units in the United States. Am J Med 1991;91((Supp 3B)):185S–191S.
12. Apelgren KN, Wilmore DW. Nutritional care of the critically ill patient. Surg Clin North Am 1983;63((2)):497–507.
13. Pingleton SK. Enteral nutrition and infection in the intensive care unit. Semin Respir Infect 1990;5:185–190.
14. Christman JW, McCain RW. A sensible approach to the nutritional support of mechanically ventilated critically ill patients. Intensive Care Med 1993;19:129–136.
15. Isaack H, Mbise RL, Hirji KF. Nosocomial bacterial infections among children with severe protein energy malnutrition. East Afr Med J 1992;69:433–436.
16. Garibaldi RA, Burke JP, Dickman ML, et al. Factors predisposing to bacteriuria during indwelling urethral catheterization. N Eng J Med 1974;291:215–219.
17. Wenzel RP, Osterman CA, Donowitz LG, et al. Identification of procedure-related nosocomial infections in high risk patients. Rev Infect Dis 1981;3:701–705.
18. Gaynes RP, Culver D, Banerjee S, et al. Meaningful interhospital comparison of infection rates in intensive care units. Am J Infect Control 1993;21:43–44.
19. Kerver AJ, Rommes JH, Mevissen Verhage EA, et al. Prevention of colonization and infection in critically ill patients: a prospective randomized study. Crit Care Med 1988;16:1087–1093.
20. Heyland DK, Cook DJ, Jaeschke R, Griffith L, Lee HN, Guyatt GH. Selective decontamination of the digestive tract: an overview. Chest 1994;105:1221–1229.
21. Flynn DM, Weinstein RA, Kabins S. Infections with gram-negative bacilli in a cardiac surgery intensive care unit: the relative role of enterobacter. J Hosp Infect 1988;11((supp A)):367–373.
22. Wey SB, Mori M, Pfaller MA, Woolson RF, Wenzel RP. Risk factors for hospital-acquired candidemia: a matched case-control study. Arch Intern Med 1989;149:2349–2353.

23. Pittet D, Garbino J. Fungal infections in the critically ill. Curr Opin Crit Care 1995;1:369–380.
24. Fridkin SF, Pear SM, Williamson TH, et al. The role of understaffing in central venous catheter-associated bloodstream infections. Infect Control Hosp Epidemiol 1996;17:150–158.
25. Haley RP, Bregman DA. The role of understaffing and overcrowding in recurrent outbreaks of staphylococcal infection in a neonatal special-care unit. J Infect Dis 1982;245:875–885.
26. Richards MJ, Edwards JR, Culver D, Gaynes RP, and the National Nosocomial Infections Surveillance System. Nosocomial infections in medical intensive care units in the United States. Crit Care Med 1999;27(5):887–854.
27. Richards MJ, Edwards JR, Culver D, Gaynes RP, and the National Nosocomial Infections Surveillance System. Nosocomial infections in coronary care units in the United States. Am J Cardiol 1998;82:789–793.
28. Centers for Disease Control and Prevention. Unpublished data 1999.
29. Richards MJ, Edwards JR, Culver D, Gaynes RP, and the National Nosocomial Infections Surveillance System. Nosocomial infections in pediatric intensive care units in the United States. Pediatrics 1999;103(4):1–7.
30. Gaynes RP, Edwards JR, Jarvis WR, Culver D, Tolson J, Martone WJ, and the National Nosocomial Infections Surveillance System. Nosocomial infections among neonates in high-risk nurseries in the United States. Pediatrics 1996;98(3):357–361.
31. Dahmash NS, Arora SC, Fayed DF, et al. Infections in critically ill patients: experience in MICU at a major teaching hospital. Infection 1994;22:264–270.
32. Torres A, Aznar R, Gatell JM. Incidence, risk, and prognosis factors of nosocomial pneumonia in mechanically ventilated patients. Am Rev Respir Dis 1990;142:523–528.
33. Rello J, Ausina V, Castella J, et al. Nosocomial respiratory tract infections in multiple trauma patients. Chest 1996;102:525–529.
34. Rello J, Quintana E, Ausina V, et al. Incidence, etiology, and outcome of nosocomial pneumonia in mechanically ventilated patients. Chest 1996;100:439–444.

2. SCOPE AND MAGNITUDE OF NOSOCOMIAL ICU INFECTIONS

MAAIKE M.S. IBELINGS, M.D. AND HAJO A. BRUINING, M.D., PH.D.

University Hospital Rotterdam Dijkzigt, PO Box 2040, 3000 CA Rotterdam, The Netherlands

INTRODUCTION

The scope and magnitude of nosocomial (ICU) infections is overwhelming, with a negative impact on both the added morbidity and the mortality, and as a consequence on the overall hospital charges and economic costs. Many studies come to similar results (1–6). This is not a special European, but also acknowledged to be a worldwide problem. It is special for the ICU, with considerably higher rates of nosocomial infection than in other hospital wards (2,7–10). Aggressive invasive diagnostics, multiple therapies and a plethora of invasive devices in combination with a temporarily compromised immunity renders the ICU patient population uniquely susceptible to nosocomial infections (11–14). Overall, intrinsic risk together with extrinsic factors make the ICU patient extremely vulnerable to nosocomial infections. As stated by Meakins et al. "Infection is their Achilles heel" (15). With the continuous recognition, the past few years, of new and more virulent organisms and with a rapid growth in antimicrobial resistance, the problem becomes even worse. Towards the year 2000 the medical profession will face the challenge of infections against which none of the current antimicrobial agents are effective; many clinicians unfortunately are not aware of this impending crisis (16).

The problem of the nosocomial ICU infections will continue to limit the potential advances to be made in critical care medicine. It is therefore of paramount concern to reduce this impact. There is still room for improvement in the control of these ICU infections. Results of the study on the Efficacy of Nosocomial Infec-

R.A. Weinstein and M.J.M. Bonten (eds.). INFECTION CONTROL IN THE ICU ENVIRONMENT.

tion Control (SENIC) have suggested that up to one third of nosocomial infections to which the modern hospital is prone should be preventable (17). An epidemiological database is needed to make a quantification of the scale of the ICU infection problem and to identificate the factors, both intrinsic and extrinsic, that affect it, highlighting the risks to which the ICU patient is exposed. Awareness of the problem of these risks has already been shown to be an important factor in successful implementation of infection control policies (17,18). Investigation of this entity of infection risk must lead to targeted surveillance programmes and the subsequent initiation of appropriate infection control measures, better prevention and appropriate therapy, hopefully resulting in lower infection rates, morbidity, mortality and substantial savings for the hospital budget.

There is a remarkable difference in the knowledge of the magnitude of the infection problem between the USA and Europe. In the United States systematized information concerning the rates of nosocomial infections, ethiological organisms and risk factors are available due to the development of various national formalized systems for ongoing surveillance. In the 1960s, the Centers for Disease Control (CDC) in Georgia began recommending that hospitals conduct surveillance over the occurrence of nosocomial infections to obtain epidemiological evidence on which to base rational control measures (19,20). After an international conference on nosocomial infections in Chicago in 1970 (21) and diverse publications (22) a nationwide movement toward the establishment of organized infection surveillance ensued, and by the end of the 1970s the majority of US nation's hospitals had jumped on the "surveillance bandwagon" (23). In January 1974, CDC initiated the SENIC Project (Study on the Efficacy of Nosocomial Infection Control, 24) to determine whether and, if so, to what extent, this control program approach was effective in reducing nosocomial infection risks (17). Of more recent date the National Nosocomial Infection Surveillance (NNIS) study was generated by 80 medical centers in the USA from 1980–1992 (25). In Europe, no such formalized systems exist, and there has been no large international study to determine the nosocomial infection rates throughout the continent, up to 1992. Only a few studies have been undertaken in individual countries (Table 1, 26–31). With relatively few hospitals taking part in each country and with very low numbers of patients, so examining only hospital-limited rates of infections. Besides, the design of the protocol of these studies differed widely (prevalence opposite incidence studies, 32). Consequently it is thus absolutely inappropriate to extrapolate the data from these studies to overall, European, epidemiological ICU settings.

THE EPIC STUDY

It was against this background that in 1992 the European Prevalence of Infection in Intensive Care (EPIC) study was undertaken,—the largest ever study of this type, conducted throughout Europ—to deal with the relative lack of information concerning nosocomial ICU infections, providing a new perspective on the scale of the problem in Europe.

Table 1. Studies before 1992 of nosocomial infection rates in Europe

Country	Reference	Type of study	Infection rate (%)	No. of ICUs surveyed	No. of patients Included
Sweden	(26), 1978	Point prevalence	72	3	29
Germany, Switzerland	(27), 1982	3-year incidence	12,5 7,2 total: 3–27	5 4	5374 1578
Italy	(28), 1986	Prevalence	6,8–12,4 (hosp-ICU)	130	34577
Italy	(29), 1987	1-year incidence	26,9	4	859
Belgium	(30), 1987	Point prevalence	9,3	106	8723
Spain	(31), 1990	Prevalence	26,8–46,6 (hosp-ICU)	33	7434

The Aims of the Study

The primary aim of the EPIC study was to determine, during exactly one day, the prevalence of ICU-acquired infections in patients on ICUs in 17 European countries. In addition, the study had a number of subsidiary aims: to differentiate the prevalence rates of specific types of nosocomial infections, to establish the microbiology and thus determining those pathogens considered to be causal of these infections, including their patterns of antimicrobial susceptibility (or resistance) to particular antibiotics, to assess the pattern of antimicrobial prescribing, to identify risk factors for infection and to establish the relative importance of these factors by correlating them with the rates and types of infection, to correlate rates of infection with the patients clinical status on admission and with their outcome (death or survival) at a predefined end point in a 6 week follow-up period, and finally to compare infection rates in different types of ICUs and to gauge the variations in infection rates between units in the 17 different countries throughout Europe. The overall key aim of the EPIC Study was to raise awareness of the problems of nosocomial infection in the ICU and to stimulate discussion, hopefully leading to better prevention, appropriate therapy and improving infection control programs.

The Protocol of the Study

This point prevalence study was conducted on a 24-hour period, 29 April 1992. On the study day, information was collected for later analysis on 10038 patients in 1417 adult, non-coronary care ICUs in 17 Western European countries, by questionnaire. Nosocomial infections in ICU were classified according to standard definitions of the Centers for Disease Control, CDC (33). Assessment of the patient's status on admission was made on the basis of his/her APACHE II score (Acute Physiology and Chronic Health Evaluation, 34,35). A logistic regression analysis was done to estimate the effects of possible risk factors, measured as odds ratios (OR, comparing relative risks), together with their 95% confidence intervals (CI). In addition multiple logistic regression analysis was done to assess which independent factors affected the overall risks of infection and death, and to investigate the relationship between these different risk factors. The complete methods have been described elsewhere (36,37). The most important reservation of the study to be mentioned, is the difficulty of identifying pathogens, who may have only reflected possible contamination or colonization in stead of represented the cause of the infection.

THE EPIC RESULTS: EUROPE OVERALL

Participation and Demographics of ICUs in Europe

Data from 1417 participating Intensive Care Units, in 17 European countries, were entered in to the study database providing a total of 10038 completed case report forms suitable for analysis. Half of these ICUs were situated in community-based hospitals (51%), 35% in university hospitals, and 14% in university-affiliated hospitals. Most units (74%) were mixed medical/surgical ICUs. The majority of ICUs (57%) were of intermediate size, consisting of 6–10 beds, though 25% were large, having 11 or more beds. Most ICUs (74%) admitted up to 14 patients per week, although a substantial number (11%) had a high admission rate of 22 or more patients per week. There was an average bed occupancy rate on the study day of 79%. The great majority of ICUs had a full-time director (67%) and/or 24-hour physician cover (72%), with consequently up to a quarter having only part-time cover. Other staff regularly joining the ICU teams included a microbiologist (overall 43%), an infection control nurse (24%), a pharmacist (20%) and an infectious diseases specialist (15%). Half of the ICUs (58%) used a written infection control policy (the others having only an informal policy), only a quarter (25%) used a written antibiotic policy, and 66% used regular bacteriological surveillance on the ICU.

Patient Demographics

The EPIC Study population was largely male (62%), and overall predominantly aged over 40 years (83%), 30% was even older than 70 years. Female patients tended to be older than men (mean age 61 and 51 years respectively). From the scored underlying conditions organ failure (of one type or another) was mostly present, in over half of the study population (57%) (Table 2). Half of the patients had undergone surgery in the month prior to the study; 32% elective surgery and 23% emergency surgery. The site of surgery most frequently performed was abdominal surgery (19%). Organ systems cited as being the most important reason for admission to the ICU were the respiratory (37%), cardiovascular (30%) and central nervous systems (23%). Of the patients 39% were admitted to the ICU for postsurgical control or surveillance. The mean APACHE II score calculated on admission was 12.7 (Figure 1). The prevalence of potential risk factors for nosocomial infection relating to the

Table 2. Patient demography: prevalence of underlying conditions

Organ failure (all types)	56,5%
Impaired respiratory reflex	21,5%
Chronic respiratory insufficiency	14,4%
Carcinoma	13,6%
Diabetes mellitus	12,6%
Multiple trauma with head injury	8,1%
Multiple trauma without head injury	4,4%
AIDS	0,8%

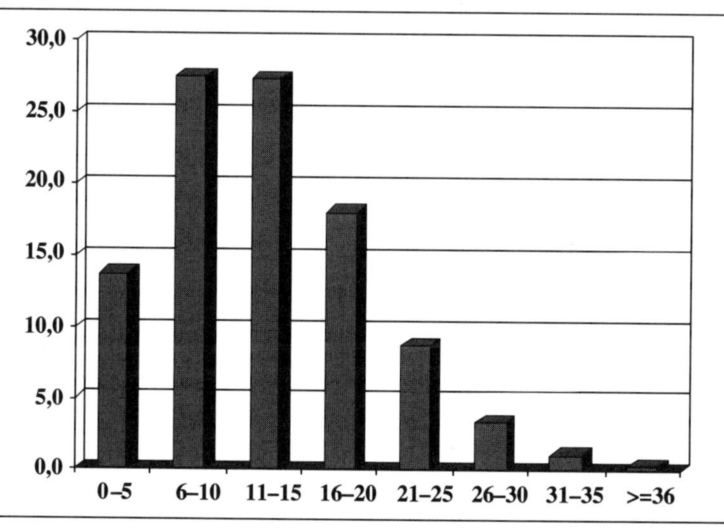

Figure 1. APACHE II scores. (% of patients)

length of ICU stay prior to 29-04-92 and certain procedural or therapeutic interventions (scored in the week prior to the study) is shown in Table 3 (SDD = selective digestive decontamination).

Prevalence of Nosocomial Infection and the Key Infection Types

On the study day a total of 4501 patients (45% of the total patient population) had one or more infections. Almost half were ICU acquired infections (21% of the total). Hospital-acquired infections were recorded in 10%, and community-acquired infections in 14%. Of those patients reported as having an ICU-acquired infection, the majority had only one such an infection, although 25% had two or more infections. Figure 2 gives the prevalence of the types of the most frequently reported ICU-acquired infections (incidence >4.0%).

Table 3. Prevalence (% patients) of reported potential risk factors for nosocomial ICU-infection, scored in the week preceding the study day

Length of ICU stay (%, days)	Diagnostic intervention	(%)	Therapeutic intervention	(%)
0–1 : 17,8	Intravenous catheter	78,3	Sedation	51,2
1–3 : 28,9	Urinary catheter	75,2	Stress ulcer prophylaxis:	
3–5 : 8,4	Central venous pressure line	63,9	H2 receptor antagonist	39,0
5–6 : 8,6	Mechanical ventilation	63,0	Sucralfate	23,5
7–13 : 13,8	Intubation	62,2	Antacids	9,2
14–20 : 8,0	Arterial catheter	44,2	Omeprazole & others	9,0
>20 : 14,5	Central iv nutrition	36,5	Prophylactic antibiotics	19,4
	Wound drain	30,6	Longterm/high dose steroids	12,9
	Chest drain	14,7	SDD	6,3
	Pulmonary artery catheter	12,8	Immunosupressive therapy	2,7
	Tracheostomy	12,6	Radiotherapy	0,3
	Peripheral iv nutrition	9,2		
	Hemodialysis	5,2		
	Atrial/ventricular pacing	4,8		
	Intracranial pressure line	2,2		
	Peritoneal dialysis	0,5		

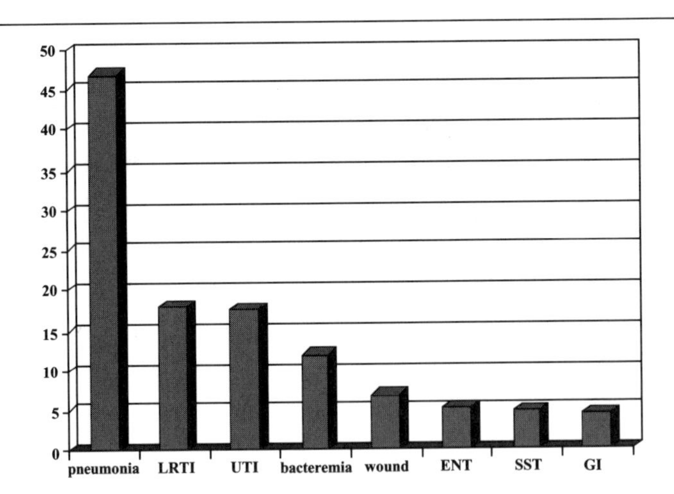

- Lrti = lower respiratory tract infection
- Uti = urinary tract infection
- Ent = ear, nose and throat
- Sst = skin and soft tissue
- Gi = gastrointestinal

Figure 2. Key infection types prevalence in ICU patients (%).

Table 4. Prevalence of reported isolates in ICU-acquired infections

Isolate	%
Staphylococcus aureus	30,1
Pseudomonas aeruginosa	28,7
Coagulase-negative staphylococci	19,1
Fungi	17,1
Escherichia coli	12,7
Enterococci	11,7
Acinetobacter spp.	9,3
Klebsiella spp.	8,1
Streptococci (other than pneumococci)	7,1
Enterobacter spp.	6,6
Proteus spp.	5,7
Other Pseudomonas spp.	4,4

The Key Types of Pathogens, Isolated from Patients with ICU-Acquired Infections

Overall, 55% of the ICU-acquired infections were polymicrobial. *Staphylococcus aureus* was the "key pathogen" most frequently isolated (30%). Only the Enterobacteriaceae were reported more often (34%), but as a class. The most commonly reported isolates acquired in the ICU infections are shown in Table 4.

From the Enterobacteriaceae, as a class within the gram-negative organisms, *E. coli* was the most commonly scored pathogen, followed by *Klebsiella spp., and Enterobacter spp.* The Enterobacteriaceae were cultured from a substantial proportion of urinary isolates, particularly *E. coli*: the most common cause of urinary tract infection—both symptomatic and asymptomatic (colonization?)—cultured in 22% of these urinary isolates. In addition, the Enterobacteriaceae were reported in 28% of the lower respiratory tract infections other than pneumonia.

As noted, *S. aureus* was the most commonly reported bacterial isolate overall. Particularly causing skin and soft tissue infections (cultured in 36% of total isolates from this type of infection), pneumonia (cultured in 32%), other lower respiratory tract infections (in 31%), wound infections (in 27%), and laboratory-confirmed bloodstream infections (in 22%).

P. aeruginosa was of substantial importance in pulmonary infections: both in pneumonia (cultured in 30% of the total pneumoniae-isolates), and in the other lower respiratory tract infections (cultured in 35%). Besides, *P. aeruginosa* was also frequently cultured from skin and soft tissue infections (in 33% of total isolates of this infection), wound infections (in 21%), and urinary tract infections (in 19%).

Coagulase-negative staphylococci (CNS) were the most frequently documented isolates in laboratory—confirmed bloodstream infections, being reported in 45% of the cultures. Overall, gram-positive organisms accounted for about 70% of the cultured isolates responsible for bacteremia: besides CNS, *S. aureus* accounted for 22% of isolates and enterococci for 11%. This result confirmed the results of other studies that have documented an increasing number of gram-positive infections, particularly CNS and enterococci in bacteremia (38). This is most probably due to the selective pressure exerted by the use of broad-spectrum antibiotics, such as the third-generation cephalosporins, which are generally more potent against gram-negative than gram-positive bacteria, and to the increasing use of intravascular devices (bearing in mind the propensity of particularly CNS to colonise vascular invasive devices). However, uncertainty exists always over whether CNS are true pathogens or merely contaminants of blood cultures, when taken from an intravascular catheter? In literature, different criteria and definitions have been used to define true bloodstream infections after isolation of CNS (39–41). The EPIC study used the CDC definitions for laboratory-confirmed primary bloodstream infection, and clinical sepsis (33).

Candida spp. are called "emerging pathogens", because over the past decades they established themselves as serious causes of infection. Many recent studies reported *Candida spp.* as a significant pathogen (42,43). This growing importance of fungal isolates is related presumably to an increasing use of broad-spectrum antibiotics, in an increasingly immunosuppressed patientpopulation (due to the primary disease and to treatment with corticosteroids). Also the EPIC results highlighted the growing prevalence of fungal pathogens, with a surprisingly high frequency of 17% (despite the low number of AIDS patients). The most common site from which fungi were cultured, was the urinary tract (isolated in 18% of urine samples, making fungi together with *E. coli* the most important pathogens in urinary tract infections). In addition, fungi were the third most frequently isolated pathogens in pneumonia (isolated in 14% of the cultures). Again here the difference between infection and colonization remains uncertain, as *Candida* pneumonia is a rare event. Yet more than 50% of patients with a positive fungal isolate were receiving antifungal treatment, indicating that these isolates were thought to be of clinical significance (36).

Other so called "emerging pathogens" are *the Acinetobacter spp.* These isolates have been cultured mostly in nosocomial pneumonia (in 10%), and in the other lower respiratory tract infections (in 11%).

With respect to the microbiological isolates reported in the EPIC study, the results are comparable with those of the NNIS study in the USA from 1980 through 1992 (25,44). One exception, being a low prevalence of *Enterobacter* species in the EPIC results (6.6%), particularly for laboratory-proven bloodstream infections. In the NNIS study the most common pathogens were *P. aeruginosa* (12%), *S. aureus* (12%), CNS (10%), *Candida spp.* (10%), *Enterobacter spp.* (9%), and enterococci (9%). The data of the NNIS documented the same increasing number of gram-positive infections, particularly CNS (with a frequency of 9% in 1989, increasing to 30% in 1992). The results of all these epidemiological studies emphasizes the need for broad-spectrum antibiotics, when starting empirical antimicrobial therapy on the ICU, being equally effective against gram-positive and gram-negative bacteria, changing to smaller specified antibiotics, effective for the causal pathogens, when culture results are positive.

Table 5. Antibiotics prescribed on the study day (% of total antibiotic use)

Antibiotic	Frequency overall (%)	Use for prophylaxis (%)	Use for treatment (%)
Cephalosporins	43,6	22,1	21,6
Aminoglycosides	23,9	5,4	18,6
Quinolones	11,9	1,6	10,4
Penicillin	10,3	4,8	5,5
Macrolides	4,4	0,8	3,6
Broad-spectrum penicillins	24,3	8,1	16,2
Imipenem	8,1	0,8	7,3
Glycopeptides	11,6	1,2	10,3
Metronidazole	17,1	7,8	9,2
Aztreonam	2,0	0,4	1,6
Other	10,3	2,6	7,7

Pattern of Antibiotic Administration

In total, 6250 patients (62%) were receiving antimicrobials on the study day, prescribed either for treatment or prophylaxis. Half of these patients (49%) were receiving single antibiotic therapy, the others receiving combination therapy with multiple antibiotics. The most frequently administered antimicrobials were the cephalosporins, used in 44% of all antibiotic treated patients, both for prophylaxis (particularly cefuroxime and cefazolin) and for treatment (particularly ceftazidime and cefotaxim). Table 5 shows the prescription policy of the scored antimicrobials. Only few patients were receiving treatment with antifungal drugs (6.6%), or antiviral drugs (1.1%). Also the (routinely) use of selective decontamination of the digestive tract (SDD) was rare (overall, 6.3% of ICUs used SDD in the week preceding the study, 5.6% used SDD on the study day). The majority of ICUs in Europe never use SDD.

Pattern of Antibiotic Resistance

Data were scored about the patterns of microbial resistance to the different types of antibiotics, of the three most frequently reported isolates in the ICU-acquired infections: *P. aeruginosa, S. aureus* and coagulase-negative staphylococci. Of the cultured *P. aeruginosa* isolates 65% were resistant to one or more antibiotics. Most common was resistance of *P. aeruginosa* to gentamicin (in 46% of resistant isolates), followed by resistance to ureidopenicillin (37%), ceftazidime (28%), ciprofloxacin (26%), and imipenem (21%). Overall, 86% of the *S. aureus* isolates were resistant to one or more antibiotics. Of these, 60% of strains of *S. aureus* were resistant to methicillin (MRSA). The most commonly recorded sites of MRSA infection were in the respiratory tract: pneumonia (52%), and lower respiratory tract infections (22%). In total 73% of the CNS isolates were resistant to one or more antibiotics. The data reported a high resistance rate of CNS to methicillin (70% of resistant isolates), cefotaxime (69%), and gentamicin (66%). Resistance of CNS to teicoplanin (9%), and vancomycin (4%) was relatively uncommon, but unfortunately does exist.

The problem of resistant pathogens is becoming worse every day, particularly in the ICU, everywhere throughout in Europe. Once we thought antibiotics to be the answer to infections, now we know they are not. The successes of the past, accomplished with the advent of (new) antibiotics, selectively eliminating of what were considered to be pathogenic microorganisms, have proved to be an illusion. On the contrary, the emergence of extremely virulent and resistant microbial strains is certainly the result of (mis)use of these antibiotics itself (45,46).

For example, the rapidity with which *methicillin-resistant S. aureus* developed in Europe after the introduction of methicillin (and cephalosporins, as cross-resistance between penicillins and fist generation cephalosporins is a common if not ever present feature). The subsequent spread of MRSA throughout Europe have created enormous problems with consequences for therapeutics and ICU-management. According to the results of the EPIC study, 60% of strains of *S. aureus* were resistant to methicillin. We evaluated, using the EPIC-data, the risk of accquisition of an infection with MRSA and the risk of death, compared with patients who developed methicillin-sensitive *S. aureus* (MSSA) infection (47). The most important risk factor was the length of stay in the ICU: the longer the stay, the higher was the risk of an MRSA rather than an MSSA infection (with an odds ratio of 4.07 for a stay longer than three weeks). MRSA infection reduced the chance of survival, particularly when it was found in lower respiratory tract infections: the risk of mortality was three times higher in patients with MRSA than in those with a MSSA infection.

The Key Risk Factors for ICU-Acquired Infection

Statistical analysis quantified the possible relationship between investigated risk factors and nosocomial infection. After univariate analysis 14 variables were identified as significant risk factors: organ failure of any type on admission, emergency surgery (but not elective), trauma, respiratory problems and mechanical ventilation, various invasive interventions (central venous, pulmonary artery and urinary catheterization, intubation, tracheostomy), stress ulcer prophylaxis, an APACHE II score of more than 6, and prolonged length of ICU stay. The most important risk factor was the length of ICU stay (up to 29.04.92, in days): compared with a length of stay of less than 1 day (odds ratio = 1), an ICU-stay of 3–4 days increased the risk of infection nine times. Those patients who had been in the ICU for 3 weeks or more, were at 76 times the risk of the one day patient. The size of the ICU was also a risk factor: patients on greater units were significantly more at risk than those on smaller units. Interestingly, cancer, an age older than 70 years, and elective surgery apparently decreased the odds ratio for infection. Also the type of ICU (medical, surgical, or mixed) and the length of stay in hospital before admission to the ICU, did not significantly affect the risk for infection. Analysing risk factors for special types of infection, also showed the length of ICU stay to be the most important risk factor. Invasive procedures to the respiratory tract (particularly tracheostomy and assisted ventilation) increased the risk of pneumonia. These interventions also

Table 6. Independent risk factors associated with ICU-acquired infection

Risk factor		Odds ratio	95% Confidence interval
Length of ICU stay:	<1 day	1	
	: 1–2 days	2,54	1,56–4,13
	: 3–4 days	8,99	5,51–14,70
	: 5–6 days	15,01	9,33–24,14
	: 7–13 days	30,75	19,43–48,67
	: 14–20 days	60,40	37,90–96,25
	: ≥21 days	76,06	48,18–120,06
Pulmonary artery catheter		1,20	1,01–1,43
Central venous pressure line		1,35	1,16–1,57
Stress ulcer prophylaxis		1,38	1,20–1,60
Urinary catheter		1,41	1,19–1,69
Mechanical ventilation		1,75	1,51–2,03
Trauma on admission		2,07	1,75–2,44

increased the risk of laboratory-confirmed bloodstream infection, together with a particular risk due to a central venous pressure line. In addition multiple logistic regression analysis was done to control for the effects of confounding variables, using all the described variables significantly associated with infection. Seven variables remained as independent risk factors, shown in Table 6. The APACHE II score was no longer a significant, independent risk factor in this analysis.

Awareness of these risk factors should promote their avoidance where possible, or at the moment the inevitable interventions are not absolutely necessary any more, one should remove them as soon as possible.

Mortality among ICU Patients, and the Relevance of Various Risk Factors

Data concerning the outcome of the ICU patients (expected, or in the case of death, actual), were recorded on discharge from the ICU, up to a follow-up period of 6 weeks after the study day. Of those patients 83.2% were discharged from the ICU alive, so the overall mortality rate was 16.8%. There was considerable variation in mortality rate by country and by ICU. This does not mean that these differences in mortality do reflect differences in level of care in the ICUs. But rather, these differences are more likely due to differences in the patientpopulation, arising from discrepancies in admission criteria, reflected in differences in the severity of illness. The patient admitted for postsurgical control or surveillance has another prognosis than the ICU patient with sepsis. Nonetheless, mortality in the EPIC study was higher in those countries with higher ICU-acquired infection rates. A significant correlation ($R^2 = 0.68$) was noted between the prevalence rate of ICU-acquired infection and the mortality rate. Again caution must be exercised in drawing any direct conclusions. The statement that intensive care patients die of, rather than with, infection is not proven (48). The question that arises is whether infection contributes to mortality? The answer remains unclear. As stated by Gross

Table 7. Independent risk factors associated with mortality

Risk factor	Odds ratio*	95% Confidence interval
Age > 60 years: 60–69 years	1,7	1,07–2,71
: ≥70 years	2,08	1,31–3,31
Organ failure on admission	1,68	1,45–19,5
APACHE II score ≥ 31	15,55	9,3–26,0
ICU stay ≥ 21 days	2,52	1,99–3,18
Carcinoma	1,48	1,23–1,79
Pneumonia	1,91	1,6–2,29
Clinical sepsis	3,5	1,71–7,18
Laboratory-confirmed Bloodstream infection	1,73	1,25–2,41

*OR's: adjusted for age.

and van Antwerpen (49) "In two groups, well matched by many criteria, differences in prognosis on admission probably accounted for the major differences in survival. Nosocomial infections may affect outcome in those whose condition is not terminal on admission". Notwithstanding that differences in mortality rate cannot be directly attributed to differences in infection rates or differences in microbial resistance, univariate analysis of the EPIC data confirmed that ICU-acquired infections are among the most important independent risk factors associated with increased mortality. According to the univariate analysis the following risk factors increased the odds of death: various ICU-acquired infection types (wound infection, laboratory-confirmed bloodstream infection, sepsis, pneumonia and lower respiratory tract infection, urinary tract infection, skin and soft tissue infection), an age older than 60 years, organ failure of any type on admission, cancer, diabetes, prolonged stay in the ICU and increasing APACHE II score. The greatest risk was associated with a high APACHE II score (which indeed reflects the risk of death), and with clinical sepsis. After using multiple logistic regression analysis, eight risk factors remained as independently associated with an increased risk of mortality (Table 7).

THE EPIC RESULTS: EUROPEAN LANDSCAPE

There were marked variations in the results of the EPIC data between the different European countries. Overall, there was a wide range in prevalence rates of ICU-acquired infections, from 10% in Switzerland to 32% in Italy. There tended to be a trend toward higher infection rates and higher overall ICU mortality rates in Southern Europe. Table 8 shows the prevalence of ICU-acquired infection and the ICU mortality rate for each country taking part in the EPIC study.It is more likely that these differences are based on differences in patient selection on admission, and in intensive care practice, rather than any real differences in quality and absolute standards of care. For example, there were substantial differences between the countries in size of the ICU. Most ICUs were of intermediate size, having 6–10 beds. France

Table 8. Prevalence of ICU-acquired infection, and mortality rate, by participating country

Country	No. of ICUs	No. of Patients	Prevalence of ICU infection (%)	ICU mortality Rate (%)
Austria	75	420	20,0	15,3
Belgium	72	669	17,2	14,9
Denmark	12	81	7,4	11,3
Eire	15	91	18,7	11,8
Finland	20	132	15,9	11,9
France	264	2359	24,2	18,7
Germany	268	2010	17,3	14,9
Greece	37	200	30,5	28,5
Italy	110	617	31,6	20,3
Luxembourg	5	29	17,2	13,0
The Netherlands	78	472	15,7	13,8
Norway	23	150	12,7	8,9
Portugal	19	120	23,3	23,9
Spain	137	1233	27,0	19,4
Sweden	39	286	7,7	8,8
Switzerland	49	329	9,7	8,4
United Kingdom	194	840	15,9	19,9
Total	1417	10038	20,6	16,8

and Spain had the largest ICUs, with 43% and 42% respectively having ≥11 beds. In contrast, in the UK only 5% of ICUs were of this size, while 48% were small ICUs, having up to 5 beds. As mentioned previously, the size of the unit is an infection risk factor it self, with significantly more infections scored in the units of 11 or more beds. There were also wide variations between countries in the ICU resources. Overall, 43% of the ICUs had a microbiologist joining the team, while Denmark, the Netherlands (both 83%) and the UK (73%) had much more often a microbiologist in the team. Discrepancies in patient selection are reflected in differences in the APACHE II scores of the patients on admission to the ICU. The average score overall in Europe was 12.7. There was a more severely ill ICU population in Eire, France, Greece, Italy, Portugal, Spain and the UK, with more than 15% of patients having an APACHE II score >20. In Norway, Sweden, Germany and Switzerland only <10% fell into this category, while >50% had an APACHE II score of 10 or less. Including in the admission criteria also patients just for post-surgical control or surveillance, decreases the average APACHE II score, and most likely decreases the average total length of stay, both with the same impact on the prevalence of ICU infections. As part of differences in intensive care practice, there were marked variations between countries with respect to the use of procedural or therapeutic interventions. Overall, the use was often highest in the UK. With respect to antibiotics most countries tended to administer single antibiotic agents for treatment. The exceptions were Eire, France, Greece, Spain and the UK where more than half of the patients with antibiotics were receiving multiple agents. The most considerable difference in the use of antibiotics was noted in the prevalence of SDD. Overall, the majority of ICUs in Europe never use SDD, the scored prevalence for

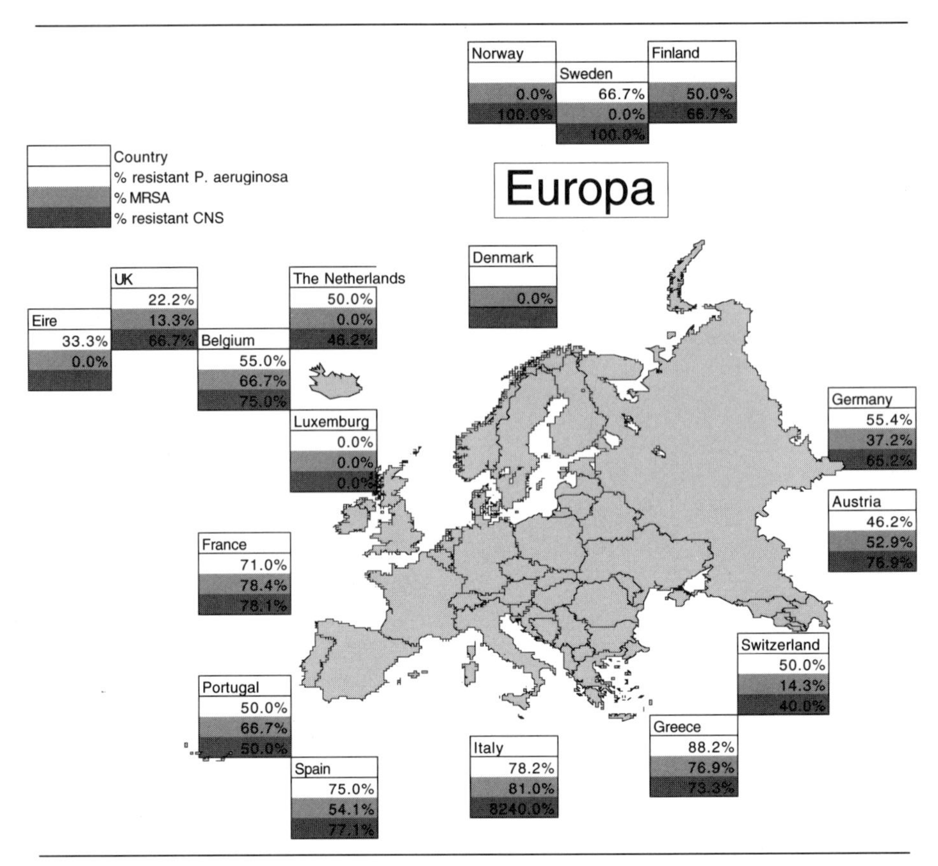

Figure 3. ••

Europe totaly was 6%, while ≥40% of units in Austria, the Netherlands and Luxembourg use SDD routinely in a selected patientpopulation.

There turned out to be an enormous intercountry variation in the prevalence of resistant *P. aeruginosa*, of MRSA, and of resistant coagulase-negative staphylococci. Figure 3 shows the frequency of resistance by European countries (taking into account the limitations of a one-day point prevalence survey, and of the sometimes low numbers of patients when analysing this item, making a surprisingly 0% sometimes possible). Apparently several countries have been able to prevent resistance problems in their ICU, by inevitable control measures and screening programs, by using antimicrobial agents only judiciously, and by reinforcing hygienic measures where necessary (47).

SUMMARY

According to the results of the EPIC study the scope and magnitude of nosocomial ICU infections in Europe is overwhelming. The highlights of the results were the prevalence of pneumonia and other lower respiratory tract infections, the importance of the Enterobacteriaceae (as a class), *S. aureus* and *P. aeruginosa* as the key pathogens, and the high prevalence of microbial resistance of these pathogens to the various antibiotics. Overall, there was a surprisingly growing significance of gram-positive pathogens, and fungi. The key risk factors associated with ICU-acquired infections were in particular a prolonged length of stay on the ICU, and various invasive interventions. Mortality rates were high, with a significant correlation between the prevalence rate of ICU-acquired infection and the mortality rate (in particular pneumonia, laboratory-confirmed bloodstream infection and sepsis were independent risk factors, associated with an increased risk of death).

Europe needs well-implemented infection control policies, to reduce these preventable infections. Data from the EPIC study are just a starting point and motivating factor to achieve this. Up to this moment there is in Europe no formalised and ongoing surveillance system (such as the NNIS in the USA), needed to establish, stimulate, up date, continuously improve the quality, and evaluate the effectiveness of such control programs. The ultimate aim for the future is more European collaborative efforts in infection control. Recently European boundaries are opened for traffic and tourism, consequently also for micro-organisms, making the task to control resistant pathogens increasingly difficult.

ACKNOWLEDGEMENT

The EPIC study was supported by a grant from Roussel Uclaf.

REFERENCES

1. Brachman PS. Nosocomial infection control: an overview. *Rev Infect Dis* 1981;3:640–648.
2. Donowitz LG, Wenzel RP, Hoyt JW. High risk of hospital-acquired infection in the ICU patient. *Crit Care Med* 1982;10:355–357.
3. Haley RW, Culver DH, White JW, Morgan WM, Emori TG. The nationwide nosocomial infection rate: a new need for vital statistics. *Am J Epidemiol* 1985;121:159–167.
4. Pittet D, Tarara D, Wenzel RP. Nosocomial bloodstream infection in critically ill patients: excess length of stay, extra costs, and attributable mortality. *JAMA* 1994;271:1598–1601.
5. Bueno-Cavanillas A, Delgado-Rodriguez M, Lopez-Luque A, et al. Influence of nosocomial infection on mortality rate in an intensive care unit. *Crit Care Med* 1994;22:55–60.
6. Harbarth S, Pittet D. Excess mortality and impact of intensive care unit-acquired infections. *Curr Opin Anaesthes* 1996;9:139–145.
7. Wenzel RP, Thompson RL, Landry SM, Russell BS, Miller PJ, Ponce de Leon S, Miller GB. Hospital acquired infections in intensive care unit patients: an overview with emphasis on epidemics. *Infect Cont* 1983;4:371–375.
8. Brown RB, Hosmer D, Chen HC, et al. A comparison of infections in different ICUs within the same hospital. *Crit Care Med* 1985;13:472–475.
9. Craven DE, Kunches LM, Lichtenberg DA, et al. Nosocomial infection and fatality in medical and surgical intensive care unit patients. *Arch Intern Med* 1988;149:1161–1168.
10. Spencer RC. Epidemiology of infection in ICUs. *Intensive Care Med* 1994;20:s2–s6.
11. Haley RW, Hooton TM, Culver DH, Stanley RC, Emori TG, Hardisson CD, Quade D, Schachtman RH, Schaberg DR, Shah BV, Schatz GD. Nosocomial infections in US hospitals 1975–76. Estimated frequency by selected characteristics of patients. *Am J Med* 1981;70:947–959.
12. Pranatharthi H, Chandrasekar MD, Kruse JA, Mathews MF. Nosocomial infection among patients in different types of intensive care units at a city hospital. *Crit Care Med* 1986;14:508–510.
13. Emmerson AM. The epidemiology of infections in intensive care units. *Intensive Care Med* 1990;16(suppl 3):s197–s200.

14. Jarvis WR, Edwards JR, Culver DH, Hughes JM, Horan T, Emori TG, Banerjee S, Tolson J, Henderson T, Gaynes RP, Martone WJ. Nosocomial infection rates in adult and pediatric intensive care units in the United States. *Am J Med* 1991;91(suppl 3B):185–191.
15. Meakins JL, Wicklund B, Forse RA, McLean AP. The surgical intensive care unit: current concepts in infection. *Surg Clin North Am* 1980;60:117–132.
16. Neu HC. The crisis in antibiotic resistance. *Science* 1992;257:1064–1073.
17. Haley RW, Culver DH, White JW, et al. The efficacy of infection surveillance and control programs in preventing nosocomial infections in US hospitals. *Am J Epidemiol* 1985;121:182–205.
18. Cruse PHE, Foord R. The epidemiology of wound infection: a 10-year prospective study of 62.939 wounds. *Surg Clin North Am* 1980;60:27–40.
19. Langmuir AD. The surveillance of communicable diseases of national importance. *N Engl J Med* 1963;268:182–192.
20. Brachman PS. Surveillance of institutionally acquired infections. In: Proceedings of the National Conference on Institutionaly acquired infections, Minneapolis, University of Minnesota School of Public Health, september 4–6, 1963. PHS publication no. 1188. Washington, DC: US GPO, 1964:138–147.
21. Garner JS, Bennett JV, Scheckler WE, et al. Surveillance of nosocomial infections. In: Proceedings of the International Conference on nosocomial infections, august 3–6, 1970. Chicago: American Hospital Association, 1971:277–281.
22. Centers for Disease Control. Outline for surveillance and control of nosocomial infections. Atlanta, GA: CDC, 1972. (reprinted september 1973, may 1974, november 1976)
23. Haley RW. Surveillance by objective: a new priority directed approach to the control of nosocomial infections. *Am J Infect Control* 1985;13:78–89.
24. Haley RW, Quade D, Freeman HE, et al. Study on the efficacy of nosocomial infection control (SENIC Project): summary of study design. *Am J Epidemiol* 1980;111:472–485.
25. Jarvis WR, Martone WJ. Predominant pathogens in hospital infections. *J Antimicrob Chemother* 1992;29(suppl A):19–24.
26. Bernander S, Hambraeus A, Myrback KE, Nystrom B, Sundelop B. Prevalence of hospital-associated infections in five Swedish hospitals in november 1975. *Scand J Infect Dis* 1978;10:66–70.
27. Daschner FD, Frey P, Wolff G, Baumann PC, Suter P. Nosocomial infections in intensive care wards: a multicenter prospective study. *Intensive Care Med* 1982;8:5–9.
28. Moro ML, Stazi MA, Marasca G, Greco D, Zampieri A. National prevalence survey of hospital-acquired infections in Italy, 1983. *J Hosp Infect* 1986;8:72–85.
29. Constantini M, Donisi PM, Turrin MG, Diana L. Hospital acquired infections surveillance and control in intensive care services. Results of an incidence study. *Eur J Epidemiol* 1987;3:347–355.
30. Mertens R, Kegels G, Stroobant A, Reybrouck G, Lamotte JM, Potvliege C, Van Casteren V, Lauwers S, Verschraegen G, Wauters G, Minne A, Thiers G. The national prevalence survey of nosocomial infections in Belgium, 1984. *J Hosp Infect* 1987;9:219–229.
31. EPINCAT Working Group. Prevalence of hospital infections in Catalonia (II). Microorganisms and antimicrobials. *Med Clinics (Barc)* 1990;95:161–168.
32. Spencer RC. Prevalence studies in nosocomial infections. *Eur J Clin Microbiol and Inf Dis* 1992;11:95–98.
33. Garner JS, Jarvis WR, Emori TG, et al. CDC definitions for nosocomial infection. *Am J Infect Control* 1988;16:128–140.
34. Knaus WA, Zimmerman JE, Wagner DP, Draper EA, Lawrence DE. APACHE—acute physiology and chronic health evaluation: a physiologically based classification system. *Crit Care Med* 1981;9:591–597.
35. Knaus WA, Draper EA, Wagner DP, Zimmerman JE. APACHE II: a severity of disease classification system. *Crit Care Med* 1985;13:818–829.
36. Vincent JL, Bihari DJ, Suter PM, et al. The prevalence of nosocomial infection in intensive care units in Europe: results of the European Prevalence of Infection in Intensive Care (EPIC) study. *JAMA* 1995;274:639–644.
37. European Report: the results of the EPIC study. Medical Action Communications Ltd, UK. 1995.
38. Wolff M, Brun-Buisson C, Lode H, Mathai D, Lewi D, Pittet D. The changing epidemiology of severe infections in the ICU. *Clin Microbiol and Infect* 1997; volume 3, suppl 1.
39. Dominiguez-de Villota E, Algora-Weber A, Millian I, Rubio JJ, Galdos P, Mosquera JM. Early evaluation of coagulase-negative staphylococcus in blood samples of intensive care unit patients: a clinically uncertain judgement. *Intensive Care Med* 1987;13:390–394.
40. Jacobson KL, Cohen SH, Inciardi JF, et al. The relationship between antecedent antibiotic use and resistance to extended-spectrum cephalosporins in group I beta-lactamase producing organisms. *Clin Infect Dis* 1995;21:1107–1113.

41. Herwaldt LA, Geiss M, Kao C, Pfaller MA. The positive predictive value of isolating coagulase-negative staphylococci from blood cultures. *Clin Infect Dis* 1996;22:14–20.
42. Colombo AL, Nucci M, Caiuby MJ, et al. High incidence of non-albicans candidemia. Nosocomial infections and surgical infections and related epidemiologic studies. 36th ICAAC Conference 1996.
43. Spencer RC, Bauernfeind A, Garcia-Rodriguez J, er al. The surveillance of the current resitance of nosocomial pathogens to antibacterials. *Clin Microbiol and Infect* 1997; volume 3, suppl 1.
44. Martone WJ, Jarvis WR, Culver DH, Haley RW. Incidence and nature of endemic and epidemic nosocomial infections. In: Bennett JV, Brachman PS, eds. *Hospital Infections*. 3rd ed. Boston, Mass: Little Brown & Co; 1992:577–596.
45. Sogaard H, Zimmermann-Nielsen C, Siboni K. Antibiotic resistant Gram-negative bacilli in a urological ward for male patients during a nine year period: relationship to antibiotic consumption. *J Infect Dis* 1974;130:646–650.
46. Mouton RP, Glerum JH, v Loenen AC. Relationship between antibiotic consumption and frequency of antibiotic resistance of four pathogens—a seven year survey. *J Antimicrob Chemother* 1976;2:9–19.
47. Ibelings MS, Bruining HA. Methicillin-resistant Staphylococcus aureus: acquisition and risk of death in patients in the Intensive Care Unit. *Eur J Surg* 1998;164:411–418.
48. Hartenauer U, Thulig B, Diemer W, Lawin P, Fegeler W, Kehrel R, Ritzerfeld W. Effect of selective flora suppression on colonization, infection, and mortality in critically ill patients: a one-year, prospective consecutive study. *Crit Care Med* 1991;19:463–473.
49. Gross PA, van Antwerpen C. Nosocomial infections and hospital deaths. A case control study. *Am J Med* 1983;75:658.

3. VANCOMYCIN-RESISTANT ENTEROCOCCI: A THREAT FOR THE ICU?

MARY K. HAYDEN, M.D.

Rush Medical College, Chicago, IL 60612 USA

INTRODUCTION

Vancomycin was used to treat serious Gram positive infections for thirty years before significant resistance to its activity developed. In 1986 vancomycin-resistance was described in two clinical isolates of *Enterococcus faecium* from France (1). Fourteen years later, vancomycin-resistance in enterococci is a worldwide problem; vancomycin-resistant enterococci (VRE) have been isolated in 18 countries on six continents. VRE are a particularly serious problem in the United States. In 1998, over 20% of enterococcal isolates reported from the Center's for Disease Control and Prevention (CDC's) National Nosocomial Infection Surveillance (NNIS) System hospitals were resistant to vancomycin, an increase of more than 50% compared to the period 1993–97 (2). The steady rise in the number of enterococci resistant to vancomycin shows no sign of slowing, despite the institution in many US hospitals of 1995 federal guidelines for decreasing the spread of VRE (3). This trend is worrisome for several reasons. First, the majority of vancomycin-resistant enterococcal isolates are concomitantly resistant to moderate- or high-levels of penicillins and to high-levels of aminoglycosides, often relegating treatment to unproven combinations of antibiotics or to investigational compounds (4). Even Synercid® (quinupristin/dalfopristin), an agent recently approved in the US for the treatment of vancomycin-resistant *E. faecium* infections, has a reported efficacy of only 52.3% (5). Second, patients who develop VRE infection tend to be those who are elderly, debilitated, who have multiple underlying medical problems, or who are immunosuppressed

R.A. Weinstein and M.J.M. Bonten (eds.). INFECTION CONTROL IN THE ICU ENVIRONMENT.

(6,7,8,9). These patient populations are expected to grow over the next decade. Third, enterococci may act as a reservoir for vancomycin resistance genes that could be transferred to more virulent bacteria, such as *Staphylococcus aureus*.

ICU patients bear a disproportionate share of the VRE burden in the US. Compared with other patients, those in ICUs have a 16-fold greater risk of acquiring a nosocomial infection due to VRE (2). This chapter will review the factors that make VRE well adapted to the ICU environment, the characteristics of ICU patients that render them especially vulnerable to colonization and infection with VRE, the effect of VRE infection on ICU patient outcomes, the epidemiology of VRE within the ICU, and strategies to control spread of this pathogen.

MECHANISMS AND GENETICS OF VANCOMYCIN RESISTANCE IN ENTEROCOCCI

Five distinct phenotypes of vancomycin resistance in enterococci have been described, designated VanA, VanB, VanC, VanD, and VanE, that are differentiated by the presence of the vanA, vanB, vanC1, vanC2/C3, vanD, and vanE genes, respectively (10,11,12,13). The mechanisms of resistance are complex and involve up to 6 gene products and multiple carefully regulated steps. In all cases, resistance to vancomycin, and sometimes to other glycopeptide antibiotics, arises because of an amino acid substitution in the peptidoglycan precursor, D-ala-D-ala, that is the binding site for vancomycin in the enterococcal cell wall. Vancomycin binds the altered target with significantly lower affinity than the wild-type. The vanA, B, C, D, and E resistance genotypes differ in the specific amino acid substitution that is made, in the regulation and genetics of resistance, and in the presence or absence of complementary gene products that enhance resistance to vancomycin and other glycopeptides. Heterogeneity exists within each genotype as well. For example, while vanB expression is most often inducible, some clinical isolates express resistance constitutively (14).

The acquired resistance genotypes vanA and vanB are the most clinically and epidemiologically important. The vanA gene cluster encodes high-level, transferable resistance to vancomycin and to the related glycopeptide antibiotic, teicoplanin. Although vanA has been identified in at least 6 different enterococcal species, *E. faecium* is most often affected. The vanB gene cluster encodes low- to high-level vancomycin resistance that is only transferable sometimes (15). Perhaps because of the more limited mobility of this resistance genotype, it has been found in only 2 enterococcal species: *E. faecium* and *Enterococcus faecalis*. VanC-type resistance is expressed as constitutive, low-level vancomycin resistance. The vanC1 gene is found in *Enterococcus gallinarum*, and the van C2/3 gene is found in *Enterococcus casseliflavus* and *Enterococcus flavescens*. Although these 3 enterococcal species may be found colonizing patients, they rarely cause infection. For example, Morris et al found that 20 (40%) of 50 patients surveyed at the University of Maryland Hospital who had rectal colonization with VRE carried *E. gallinarum*. Over that same period, none of 63 vancomycin-resistant enterococcal infections were caused by *E. gallinarum* (14). Enterococcal isolates harbouring vanD or vanE have been identified in only a handful of patients thus far (12,13).

VRE ARE WELL ADAPTED TO THE ICU ENVIRONMENT

The explosive increase of VRE in ICUs may be explained partly by the remarkable ability of VRE to thrive in an environment that many other bacteria find hostile. Perhaps the greatest selective advantage held by VRE is its resistance to multiple antibiotics. In addition to vancomycin resistance, VRE, like all enterococci, express resistance to cephalosporins, to trimethoprim-sulfamethoxazole, and to clindamycin. The majority of VRE are also highly resistant to penicillin, usually due to modification or over-production of penicillin binding proteins (17). These penicillin binding protein changes render the enterococcus resistant to all β-lactams, β-lactam-β-lactamase inhibitor compounds, and to carbapenems. Data from the US Project ICARE, a study assessing antimicrobial use and resistance in a subset of 41 hospitals participating in the NNIS system, show that many of these drugs are used more intensively in ICU settings than in other inpatient wards (2).

In addition to the survival advantage conferred by resistance to antibiotics, enterococci possess the ability to grow in the presence of bile and in high concentrations of salt (18). Enterococci are relatively resistant to heat and to removal by washing with bland soap (19,20). After inoculation onto bed rails and other inanimate environmental surfaces, VRE can survive for up to 24 hours with minimal reductions in colony counts (21). VRE have been found to persistently colonize the intact skin on the upper extremities of ICU patients for over a week (22); rectal colonization with VRE has been documented to persist for up to 19 months (23). Clearly, these nosocomial pathogens are well adapted to ICU life.

ICU PATIENTS ARE VULNERABLE TO COLONIZATION AND INFECTION WITH VRE

ICU patients are especially vulnerable to colonization and infection with VRE. Many of the risk factors that have been associated with VRE acquisition are common in patients in ICUs. These include advanced age, severity of underlying illness, hematologic malignancy, neutropenia, cirrhosis, recent intraabdominal surgery, renal dialysis, prior nosocomial infection, and the presence of pressure sores (6,7,8,9). Risk factors for children in pediatric ICUs are similar (24). In addition, low birth weight was found to be a risk factor for VRE colonization in one neonatal ICU (25). When multivariate analysis has been done, the most common host factor associated with VRE infection has been severe underlying illness, a condition almost universally present among ICU patients.

Antibiotic exposure has often been found to be a risk factor for acquisition of VRE. Receipt of vancomycin, cephalosporins, or drugs with anti-anaerobic activity has been linked to VRE colonization or infection (16,22,26,27). Project ICARE data show that for all types of ICUs, the defined daily dose of most of these antibiotics administered per 1000-patient days is greater than that administered in other inpatient units (2). In addition to antibiotics, other exposures that have been found to be risk factors for VRE acquisition include length of hospital stay, transfer from another hospital, transfer between hospital floors, proximity to a known infected or colonized patient, receipt of enteral feedings, and receipt of sucralfate (24,27,28,29,30,31). Most of these exposures are common among ICU patients. In multivariate analyses, the most significant risk factors for VRE acquisition include length of hospital stay, proximity to another VRE-positive patient, and transfer within a hospital.

DOES INFECTION WITH VRE POSE A SIGNIFICANT THREAT TO ICU PATIENTS?

The marginal activity of even "effective" antibiotics against multidrug resistant VRE implies that patients with serious VRE infections will have worse outcomes than patients with infections due to vancomycin-susceptible enterococci. It is not surprising, then, that a number of studies have found that infection with VRE portends a poor prognosis (7,31,32). However, the severe underlying illnesses of most of the affected patients, as well as the inclusion of those who were only colonized or transiently infected, makes determination of attributable morbidity or mortality difficult. This has led some investigators to conclude that VRE is a surrogate marker for disease severity but that in and of itself it is of little clinical consequence (32,33). If vancomycin resistance were clinically significant, one would expect that this would be most easily demonstrated in a study of bloodstream infections. One such study was conducted by Mainous et al, who looked at 41 episodes of nosocomial enterococcal bacteremia in 39 patients in a surgical ICU; 24.4% of the episodes of bacteremia were due to VRE (33). Mortality within 72 hours of the onset of bacteremia was the same for patients with infections due to vancomycin-resistant and vancomycin-susceptible enterococci: 38.7% and 40%, respectively. However, the authors included patients with even a single, positive enterococcal blood culture in the study, and a source of bacteremia could not be identified for 20% of cases. Since it is well documented that a single blood culture growing enterococcus may merely represent transient bacteremia or blood culture contamination (26), it is likely that cases of clinically inconsequential bacteremia were included in this investigation. Finally, the small sample size limited the power to detect a difference in mortality between the two patient groups.

The conclusions of other studies that compared the outcomes of patients with vancomycin-resistant and vancomycin-susceptible enterococcal bacteremia had similar limitations. These included small sample size (32,34,35), the inclusion of patients with only a single blood culture positive for enterococcus (32,35,37), or failure to use a validated severity of disease scoring system, such as APACHE II, to account for differences in comorbid factors between cases and controls (9). Finally, none of these studies differentiated between infection with multidrug-resistant VRE, for which no proven therapy exists, and infection with VRE that remain susceptible to an effective antibiotic. This last point is important because one would expect that the outcome of a patient with bacteremia due to an ampicillin-susceptible *E. faecalis* strain would be better than that of a patient infected with a strain of *E. faecium* that was resistant to all established agents.

Vergis et al conducted a prospective, multicenter, observational study of the outcomes of patients with enterococcal bacteremia that attempted to overcome the shortcomings of the previously mentioned investigations. Over a 24-month period,

391 consecutive adult patients with clinically significant enterococcal bacteremia were enrolled from 5 US hospitals (38). Clinically significant bacteremia was defined as 2 or more separately drawn blood cultures growing an enterococcal isolate or isolation of enterococcus from a single antemortem blood culture and from a concomitant site of infection in the presence of clinical signs and symptoms compatible with bloodstream infection (39). Data collected included APACHE II scores and appropriateness of antibiotic therapy, as defined by treatment for at least 72 hours with at least one antibiotic that the enterococcal isolate was susceptible to in vitro and that was initiated within 48 hours of the onset of bacteremia. One hundred forty-seven patients (37%) were infected with VRE and 76 of these (52%) were housed in the ICU. In multivariate analysis, the total APACHE II score was the single best independent predictor of 14- and 30-day mortality, with an increase in the odds ratio of 1.10 for each incremental increase in the score. However, vancomycin resistance was also a significant risk factor for mortality, with an odds ratio of 2.10 (95% confidence interval, 1.14 to 3.88; *P*, 0.02). In the subset of 174 patients alive 48 hours after the onset of monomicrobial enterococcal bacteremia, appropriate antibiotic therapy had a statistically significant protective effect, with an odds ratio of 0.21 (95% confidence intervals, 0.06 to 0.80; *P*, 0.02). These data strongly suggest that VRE can cause significant, life-threatening disease, and that effective antibiotic treatment of VRE bacteremia can save patient lives.

EPIDEMIOLOGY OF VRE SPREAD WITHIN THE ICU

The paucity of effective antibiotic therapy for treatment of serious VRE infections makes prevention of VRE acquisition imperative. In order to control VRE, one must first have a thorough understanding of the epidemiology of its spread. Vancomycin resistance does not emerge de novo in susceptible enterococci exposed to vancomycin. Therefore, the first step towards infection with VRE must be exposure to a resistant enterococcal strain. A number of epidemiological studies have attempted to delineate the ways in which ICU patients come in contact with VRE. When interpreting these studies, it is important to keep two concepts in mind. First, because colonization with VRE generally precedes infection, and because the number of colonized patients may be 10-times that of those infected (28), the most illuminating studies are those that investigate the epidemiology of VRE colonization. Second, the epidemiology of VRE spread may be different during an epidemic caused by a single strain of VRE and in a setting where VRE are endemic and many different strains are circulating.

Boyce et al published an investigation of a monoclonal vanB *E. faecium* outbreak in an ICU (29). Comparison of 12 case-patients with matched controls revealed that the primary risk factors for VRE colonization were proximity to a case patient (*P*, 0.0005) or exposure to a nurse who cared on the same shift for a case patient (*P*, 0.0007). The authors found no significant difference between case and control patients in APACHE II scores or in length of previous ICU stay. The epidemic strain was recovered from 26 (28%) of 92 environmental surfaces cultured in case-patient rooms; environmental contamination was significantly more likely to be detected if the case-patient had diarrhea. These results suggest that cross-contamination of VRE within the ICU was the primary means of VRE spread. The relative importance of case-patients and of the environment as reservoirs for VRE was not determined, however.

Bonten et al expanded on these findings in a prospective cohort study of patient colonization and environmental contamination with VRE in a 16 bed MICU (22). Thirty-eight mechanically ventilated patients were studied over a 7-week period. Nine (24%) patients were already colonized with VRE when they were admitted to the MICU. Of the remaining 29 patients, 12 (41%) acquired VRE colonization during their ICU stay. Risk factors for VRE acquisition on univariate analysis included older age and receipt of a third generation cephalosporin. Colonization of patient body sites was persistent, even on the intact skin of upper extremities; 75% of cultures remained positive for VRE after the first positive culture. Environmental contamination was common, although it was found in smaller amount and was more transient than was patient body site colonization. Molecular epidemiological analysis revealed that, as in the Boyce study (29), cross-colonization appeared to be the primary means of spread of VRE within the MICU, accounting for 85% of cases of VRE acquisition. Unlike the situation described by Boyce et al, however, VRE were endemic at this hospital. Twenty different strains of VRE were identified in the MICU during the study period. Another important observation of this study was that only 5 patients grew VRE from clinical cultures. Thus, the majority of colonized patients would have gone undetected if active screening for VRE had not been done.

The epidemiology of VRE in this endemic setting was more complex than in the monoclonal epidemic. The primary complication was admission to the MICU of patients who were already colonized with VRE, which added as many new cases as did cross-transmission. In another study that evaluated these patients as well as patients enrolled in an earlier investigation in the same MICU (28), 43 (14%) of 301 patients were already colonized with VRE at the time of MICU admission (40). Of particular interest is the authors' observation that 3 (7%) of the 43 patients were admitted directly from the community without demonstrable prior hospital contact. In the US, a community reservoir for VRE has never been identified. Given that rectal colonization with VRE can persist for a prolonged period, it is most likely that these 3 patients acquired VRE colonization during a hospital contact in the distant past. Transmission of VRE outside of healthcare institutions is rare (41), but may become more common as the care of chronically ill patients in outpatient settings increases.

The admission of patients to the ICU who are already colonized with VRE has been shown to be important in other studies as well. Ostrowski et al found that 12% of 290 patients admitted to 2 surgical ICUs at one hospital were already colonized with VRE at the time of admission, while 12.8% of the remaining patients became colonized with VRE sometime during their ICU stay. Prior to this investigation, few patients at the study hospital were known to carry VRE; on average, only 2 cases of VRE were detected by clinical cultures each month (30). Thus, even when the hospital-wide incidence of VRE in clinical cultures is low, the prevalence of VRE colonization in an ICU can be high. Finally, both of these studies demonstrate that the transfer of patients who are already colonized with VRE to the ICU can have a substantial impact on the epidemiology of VRE within the unit.

In another study, Bonten et al identified an additional variable important to the epidemiology of VRE in ICUs: "colonization pressure". This was defined as the proportion of patients colonized with VRE during a given time (42). The investigators studied 181 patients who were admitted for 48 hours or more over a 19-week period to an MICU where VRE were endemic, and where multiple different strain types were circulating. One hundred-fifty three patients were not colonized with VRE at the time of ICU admission, and 45 of them (29%) acquired rectal colonization with VRE. Twelve variables were entered separately into a Cox proportional hazards regression model in which the number of days until acquisition of VRE was the dependent variable. The independent variables included antibiotic use, enteral feeding, receipt of sucralfate, APACHE II score, compliance of health care workers with infection control measures, and the daily point prevalence of VRE colonized patients ("colonization pressure"). When all variables were tested as covariates, the best model included the colonization pressure, the proportion of days with enteral feeding, and the proportion of days of cephalosporin use. When the model (colonization pressure and either cephalosporin use or enteral feeding) was used to calculate the median time until acquisition of VRE, colonization pressure had the greatest effect. In fact, once the colonization pressure was greater than 50%, the other variables had only a slight effect on time to acquisition of VRE. The authors reasoned that in an ICU where the majority of patients were colonized with VRE, a lapse in infection control practices was more likely to result in cross-transmission of VRE than in an ICU where few patients were colonized. A limitation of this study was that compliance rates were ICU specific, not patient specific. The resultant small range of compliance rates may have masked the importance of compliance with infection control measures in preventing cross transmission of VRE.

The Importance of Hand Contamination

Most hospital patients acquire VRE from another patient, presumably via the contaminated hands of a healthcare worker. This presumption is based primarily on the isolation of identical VRE strains from patient specimens and from health care workers' hands. In epidemiological investigations in which VRE contamination of healthcare worker hands has been sought, it has been found in 0% to 41% of hands sampled (43,44,45,46). While VRE have been isolated from the fingers of volunteers 60 minutes after inoculation (21), it is not known whether VRE can colonize the hands of healthcare workers for prolonged periods. However, the fact that handwashing is effective in removing VRE suggests that if colonization occurs, it is transient.

In a clinical and epidemiological study carried out by Bonilla et al, a 15 second wash with 0.6% parachlorometaxylenol (Medi-Scrub, Huntington Laboratory, Huntington, IN) removed VRE from the majority of healthcare worker hands cultured

(43). VRE could still be recovered from 3 of 60 (5%) healthcare workers after handwashing, however. When tested formally in the laboratory, a 30 second scrub with either Medi-Scrub or a bland soap preparation (Germa-care, Huntington Laboratories) effectively removed 10^2 cfu of VRE that had been inoculated onto volunteers' hands, while a 5 second scrub with the same agents eliminated 99% of the organisms (21). In contrast, another study found that a 30 second wash with a disinfectant product—60% isopropyl alcohol, alcoholic chlorhexidine, chlorhexidine skin cleanser, or povidone-iodine—was more effective at eliminating 10^4 cfu of VRE from subjects' hands than was bland soap and water (19). These findings suggest that length of contact with the cleansing agent is important in removing VRE from hands, and that disinfectants may be more effective than bland soap in cleaning hands that are heavily contaminated with VRE. Finally, it appears to be necessary for healthcare workers to wash their hands after contact with a VRE colonized or infected patient even if gloves are worn during the contact. This was demonstrated in a study in which 17 of 50 (39%) healthcare givers who had contact with a VRE-positive patient acquired the patient's VRE strain on their gloves; 5 of the 17 were also found to have VRE on their hands after glove removal (46). In this study, glove contamination was associated with duration of patient contact, contact with a patient's bodily fluids, patient skin contamination with VRE, and diarrhea.

Is the Hospital Environment an Important Reservoir for VRE?

The significance of the inanimate environment as a source for VRE transmission is less well defined than that of contaminated healthcare worker hands. Evidence favoring the environment as an important reservoir for VRE includes the following: 1) After inoculation onto bedrails and other surfaces, VRE are able to survive for up to 24 hours with minimal reduction in colony counts (21). 2) Enterococci, including VRE, are relatively resistant to killing by heat and to removal by washing with bland soap (19,20,21). 3) In a number of epidemiological investigations, VRE have been isolated from environmental surfaces in patient rooms, including patient and health care worker gowns, door handles, cabinets, overbed tables, floors, intravenous fluid pumps, EKG monitors, bedrails, blood pressure cuffs, urinals, bedpans, toilet seats, and bed linen (5,8,11,14,16,17,18,27). In the Boyce study discussed earlier (29), a VRE outbreak was not controlled until all health care workers entering the rooms of patients who were infected or colonized with VRE donned cover gowns as well as gloves. This intervention may have decreased contact between healthcare workers and VRE in the patient's environment. 4) In the study by Bonten et al, 23% of patients whose rooms became contaminated with VRE became colonized with the environmental strain (22). 5) Two retrospective, case-control studies implicated contaminated fomites as the source of VRE outbreaks (47,48). In a third study, cross-transmission of VRE was linked to a contaminated fluidized bed (49).

None of these investigations provides incontrovertible evidence that hospitalized patients acquire VRE from the environment. In fact, there are data that implicate a minor role for this mode of transmission. Only the study cited above by Bonten et al was designed specifically to evaluate the contribution of environmental contamination to transmission of VRE (22). Therefore, the significance of finding VRE in the environment in the other investigations is uncertain. Even in the Bonten study, VRE contamination was present transiently and in low numbers at most environmental sites. Moreover, all of the patients who acquired VRE after their rooms became contaminated were colonized with a strain that was simultaneously present in other patients in the MICU; these other patients were therefore also potential sources of cross-colonization. Furthermore, the number of patient body sites colonized with VRE was highly associated with environmental contamination in a patient's room, suggesting that the patient contaminated the environment and not visa versa.

VRE commonly contaminate environmental surfaces on hospital wards that house VRE colonized or infected patients. Whether patients can acquire VRE from the contaminated surfaces, either directly or via the hands of healthcare workers, remains unclear. Until the importance of the hospital environment as a reservoir for VRE can be determined with certainty, it is probably safest to assume that transmission from the environment to patients can occur, and to take precautions to prevent such spread.

A Mathematical Model to Describe the Spread of VRE within the ICU

Using data from an earlier study (28), Austin, Bonten and other investigators created a mathematical description of the spread of VRE in the ICU (Figure 1) (50). They extrapolated the Ross-Macdonald model of vector-borne disease transmission, assuming that healthcare workers were "vectors" who transmitted VRE indirectly from one patient ("host") to another. Because environmental contamination had been found to be low-level and transient in their previous studies, and in order to simplify the model, environmental contamination was not considered.

A set of differential equations was used to describe the dynamics of cross transmission of VRE in the ICU. The authors first defined R_o, the basic reproductive number, as the average number of secondary colonized patients generated by a primary case in a formerly VRE-free ICU. If R_o is greater than 1, each colonized patient can generate at least one subsequent case and an epidemic can occur. If R_o is less than one, an outbreak cannot be sustained. They then assumed that R_o was comprised of 2 components: R_p, transmission of VRE from patient to healthcare worker and R_h, transmission of VRE from healthcare worker to patient. The authors assumed further that patients remained colonized with VRE for the duration of their ICU stay, but that healthcare workers were contaminated with VRE only transiently. Therefore, each colonized patient was thought to contaminate many healthcare workers, but each healthcare worker was expected to transmit VRE to few patients. From these variables, they derived y_p, the endemic VRE colonization prevalence in patients, and y_h, the VRE contamination rate among healthcare workers. They assumed that the prevalence of VRE among newly admitted patients provided a lower limit for y_p. Prevalence above this value was felt to reflect the impact of cross transmission of VRE.

The investigators then examined the effect on the model of antibiotic restriction,

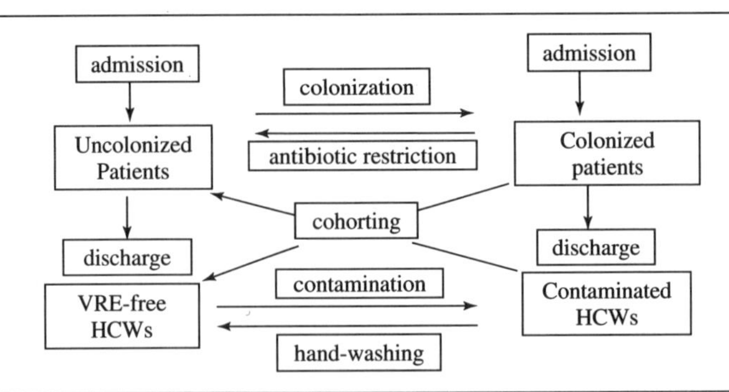

Figure 1. Ross-Macdonald model of indirect patient-healthcare worker-patient transmission of vancomycin-resistant enterococci in an intensive care unit showing the possible effect of infection control measures (50).

handwashing, and cohorting of patients. They calculated that given published compliance rates with handwashing of only 20% to 40%, this intervention alone was unlikely to be effective in controlling the spread of VRE in an ICU where R_0 was high. However, cohorting of nursing contacts had a very high theoretical chance of controlling cross transmission; if the majority of a nurse's contacts were with a single VRE-colonized patient, the chance that the nurse would transmit VRE from this patient to another would be small. A high rate of antibiotic exposure was assumed to provide a selective advantage for the survival of VRE. Antibiotic restriction would then be expected to decrease the selective advantage, and by extrapolation, the probability of VRE transmission.

The equations were then used to calculate R_0 for a single MICU where detailed clinical, demographic, and microbiological data related to VRE colonization had been collected (28). For the MICU analyzed, R_0 was calculated to be between 3 and 4, which should have resulted in a prevalence of VRE colonization of almost 80%. The observed prevalence was approximately 36%. The difference in these values was attributed to a reduction in transmission effected by implementation of infection control measures. The frequent admission to the MICU of patients who were already colonized with VRE was felt to stabilize the prevalence further.

This model makes several assumptions that require further testing. Nevertheless, its provision of a mathematical framework to describe the transmission of VRE in the ICU setting may allow more accurate determination of the effect of control strategies in the future.

CONTROL MEASURES

The ability of VRE to survive in hospitals may be unique among nosocomial bacterial pathogens. Weinstein et al noted that VRE poses a "triple threat" to hospitalized patients (22). It is able to colonize patients' gastrointestinal tract and skin, thus posing a risk similar to that of antibiotic resistant gram-negative rods and methicillin-resistant S. aureus combined. It also colonizes the hospital environment, which presents a risk similar to *Clostridium difficile*. Control of VRE therefore presents a special challenge to hospitals. The steady increase in the number of clinical isolates of VRE reported from US hospitals suggests that this challenge has yet to be confronted successfully.

In 1995, the CDC's Hospital Infection Control Practices Advisory Committee published recommendations for preventing the spread of vancomycin resistance (3); these recommendations are currently under revision. They included more prudent vancomycin use, education of hospital staff about the problem of VRE, guidelines for accurate detection of VRE by the clinical microbiology laboratory, guidelines for active screening for VRE carriage, implementation of contact precautions for patients who are known to be infected or colonized with VRE, and cohorting of VRE-positive patients and the healthcare workers caring for them. Since their publication, the efficacy of several of the interventions has been tested, and the results of these evaluations have been published (16,28,52).

Two investigators studied restriction of vancomycin use as a means of controlling VRE. Morris et al restricted intravenous and oral vancomycin use over a 7 month period at a large university hospital where serial point prevalence surveys revealed the endemic prevalence of VRE to be 20% (16). Infection control measures, including physical separation of VRE-positive patients and cohorting, were also implemented. During the study, intravenous vancomycin use fell by 59%, and use of oral vancomycin declined by 85%. However, the prevalence of VRE colonization among patients remained unchanged. The authors speculated that the interventions may have prevented an increase in colonization prevalence, and that a decrease in prevalence may have been seen if the study were carried out longer.

In contrast, Quale et al found that restriction of cefotaxime, clindamycin, and vancomycin resulted in a decrease in VRE rectal colonization and infection among patients at a Veterans Administration hospital where VRE were endemic (51). Infection control measures implemented earlier had failed to decrease the prevalence of VRE among clinical isolates. However, these measures were continued during the antibiotic restriction period. Interpretation of these findings is made difficult by several factors. First, the extent of compliance with infection control interventions was not reported. Second, antibiotic consumption was not normalized for total patient days or number of admissions. Third, the reported fall in mean number of clinical cases of VRE was moderate, with a large standard deviation that overlapped with that of the mean number of cases reported prior to antibiotic restriction. Finally, the decrease in rectal colonization reported was based on results of a single point prevalence survey. Given the natural variability in colonization rates that has been reported in studies done in other endemic settings (22,28), this difference may not have been significant. Even if one assumes that the intervention was effective, the prevalence of VRE colonization among patients remained 15%, illustrating the difficulty of eradicating VRE in an endemic setting.

The recommended isolation precautions for patients known to be infected or colonized with VRE include wearing clean, nonsterile gloves when entering the patient's room and wearing a clean nonsterile cover gown if extensive contact with the patient or the environment is anticipated, or if the patient has diarrhea, fecal incontinence, an ileostomy, a colostomy, or wound drainage not covered by a dressing (3). These recommendations are based on the finding of extensive environmental contamination in several studies (29,47), as well as the failure to control a monoclonal VRE outbreak until gowning was mandated for all contacts with VRE-positive patients (29). Slaughter et al tested the efficacy of this recommendation in a comparative study of the effect of universal use of gloves and gowns with that of glove use alone in a medical ICU where VRE were endemic (28). One hundred eighty-one consecutive patients admitted to the ICU for more than 48 hours were studied. Rectal cultures were obtained daily from all patients, and compliance with precautions—4363 total observations—was monitored weekly. Fifteen percent of patients were already colonized with VRE at the time of ICU admission, and 25% of the remaining patients acquired VRE. Although there was no difference between the 2 groups in acquisition of rectal colonization with VRE, compliance with gloving and handwashing was significantly better in the glove and gown cohort than in the cohort where only gloves were worn (overall compliance, 78.9% versus 62.1%, $P < 0.001$). In this setting, gowns seemed to increase healthcare worker awareness of the infection control problem and of the need for isolation precautions. Furthermore, when these data were analyzed in the transmission model of Austin et al, implementation of infection control measures was calculated to have decreased transmission of VRE (50).

What measures can be recommended to control VRE in the ICU? The most successful reports have come from single units where one predominant strain of VRE was colonizing or infecting patients (25,29). In these situations, aggressive use of barrier precautions, prospective surveillance, and placing patients in private rooms have successfully contained outbreaks. In a monoclonal outbreak in a neonatal ICU, cohorting of colonized babies and of babies who had been exposed to a colonized patient played a major role in controlling the epidemic strain (25). Control in hospitals where VRE are endemic is more problematic. Eradication of VRE from ICUs in these settings may not be realistic, especially given the likely ongoing importation of positive cases from outside of the unit. However, some investigators have been successful in decreasing the transmission of VRE in endemic settings. For example, Montecalvo et al reported that institution of a comprehensive program of enhanced infection control measures, coupled with an overall decrease in antibiotic use, resulted in a 50% reduction in VRE colonization and a 4.7-fold decrease in VRE bacteremia on an oncology ward where VRE were endemic (52). Bodnar et al reported a novel strategy of molecular epidemiological analysis of apparent clusters of VRE that appeared against a background of endemicity (53). In that study, identification of a single clone infecting 12 seemingly unrelated patients prompted an in depth chart review that revealed common links among them. Targeted infection control measures were then instituted and further transmission of the epidemic strain was halted.

VRE will likely continue to be problem pathogens for US ICUs. While eradication of VRE may not be possible in ICUs where VRE are endemic, efforts to reduce the prevalence of colonization and infection should continue. Innovative intervention strategies and multifaceted programs that include antibiotic restriction with infection control measures may yield the best outcomes.

REFERENCES

1. Leclerq R, Derlot E, Duval J, Courvalin P. Plasmid-mediated resistance to vancomycin and teicoplanin in *Enterococcus faecium*. N Engl J Med 1988;319:157–161.
2. Fridkin SK, Gaynes RP. Antimicrobial resistance in intensive care units. Clinics in Chest Medicine 1999;20:303–316.
3. Centers for Disease Control and Prevention. Recommendations for preventing the spread of vancomycin resistance: recommendations of the Hospital Infection Control Practices Advisory Committee (HICPAC). MMWR. 1995;44(RR-12):1–13.
4. Centers for Disease Control and Prevention. Nosocomial enterococci resistant to vancomycin-United States, 1989–1993. MMWR Morb Mortal Wkly Rep 1993;42:597–599.
5. Synercid® I.V. (quinupristin/dalfopristin), package insert.
6. Montecalvo MA, Horowitz H, Gedris C, Carbonaro C, Tenover FC, Issah Abdul, Cook Perry, Wormser GP. Outbreak of vancomycin-, ampicillin-, and aminoglycoside-resistant *Enterococcus faecium* bacteremia in an adult Oncology unit. Antimicrob Agents Chemother 1994;38:1363–1367.
7. Edmond MB, Ober JF, Weinbaum DL, Pfaller MA, Hwang T, Sanford MD, Wenzel RP. Vancomycin-resistant *Enterococcus faecium* bacteremia: risk factors for infection. Clin Infect Dis 1996;20:1126–1133.
8. Henning KJ, Delencastre H, Eagan J, Boone N, Brown A, Chung M, Wollner N, Armstrong D. Vancomycin-resistant *Enterococcus faecium* on a pediatric oncology ward: Duration of stool shedding and incidence of clinical infection. Pediatr Infect Dis J 1996;15:848–854.
9. Linden PK, Pasculle AW, Manez R, Kramer DJ, Fung JJ, Pinna AD, Kusne S. Difference in outcomes for patients with bacteremia due to vancomycin-resistant *Enterococcus faecium* or vancomycin-susceptible *E. faecium*. Clin Infect Dis 1996;22:663–670.
10. Arthur M, Courvalin P. Genetics and mechanisms of glycopeptide resistance in enterococci. Antimicrob Agents Chemother 1993;37:1563–1571.
11. Navarro F, Courvalin P. Analysis of genes encoding D-alanine-D-alanine ligase-related enzymes in *Enterococcus casseliflavus* and *Enterococcus flavescens* Antimicrob Agents Chemother 1994;38:1788–1793.
12. Fines M, Perichon B, Reynolds P, Sahm DF, Courvalin P. VanE, a new type of acquired glycopeptide resistance in *Enterococcus faecalis* BM 4405. Antimicrob Agents Chemother 1999;43:2162–2164.
13. Perichon B, Reynolds P, Courvalin P. VanD-type glycopeptide-resistant *Enterococcus faecalis* BM 4339. Antimicrob Agents Chemother 1997;41:2016–2018.
14. Hayden MK, Trenholme GM, Schultz JE, Sahm DF. In vivo development of teicoplanin resistance in a VanB *Enterococcus faecium* isolate. J Infect Dis 1993;167:1224–1227.
15. Quintiliani R Jr., Courvalin P. Conjugal transfer of the vancomycin-resistance determinant vanB between enterococci involves movement of large genetic elements from chromosome to chromosome. FEMS Microbiol Lett 1994;119:359–364.
16. Morris JG, Shay DK, Hebden JN, McCarter RJ, Perdue BE, Jarvis W, Johnson JA, Dowling TC, Polish LB, Schwalbe RS. Enterococci resistant to multiple antimicrobial agents, including vancomycin: Establishment of endemicity in a University Medical Center. Ann Intern Med 1995;123:250–259.
17. Klare I, Rodloff AC, Wagner J, Witte W, Hakenbeck. Overproduction of a penicillin-binding protein is not the only mechanism of penicillin resistance in *Enterococcus faecium*. Antimicrob Agent and Chemother 1992;36:783–787.
18. Murray PR, Baron EJ, Pfaller MA, Tenover FC, Yolken RH, editors. Manual of Clinical Microbiology. 7th ed. ASM Press, Washington, D.C., 1999.
19. Wade JJ, Desai N, Casewell MW. Hygienic hand disinfection for the removal of epidemic vancomycin-resistant *Enterococcus faecium* and gentamicin-resistant *Enterobacter cloacae*. J Hosp Infect 1991;18:211–218.
20. Gordon CLA, Ahmad MH. Thermal susceptibility of *Streptococcus faecium* strains isolated from frankfurters. Can J Microbiol 1991;37:609–612.
21. Noskin GA, Stoser V, Cooper I, Peterson LR. Recovery of vancomycin-resistant enterococci on fingertips and environmental surfaces. Infect Control Hosp Epidemiol 1996;17:770–771.
22. Bonten MJM, Hayden MK, Nathan C, van Voorhis RN, Matushek M, Slaughter S, Rice T, Weinstein RA. The epidemiology of patient colonization and environmental contamination

with vancomycin-resistant enterococci: the challenge for infection control. Lancet 1996;348:1615–1619.
23. Montecalvo MA, de Lencastre H, Carraher M, Gedris C, Chung M, VanHorn K, Wormser GP. Natural history of colonization with vancomycin-resistant *Enterococcus faecium*. Infect Control and Hosp Epidem 16:680–685.
24. McNeeley DF, Brown AE, Noel GJ, Chung M, de Lencastre H. An investigation of vancomycin-resistant *Enterococcus faecium* within the pediatric service of a large urban medical center. Ped Infect Dis J 1998;17:184–188.
25. Malik RK, Montecalvo MA, Reale MR, Li K, Maw M, Munoz JL, Gedris C, VanHorn K, Carnevale KA, Levi MH, Dweck HS. Epidemiology and control of vancomycin-resistant enterococci in a regional neonatal intensive care unit. Ped Infect Dis J 1999;18:352–356.
26. Beezhold DW, Slaughter S, Hayden MK, Matushek M, Nathan C, Trenholme GM, Weinstein RA. Skin colonization with vancomycin-resistant enterococci among hospitalized patients with bacteremia. Clin Infect Dis 1997;24:704–706.
27. Tornieporth NG, Roberts RB, John Joylene, Hafner A, Riley LW. Risk factors associated with vancomycin-resistant *Enterococcus faecium* infection or colonization in 145 matched case patients and control patients. Clin Infect Dis 1996;23:767–772.
28. Slaughter S, Hayden MK, Nathan C, Hu TC, Rice T, van Voorhis J, Matushek M, Franklin C, Weinstein RA. A comparison of the effect of universal glove and gown use with glove use alone in the acquisition of vancomycin-resistant enterococci in a medical intensive care unit. Ann Intern Med 1996;125:448–456.
29. Boyce JM, Opal SM, Chow JW, Zervos MJ, Potter-Bynoe G, Sherman CB, Romulo RL, Fortna S, Medeiros AA. Outbreak of multidrug-resistant *Enterococcus faecium*_with transferable vanB class vancomycin resistance. J Clin Microbiol 1994;32:1148–1153.
30. Ostrowsky BE, Venkataraman L, D'Agata EMC, Gold HS, DeGirolami PC, Samore MH. Vancomycin-resistant enterococci in intensive care units: high frequency of stool carriage during a non-outbreak period. Arch Intern Med 1999;159:1467–1472.
31. Papanicolaou GA, Meyers BR, Meyers J, Mendeson MH, Lou W, Emre S, Sheiner P, Miller C. Nosocomial infection with vancomycin-resistant *Enterococcus faecium* in liver transplant recipients: risk factors for acquisition and mortality. Clin Infect Dis 1996;23:760–766.
32. Shay DK, Maloney SA, Montecalvo M, et al. Epidemiology and mortality risk of vancomycin-resistant enterococcal bloodstream infections. J Infect Dis 1995;172:993–1000.
33. Mainous MR, Lipsett PA, O'Brien M, and The Johns Hopkins SICU Study Group. Enterococcal bacteremia in the surgical intensive care unit: does vancomycin resistance affect mortality? Arch Surg 1997;132;76–81.
34. Stroud L, Edwards J, Danzig L, Culver D, Gaynes R. Risk factors for mortality associated with enterococcal bloodstream infections. Infect Control Hosp Epidemiol 1996;17:576080.
35. Edmond MB, Ober JF, Dawson JD, Weinbaum DL, Wenzel RP. Vancomycin-resistant enterococcal bacteremia: natural history and attributable mortality. Clin Infect Dis 1996;23:1234–1239.
36. Montecalvo MA, Shay DK, Patel P, Tacsa L, Maloney SA, Jarvis WR, Wormser GP. Bloodstream infections with vancomycin-resistant enterococci. Arch Intern Med 1996;156:1458–1462.
37. Lucas GM, Lechtzin N, Puryear DW, Yau LL, Flexner CW, Moore RD. Vancomycin-resistant and vancomycin-susceptible enterococcal bacteremia: comparison of clinical features and outcomes. Clin Infect Dis 1998;26:1127–1133.
38. Vergis EN, Chow JW, Hayden MK, Snydman DR, Zervos MZ, Linden PK, Wagener MM, Muder RR. Vancomycin resistance predicts mortality in enterococcal bacteremia: a prospective, multicenter study of 375 patients. 37th Interscience Conference on Antimicrobial Agents and Chemotherapy, Toronto, Ontario, Canada, September 28–October 1, 1997, Abstract No. J-6, p. 289.
39. Maki DG, Agger WA. Enterococcal bacteremia: clinical features, the risk of endocarditis, and management. Medicine 1988;67:248–269.
40. Bonten MJM, Slaughter S, Hayden MK, Nathan C, van Voorhis J, Weinstein RA. External sources of vancomycin-resistant enterococci for intensive care units. Crit Care Med 1998;26:2001–2004.
41. Shekar R, Chico G, Bass SN, Strozewski K, Biddle J. Household transmission of vancomycin-resistant *Enterococcus faecium*. Clin Infect Dis 1995;21:1511–1512.
42. Bonten MJM, Slaughter S, Ambergen AW, Hayden MK, van Voorhis J, Nathan C, Weinstein RA. The role of "colonization pressure" in the spread of vancomycin-resistant enterococci: an important infection control variable. Archives Int Med 1998;158:1127–1132.
43. Bonilla HF, Zervos MA, Lyons MJ, Bradley SF, Hedderwick SA, Ramsey MA, Paul LK, Kauffman

CA. Colonization with vancomycin-resistant *Enterococcus faecium*: comparison of a long-term-care unit with an acute-care hospital. Infection Control & Hospital Epidemiology 1997;18:333–339.

44. Boyce JM, Mermel LA, Zervos MJ, Rice LB, Potter-Bynoe G, Giorgio C, Medeiros AA. Controlling vancomycin-resistant enterococci. Infect Control Hosp Epidem 1995;16:634–637.
45. Rubin LG, Tucci V, Cercenado E, Eliopoulos G, Isenberg HD. Vancomycin-resistant *Enterococcus faecium* in hospitalized children. Infect Control Hosp Epidem 1992;13:700–705.
46. Badri SM, Sahgal NB, Tenorio AR, Law K, Hota B, Matushek M, Hayden MK, Trenholme GM, Weinstein RA. Effectiveness of gloves in preventing transmission of vancomycin-resistant enterococcus (VRE) during patient care activities. 36th Annual Meeting of the Infectious Diseases Society of America, November 12–15, 1998, Denver, CO, Abstract No. 599 Fr, p. 189.
47. Livornese LL Jr., Dias S, Samel C, Romanowski B, Taylor S, May P, Pitsakis P, Woods G, Kaye D, Levison ME, Johnson CC. Hospital-acquired infection with vancomycin-resistant *Enterococcus faecium* transmitted by electronic thermometers. Ann Int Med 1992;117:112–116.
48. Porwacher R, Sheth A, Remphrey S, Taylor E, Hinkle C, Zervos M. Epidemiological study of hospital-acquired infection with vancomycin-resistant *Enterococcus faecium*: Possible transmission by an electronic ear-probe thermometer. Infect Control Hosp Epidemiol 1997;18:771–772.
49. Wilcox JH, Jones BL. Enterococci and hospital laundry. Lancet 1995;345:594.
50. Austin DJ, Bonten MJM, Weinstein RA, Slaughter S, Anderson RM. Vancomycin-resistant enterococci in intensive-care hospital settings: tranmsission dynamics, persistence, and the impact of infection control programs. Proc Natl Acad Sci USA 1999;96:6908–6913.
51. Quale J, Landman D, Saurina G, Atwood E, DiTore V, Patel K. Manipulation of a hospital antimicrobial formulary to control an outbreak of vancomycin-resistant enterococci. Clin Infect Dis 1996;23:1020–1025.
52. Montecalvo MA, Jarvis WR, Uman J, Shay DK, Petrullo C, Rodney K, Gedris C, Horowitz HW, Wormser GP. Infection-control measures reduce transmission of vancomycin-resistant enterococci in an endemic setting. Ann Intern Med 1999;269–272.
53. Bodnar UR, Noskin GA, Suriano T, Cooper I, Reisberg BE, Peterson LR. Use of in-house studies of molecular epidemiology and full species identification for controlling spread of vancomycin-resistant *Enterococcus faecalis* isolates. J Clin Microbiol 1996;34:2129–2132.

4. VANCOMYCIN-RESISTANT ENTEROCOCCI IN EUROPE: A CHANGING EPIDEMIOLOGY?

MARC J.M. BONTEN, M.D., PHD

University Medical Center Utrecht, Utrecht, The Netherlands

INTRODUCTION

The recent emergence of infections caused by vancomycin-resistant enterococci (VRE) has created worldwide interest in these bacteria, which were, until ten years, considered to be relatively avirulent. The clinical problems with VRE have occurred primarily in the United States of America (1). Here, VRE have become endemic colonizers in many ICUs, whereas colonization outside hospitals is absent. The European epidemiology, however, is completely different. In Europe, VRE have been demonstrated in feces of healthy persons, whereas infections in ICU-patients remain extremely rare. So far, outbreaks with VRE have been reported only sporadically, but from at least eight countries (Table 1). In 1999–2000 three outbreaks of VRE occurred in Dutch hospitals. The first outbreak (*van*A *Enterococcus faecium*) occurred on a hematology ward (2) and the second (also *van*A *E. faecium*) on a renal and dialysis ward (3). Both outbreaks could be controlled with extensive infection control measures. Epidemiological analysis of the second outbreak identified a clear association with a nearby university hospital. Here, surveillance demonstrated hospital-wide spread of colonization with VRE and control of spread proved to be very difficult (4). The question is whether these three outbreaks represent a significant change in the epidemiology of VRE in the Netherlands and Europe, which could eventually lead to endemicity of colonization with VRE in European ICUs.

In the Netherlands, similar concerns were raised in the eighties when the first cases of colonization and infection with methicillin-resistant *Staphylococcus aureus*

R.A. Weinstein and M.J.M. Bonten (eds.). INFECTION CONTROL IN THE ICU ENVIRONMENT.

Table 1. Reported outbreaks caused by VRE in Europe

First author	Year of publication	Country	Setting	Number of patients	Type of VRE	Infection control successful
Jordens (25)	1994	Great Britain	Multiple wards, mainly renal	22	*Van*A *E. faecium*	?
Biavasco (26)	1996	Italy	Neurosurgical ICU	8	*Van*A *E. faecalis*	Yes
Torell (27)	1997	Sweden	?	4	*Van*A *E. faecium*	Yes
Brown (28)	1998	Great Britain	Renal ward	29	*Van*A *E. faecium*	Yes
Schuster (29)	1998	Germany	Pediatric oncology ward	24	?	Yes
Suppola (30)	1999	Finland	6 hospitals	156	Mainly *Van*A *E. faecium*	Yes
Kawalec (31)	2000	Poland	Haematology ward	128	*Van*A *E. faecium*	Yes
Nourse (32)	2000	Ireland	Pediatric oncology ward	16	*Van*A *E. faecium*	Yes
Vandenbroucke-Grauls (2)	2000	The Netherlands	Haematology ward	14	*Van*A *E. faecium*	Yes
Van der Steen (3)	2000	The Netherlands	Renal ward	12	*Van*A *E. faecium*	Yes
Mascini (4)	2000	The Netherlands	Multiple hospital wards	26	*Van*A *E. faecium*	?

(MRSA) occurred. Since then, patients suspected for colonization with MRSA, mainly patients transferred from hospitals abroad, are treated in isolation until colonization with MRSA is excluded or eradicated. Using this strategy, infections and colonization with MRSA have remained extremely rare in Dutch hospitals, despite endemicity in all surrounding countries (5). The considerations regarding the control of VRE, as described in this chapter, have been published partly elsewhere (6).

THE ENTEROCOCCUS AS A PATHOGEN

Enterococci are usually avirulent commensals of the human intestinal tract. Severe infections, such as bacteraemias, abdominal infections, urinary tract infections, intravascular line infections and endocarditis, occur almost exclusively in immunocompromised patients (7). Exact incidences of these infections, however, are unknown. Enterocooci are intrinsically resistant to many antibiotics, and have, parallel to the clinical use of other classes of antibiotics, acquired resistance. For some enterococci, vancomycin remained the last therapeutic resort. VRE were first described in the eighties and in 1993 researchers demonstrated that the genetic code for resistance was located on a transposon, which could easily be transferred to susceptible enterococci (8,9). By now, five different genetic mechanisms for vancomycin-resistance have been identified (*van*A-*van*E), of which the *van*A-type is most prevalent.

THE EPIDEMIOLOGY OF VRE IN THE NETHERLANDS

VRE are widely distributed in the Dutch community. Prevalences of colonization among healthy subjets range from 2% (10) to 15% (11). In the last study, more than 50% of VRE belonged to the *van*A-type (11). In addition, VRE have been isolated in large amounts among calves, pigs, broilers and meat (12). It is very suggestive that the use of avoparcin, which was used as a growth promoter in the veterinary industry during the last 25 years, has selected VRE. From this reservoir VRE or the transposon coding for vancomycin resistance may have been transmitted to healthy people. The European Community prohibited the use of avoparcine as a growth promoter in 1997. This ban has already resulted in a decrease in the prevalence of VRE among healthy subjects, both in the Netherlands and in Germany (13,14). In the Netherlands the prevalence among pigs, broilers and healthy humans decreased from 34%, 80% and 12 % respectively in 1997 to 17%, 21% and 6% respectively in 1999 (13).

The widespread distribution of VRE in the community did, until 2000, not create clinical problems within Dutch hospitals. In a large survey among patients treated in ICUs and hematology wards in nine hospitals revealed an overall prevalence of colonization of 2% (10). Although an estimated proportion of the total population of 2–15% is colonized with VRE, the number of infections caused by VRE is extremely low. Moreover, there are no identified risk factors for VRE-colonizers. In Belgium, the prevalence of VRE-colonization among patients requiring haemodialysis is 14%, which is higher than the prevalence among healthy subjects (15). Although comparable prevalence rates were reported from dialysis patients in two Dutch hospitals (10% and 23%) (3,4), data from other Dutch centers are lacking. Since many different genotypes were isolated among the Belgium dialysis patients, it is likely that resistance was acquired through selection by antibiotic use rather than via cross-transmission from patient to patient. The fact that no risk groups for VRE-carriership can be identified hampers institution of infection control measures, once VRE-carriers are admitted to hospital. This is in contrast to the epidemiology of MRSA in the Netherlands. Colonization with MRSA among healthy Dutch subjects is extremely rare and only patients admitted from hospitals abroad must be considered as potential sources for MRSA. These patients can be treated in isolation until colonization with MRSA is excluded or eradicated.

RISKS OF VRE-COLONIZATION IN INDIVIDUAL PATIENTS

Usually, enterococci only cause infections in immunocompromised patients, who are at risk for infections with intestinal bacteria or bacteria associated with intravascular devices, such as patients who underwent bone marrow or solid organ transplantation or those treated in intensive care units. However, it is unknown whether infections caused by VRE, as compared to infections caused by vancomycin-susceptible enterococci, influence patient survival. Attributable mortality due to VRE has been reported for hematological patients and patients with liver transplantation (16,17). Other investigators, however, failed to confirm this association (18). Moreover, some new antibiotics covering VRE have been introduced, but clinical experience with these agents is sparse and resistance has already been reported.

Although infections are almost always preceded by colonization, it is unknown to what extent colonization with VRE increases the risk for infection. However, once colonized, patients frequently remain colonized for prolonged periods of time (19). Attempts to eradicate VRE-colonization by antibiotics have not been successful. An effective measure to eradicate VRE could significantly contribute to future control of the spread of VRE.

RISKS OF VRE-COLONIZATION FOR OTHER PATIENTS

Detailed studies combining epidemiological investigations and molecular biological typing methods have demonstrated how rapidly VRE can be transmitted from patient to patient (20,21). These transmissions usually occur via the hands of health care workers. The possibility of the transposon coding for vancomycin-resistance to be transferred to staphylococci has been feared, but has, up till now, not been demonstrated in human subjects. In contrast, such a transfer has been demonstrated in an experimental mice model (22).

HOW DOES VRE SPREAD?

As stated above transfer from patient to patient mostly occurs via the temporarily contaminated hands of health care workers. Although enterococci usually colonize the gastrointestinal tract, they can also persistently colonize the skin of critically ill patient (21,23). In addition, contamination of the environment of colonized patients frequently occurs and seems to be related to the number of body sites that a patient is colonized with VRE (21). From these sources, other non-colonized patients may become colonized. Therefore, each contact with a patient or his or hers direct environment contains a risk for bacterial spread. Furthermore, colonization is stimulated by antibiotic use. Especially, third-generation cephalosporins, vancomycin and anti-anaerobic agents have been associated with increased risks on colonization (1). High compliance with infection control measures (especially disinfecting of hands) and restrictive use of antibiotics are the cornerstones of infection prevention.

Based on epidemiological investigations, 2–15% of health care workers in Western Europe will be colonized with VRE, but it is unknown if, and to what extent, physicians and nurses colonized with VRE participate in the epidemiology of VRE.

WHY OCCURRED VRE-OUTBREAKS SO SPORADICALLY IN EUROPE?

So far, approximately ten VRE-outbreaks have been reported from Europe, although this list may not be exhaustive (Table). Most outbreaks were caused by *van*A *E. faecium* strains, and oncology, hematology and renal wards were frequently involved.

Transmission of VRE is influenced by variables such as compliance with infection control procedures on hospital wards, the amounts of antibiotics prescribed, the capacity of bacteria for spread, and the susceptibility of patients to acquire colonization. It is very likely that introduction of VRE into all kind of hospital wards has occurred on a daily basis in the last twenty years. However, it is unknown why epidemics with VRE have occurred so rarely in Western Europe, despite an enormous reservoir of VRE in the community. The recent occurrence of epidemics, therefore, suggests that several types of VRE with specific capacities for spread have emerged.

WHAT TO DO WITH VRE IN THE NETHERLANDS?

The occurrence of the first three VRE-outbreaks in The Netherlands has created a large dilemma about how to cope with similar outbreaks in the future. Two of the three outbreaks, both located in a single hospital ward, could be controlled with extensive infection control measures. The third outbreak was hospital wide and was much harder to control. Until now, active surveillance for VRE-colonization is not performed routinely in the Netherlands. The outbreaks were discovered by the remarkable occurrence of two clinical isolates (blood cultures in one and urine cultures in the other hospital) with an abnormal susceptibility profile. As for most pathogens isolation of VRE from clinical samples represents the tip of an iceberg, and in both cases much more patients proved to be colonized without any symptoms of infection. The question, therefore, is whether extensive surveillance should be performed when VRE are isolated from clinical cultures.

One may argue not to search actively for VRE, for several reasons. So far, in the Netherlands only few infections with VRE have been documented, the incidence of infections with enterococci is low anyhow, it is unknown whether infections with VRE have an attributable mortality as compared to infections with vancomycin-susceptible enterococci, and the pharmaceutical industry will probably develop new and active antibiotics before severe clinical problems emerge. Moreover, the ban of avoparcine use in the veterinary industry has already resulted in a decrease of VRE-colonization in the community, suggesting that this problem will disappear spontaneously.

On the contrary, the recent epidemics suggest that the epidemiology of VRE in the Netherlands is changing. In analogy to other pathogenic and multi-resistant microorganisms this will ultimately result in infections. For VRE this means infections with a relatively avirulent bacteria, which may life-threatening in critically ill or immunocompromised patients and which may be difficult to treat In addition, a genetic reservoir of vancomycin-resistance will develop from where transfer of resistance to more pathogenic bacteria may occur. From this viewpoint a proactive approach towards surveillance of VRE-colonization and limitation of spread in hospitals seems to be justified. The question is, how proactive?

One option would be to react similarly as in the first VRE-outbreaks. Only when VRE are isolated from clinical cultures, surveillance for colonization is initiated. When spread of a single genotype has been demonstrated appropriate measures for infection control should be implemented, such as contact isolation of colonized patients to limit further spread. Needless to say that compliance with basic infection control measures (hand disinfection) and restrictive use of antibiotics should be pursued under these circumstances. This strategy has been successful in most monoclonal VRE-outbreaks, so far.

Another option would be to prevent the spread of VRE to high-risk patients, such as those receiving bone marrow and solid organ transplantation and those treated in ICUs. Patients newly admitted to these wards should be screened for VRE-colonization. If positive, a patient should be cared for in isolation in order to prevent spread to other susceptible patients. The danger of this strategy is the development of endemicity of VRE-colonization on other hospital wards, from where patients will be transferred to the wards with high-risk patients. After some time the number of VRE-positive patients on admission to these wards may be so high that effective control becomes impossible. This seemed to be an important reason for the development and persistence of endemicity of VRE in ICUs in the U.S. (24).

Finally, one might aim to prevent any transmission of VRE within hospitals. This policy resembles the so far very successful "search and destroy" policy, that was adapted to control MRSA in the Netherlands. However, this policy seems to be impossible for VRE. There is no clear risk profile for VRE-carriership, and, therefore, each patient admitted should be considered VRE-positive. As for patients suspected of colonization with MRSA, these patients should be screened and be treated in strict isolation until proven negative for VRE. Since colonization cannot be eradicated, approximately 2–15% of all patients should be treated in isolation. This would be impossible, both for patients as well as for health care workers.

CONCLUSION

It will be clear that many questions regarding the optimal strategy to control the spread of VRE remain unanswered. Although even the incidence of enterococcal infections in The Netherlands is unknown, endemicity with easily transmissible VRE should, to my opinion, be prevented for three reasons: A high prevalence of colonization will, sooner or later, result in infections caused by VRE, most likely among the most critical and vulnerable patients. The size of this patient group will increase in the years to come. Finally, a genetic reservoir may lead to transfer of resistance to other, more virulent, bacteria. Large extramural and intramural studies have demonstrated that low prevalences of VRE have been present in the Netherlands for years without the development of outbreaks. The recent outbreaks, however, may have resulted from the development and introduction of specific clones of VRE, which may have special characteristics making them more suitable for nosocomial spread.

REFERENCES

1. Murray BE. Vancomycin-resistant enterococcal infections. *New England Journal of Medicine.* 2000;342:710–721.
2. Vandenbroucke-Grauls CMJE, Meester HHM, Donkers LEA, et al. Succesvolle bestrijding van een

epidemie met vancomycineresistente Enterococcus faecium op een hematologische afdeling. *Nederlands Tijdschrift voor Medische Microbiologie*. 2000;8:S28.
3. Steen Fvd, Bonten M, Kregten Ev, Willems R, Gaillard CA. Epidemie veroorzaakt door vancomycine-resistente Enterococcus faecium op een afdeling inwendige geneeskunde/nefrologie. *Nederlands Tijdschrift voor geneeskunde*. 2000 (in press).
4. Mascini EM, Gigengack-Baars ACM, Hené R, Kamp-Hopmans TEM, Weersink AJL, Bonten MJM. Epidemie veroorzaakt door verscheidene genotypen van vancomycine-resistente Enterococcus faecium in een Academisch Ziekenhuis. *Nederlands Tijdschrift voor geneeskunde*. 2000 (in press).
5. Ibelings MMS, Bruining HA. Methicillin-resistant Staphylocuccus aureus: Acquisition and risk of death in patients in the Intensive Care Unit. *Eur J Surg*. 1998;164:411–418.
6. Bonten MJM, Mascini EM, Willems R, et al. Wat te doen bij epidemieën veroorzaakt door vancomycine-resistente enterokokken. *Nederlands Tijdschrift voor Geneeskunde*. 2000 (in press).
7. Moellering RC. Emergence of Enterococcus as a significant pathogen. *Clin Infect Dis*. 1992;14:1173–1178.
8. Leclercq R, Derlot E, Duval J, Courvalin P. Plasmid-mediated resistance to vancomycin and teicoplanin in Enterococcus faecium. *New Engl J Med*. 1988;319:157–161.
9. Arthur M, Molinas C, Depardieu F, Courvalin P. Characterization of Tn1546, a Tn3-related transposon conferring glycopeptide resistance by synthesis of depsipeptide peptidoglycan precursors in Enterococcus faecium BM4147. *Journal of Bacteriology*. 1993;175:117–127.
10. Endtz HP, van den Braak N, van Belkum A, et al. Fecal carrigae of vancomycin-resistant enterococci in hospitalized patients and those living in the community in The Netherlands. *J Clin Microbiol*. 1997;35:3026–3031.
11. Willems R. Vancomycineresistente enterokokken: epidemiologie en transmissie van resistentie. *Nederlands Tijdschrift voor Medische Microbiologie*. 1999;7:5–8.
12. van den Bogaard AE, Mertens P, London NH, Stobberingh EE. High prevalence of colonization with vancomycin- and pristinamycin-resistant enterococci in healthy humans and pigs in The Netherlands: is the addition of antibiotics to animal feeds to blame? *Journal of Antimicrobial Chemotherapy*. 2000;40:454–456.
13. van den Bogaard AE, Bruinsma N, Stobberingh EE. The effect of banning avoparcin on VRE carriage in The Netherlands. *Journal of Antimicrobial Chemotherapy*. 2000;46:146–147.
14. Klare I, Badstübner D, Konstabel C, Böhme G, Claus H, Witte W. Decreased incidence of vanA-type vancomycin-resistant enterococci isolated from poultry meat and from fecal samples of humans in the community after discontinuation of avoparcin usage in animal husbandry. *Microbial Drug Resistance*. 1999;5:45–52.
15. Descheemaeker P, Ieven M, Chapelle S, et al. Prevalence and molecular epidemiology of glycopeptide-resistant enterococci in Belgian renal dialysis units. *Journal of Infectious Diseases*. 2000;181:235–241.
16. Edmond MB, Ober JF, Dawson JD, Weinbaum DL, Wenzel RP. Vancomycin-resistant enterococcal bacteremia: Natural history and attributable mortality. *Clin Infect Dis*. 1996;23:1234–1239.
17. Linden PK, Pasculle AW, Manez R, et al. Differences in outcomes for patients with bacteremia due to vancomycin-resistant Enterococcus faecium or vancomycin-susceptible E. faecium. *Clin Infect Dis*. 1996;22:663–670.
18. Garbutt JM, Ventrapragada M, Littenebrg B, Mundy LM. Association between resistance to vancomycine and death in cases of Enterococcus faecium bacteremia. *Clinical Infectious Diseases*. 2000; 30:466–472.
19. Roghmann M, Qaiyumi S, Johnson JA, Schwalbe R, Morris JG. Recurrent vancomycin-resistant Enterococcus faecium bacteremia in a leukemia patient who was persistently colonized with vancomycin-resistant enterococci for two years. *Clin Infect Dis*. 1997;24:514–515.
20. Slaughter S, Hayden MK, Nathan C, et al. A comparison of the effect of universal use of gloves and gowns with that of glove use alone on acquisition of vancomycin-resistant enterococci in a medical intensive care unit. *Ann Intern Med*. 1996;125:448–456.
21. Bonten M, Hayden MK, Nathan C, et al. Epidemiology of colonisation of patients and environment with vancomycin-resistant enterococci. *Lancet*. 1996;348:1615–1619.
22. Noble WC, Virani A, Cree R. Cotransfer of vancomycin and other resistance genes from Enterococcus faecalis NCTC 12201 to Staphylococcus aureus. *FEMS Microbiol Lett*. 1992;93:195–198.
23. Beezhold DW, Slaughter S, Hayden MK, et al. Skin colonization with Vancomycin-resistant enterococci among hospitalized patients with bactermia. *Clin Infect Dis*. 1997;24:704–706.
24. Austin DA, Bonten MJM, Slaughter S, Weinstein RA, Anderson RM. Vancomycin-resistant entero-

cocci in Intensive Care hospital settings: Transmission dynamics, persistence and the impact of infection control programs. *Proceedings of the National Academy of Sciences USA*. 1999;96:6908–6913.

25. Jordens JZ, Bates J, Griffiths DT. Faecal carriage and nosocomial spread of vancomycin-resistant Enterococcus faecium. *J Antimicrob Chemother*. 1994;34:515–528.
26. Biavasco F, Miele A, Vignaroli C, Manso E, Lupidi R, Varaldo PE. Genotypic characterization of a nosocomial outbreak of VanA Enterococcus faecalis. *Microbial Drug Res*. 1996;2:231–237.
27. Torell E, Fredlund H, Tornquist E, Myhre EB, Sjoberg L, Sundsfjord A. Intrahospital spread of vancomycin-resistant Enterococcus faecium in Sweden. *Scandinavian Journal of Infectious Diseases*. 1997;29:259–263.
28. Brown AR, Amyes SGB, Paton R, et al. Epidemiology and control of vancomycin-resistant enterococci in a renal unit. *J Hosp Infection*. 1998;40:115–124.
29. Schuster F, Graubner UB, Schmid I, Weiss M, Belohradsky BH. vancomycin-resistant enterococci colonization of 24 patients on a pediatric oncology unit. *klinische Padiatrie*. 1998;210:261–263.
30. Suppola JP, Kolho E, Salmenlinna S, Tarkka E, Vuopio-Varkila J, Vaara M. vanA and vanB incorporate into an endemic ampicillin-resistant vancomycin-sensitive Enterococcus faecium strain: effect on interpretation of clonality. *Journal of Clinical Microbiology*. 1999;37:3934–3939.
31. Kawalec M, Gniadkowski M, Hryniewicz W. Outbreak of vancomycin-resistant enterococci in a hospital in Gdansk, Poland, due to horizontal transfer of different Tn1546-like transposon variants and clonal spread of several strains. *Journal of Clinical microbiology*. 2000;38:3317–3322.
32. Nourse C, Byrne C, Murphy H, Kaufmann ME, Clarke A, Butler K. Eradication of vancomycin resistant Enterococcus faecium from a paediatric oncology unit and prevalence of colonization in hospitalized and community-based children. *Epidemiology and Infection*. 2000;124:53–59.

5. METHICILLIN-RESISTANT STAPHYLOCOCCUS AUREUS: IS CONTROL NECESSARY?

JOHN M. BOYCE, M.D.

Hospital of Saint Raphael, New Haven, CT 06511 USA

INTRODUCTION

Methicillin-resistant strains of *Staphylococcus aureus* (MRSA) first emerged as important nosocomial pathogens in the United States in the 1980s, and have continued to increase in frequency in subsequent years (Figure 1). By 1997, MRSA caused more than 35 percent of nosocomial *S. aureus* infections in hospitals with more than 500 beds, and caused 25% to 30% of such infections in small and medium-sized hospitals, respectively (1). Since the earliest reports of MRSA outbreaks in United States, it has been clear that patients in intensive care units (ICUs) have been at increased risk for developing nosocomial MRSA infections. Many of the early MRSA outbreaks affected patients in the burn units, surgical intensive care units, and neonatal ICUs (2). Recent data from the Centers for Disease Control and Prevention (CDC) National Nosocomial Infection Surveillance (NNIS) system demonstrate that the prevalence of MRSA infections continues to be higher in ICUs than on non-ICU wards (3). In 1999, MRSA accounted for 52 percent of nosocomial *S. aureus* infections in the ICU patients in NNIS hospitals (4).

Risk factors. Factors associated with acquiring MRSA in ICUs include high severity of illness scores, longer stays in the ICU, preceding surgery, greater intravascular device use, preceding antimicrobial therapy, and mechanical ventilation (5). Overcrowding of patients and understaffing have contributed to transmission of MRSA in several ICUs (6,7). Although selective digestive tract decolonization (SDD) regimens have been identified as a risk factor for acquisition of MRSA in

R.A. Weinstein and M.J.M. Bonten (eds.). INFECTION CONTROL IN THE ICU ENVIRONMENT.

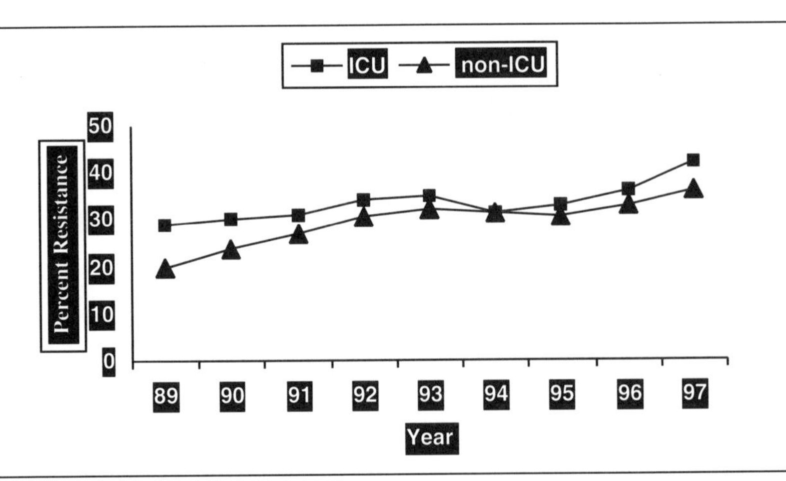

Figure 1. Percent of Nosocomial *Staphylococcus aureus* Infection on ICU and non-ICU Wards, NNIS, 1987–1999.

some intensive care units in Europe, such regimens have not been documented as being an important risk factor for MRSA in ICUs in United States.

Frequency of MRSA in ICUs. The prevalence of MRSA colonization and infection varies considerably among hospitals. The organisms have become highly endemic or epidemic in some ICUs, while in other hospitals, the incidence of MRSA infections remains relatively low. For example, in a hospital where MRSA accounted for less than 20 percent of all *S. aureus* isolated by the clinical microbiology laboratory, cultures obtained by physicians for clinical purposes detected new hospital-acquired MRSA colonization or infection in only 0.6 percent of patients admitted to a medical-surgical ICU over a seven-year period. Patients with colonization undetected by clinical cultures may not have been recognized. However, periodic point prevalence culture surveys performed on 19 occasions over 4 years in the ICU detected unsuspected MRSA colonization in only two of 176 patients (8). During this time, MRSA infections occurred in 17 patients, an incidence rate of 0.3 nosocomial MRSA infections per 100 ICU admissions.

No widely accepted criteria have been adopted for defining what constitutes an outbreak of MRSA in an ICU. In a recent consensus statement, a number of experts in the United States felt that in some high-risk units where the organism is not endemic, a single new MRSA case might be considered an outbreak (9). No criteria could be agreed-upon for defining an outbreak in ICUs where MRSA is endemic.

Patterns of Transmission. MRSA outbreaks in ICUs often have followed unsuspected introduction of the organism into the unit by transfer of a colonized or infected patient (10,11). In some facilities, such index patients have acquired MRSA on another ward of the same hospital, and in other situations, at nearby facilities or in high-risk units located in another state.

In most ICUs where MRSA is endemic or epidemic, spread of the organism via the hands of health-care workers is likely to be the most common form of transmission (12,13). Some outbreaks have been due to transmission of an epidemic strain from one or more personnel who are have persistent nasal carriage of MRSA or have areas of dermatitis colonized or infected with MRSA (14,6,15,16,17,18). The role of contaminated environmental surfaces in transmission of MRSA is not clear. Prospective studies of patients colonized or infected with MRSA have revealed that environmental surfaces in the rooms of affected patients may become contaminated, particularly if the patient has MRSA in a wound, urine, or at the site of the a tracheostomy (19,20). Nurses who have had no direct patient contact may contaminate their gloves or hands by touching contaminated surfaces (20). Further studies are necessary to determine the relative importance of environmental contamination in transmission of MRSA in ICUs. Airborne transmission of MRSA may occur in some high-risk units, such as burn units (19).

Strain Typing. Molecular typing of MRSA isolates has confirmed that such epidemics often have been due to transmission of a single clone (16,13,17,18). In some ICUs, pulsed-field gel electrophoresis of isolates has documented that MRSA outbreaks involving primarily ICUs have resulted from simultaneous transmission of two or more clones (Boyce JM, unpublished data).

Transmission of MRSA in ICUs not only affects patients within the unit, but often results in spread of the organism to other wards following transfer of ICU patients to other areas of the hospital (21,22,23,24). For this reason, controlling transmission of MRSA in high-risk units may have a beneficial effect on the prevalence of MRSA hospital-wide.

MRSA INFECTIONS

Data from early MRSA outbreaks in the United States revealed that about 55% of ICU patients who acquired MRSA subsequently developed clinically significant infections (2). The types of MRSA infections seen most frequently in ICU patients in the United States involve the bloodstream, postoperative or burn wounds, lower respiratory tract, cutaneous sites, urinary tract, or other body sites (22,2,25). The relative frequency of the various types of infection depends to some extent on the type of ICU. Bloodstream infections have predominated in some NICUs and in a liver transplant unit (7,26). In surgical ICUs and burn units, wound infections and bacteremias often predominate (25,10,22,27,14,28,29). In some medical-surgical ICUs, lower respiratory infections have been the most common form of MRSA infection.

Adverse Outcomes Associated with MRSA. Allowing MRSA to become endemic or epidemic in ICUs should be avoided whenever possible, for several reasons. First, MRSA infections are often associated with considerable morbidity among affected patients, and often increase the length of stay of affected ICU patients (12,30,6,31). Second, MRSA isolates are as virulent as methicillin-susceptible *S. aureus* strains and are associated with significant mortality in high-risk patients. Crude mortality rates among ICU patients with MRSA infections average 25% (23,6,10,22,12,25,32,11,33,7,18). In a few studies where attributable mortality rates were given, MRSA infection was considered to be the primary or contributing cause of death in 10% to 15% of affected ICU patients. Mortality rates vary considerably, based on the body site affected. Singh et al. found that crude mortality rates were 86% in liver transplant patients with bacteremic MRSA pneumonia or abdominal infections, but the mortality rate was only 6% in those with catheter-related MRSA bacteremia (26).

Third, several studies in the United States have shown that hospital charges or costs associated with MRSA infections are often $3,200 to $17,000 greater than those attributable to methicillin-susceptible *S. aureus* infections (22,34,35,36). Importantly, under the Prospective Payment System in the United States, hospitals are seldom reimbursed adequately for such additional costs. Studies in Europe have confirmed that MRSA infections often generate excess hospital costs (37).

Impact on Vancomycin Use. Finally, allowing MRSA to become endemic or epidemic in ICUs promotes frequent use of vancomycin. For example, data from 108 ICUs in 41 hospitals participating in Project ICARE have documented that vancomycin usage correlated with the proportion of S. aureus isolates that were MRSA and with the incidence of central line-associated bloodstream infections (38). MRSA rates in the ICUs were an independent predictor of the amount of vancomycin used, when expressed as defined daily doses/1000 patient-days. Little has been published regarding the proportion of all vancomycin courses administered in ICUs that is attributable to therapy of MRSA infections. In a study supported by the CDC Prevention Epicenter program, analysis of intravenous vancomycin used in a medical-surgical ICU during a one-year period revealed that 11 (16%) of 70 courses of vancomycin therapy were administered for treatment of MRSA infections (Boyce JM et al., unpublished data). The relatively low percentage of vancomycin used for treatment of MRSA infections in this unit may be related to the fact that the incidence of MRSA infections (community-acquired and nosocomial cases) was relatively low (3.2/1000 patient-days) in the unit. In many ICUs, where MRSA account for up to 50% of *S. aureus* infections, vancomycin use related to treatment of MRSA infections is likely to account for a substantially larger percent of all vancomycin usage. There is little doubt that high vancomycin usage in the United States has promoted the emergence of vancomycin-resistant enterococci and will likely foster emergence of vancomycin-intermediate *S. aureus* (39,40).

CONTROL MEASURES

During the years when MRSA emerged as important pathogens in the United States, there was no universally accepted approach to prevention and control of these pathogens in hospitals. In 1995, the Hospital Infection Control Practices Advisory Committee (HICPAC) published general guidelines for preventing nosocomial transmission of multidrug pathogens, including MRSA (41). Recommendations included in the guidelines are summarized briefly below.

1) Place patients with MRSA in a private room, or cohort patients.
2) Wear gloves whenever entering an MRSA patient's room.

3) Wear a gown if substantial contact with the patient or the patient's environment is anticipated.
4) Remove gloves (and gown) upon leaving the patient's room.
5) Wash hands with an antimicrobial soap or with a waterless antiseptic agent.
6) Whenever possible, dedicate non-critical medical equipment to the patient's room. If equipment must be shared, items should be sterilized or disinfected before use on other patients.
7) Limit transport of patients to essential purposes.

Although many hospitals have adopted the HICPAC guidelines, compliance with recommended measures appears to vary substantially among hospitals. For example, failure of personnel to remove their gloves following contact with known MRSA patients was felt to contribute to transmission of the organism in an ICU (42). Although some hospitals question the efficacy and cost-effectiveness of infection control measures, careful epidemiological studies in the United States and Europe have demonstrated that implementation of appropriate control measures can reduce transmission of MRSA in ICU settings and can be cost-effective in many settings (43,37).

A number of studies have shown that nurses and physicians working in ICUs often fail to wash their hands as frequently as recommended (Table 1) (44,45,46,47,48,49,50,51). Although one might predict that compliance would be better in ICUs where high-risk patients receive care, Pittet et al. (51) found that the compliance rate in ICUs was only 36%, compared to 47% to 59% on other wards. The lower compliance noted in ICUs is presumably related to the heavy workloads experienced by personnel working in such high-risk units (51). Since MRSA is most frequently transmitted on the hands of personnel, renewed efforts to improve hand hygiene among ICU personnel are warranted. A multidisciplinary approach, which includes educational and motivational strategies as well as reducing logistic barriers to frequent handwashing, is required (51,52). Placing an alcohol-based waterless antiseptic agent at each patient's bedside improves access to hand hygiene materials, and takes less time than standard soap and water handwashing (53). At least one study has demonstrated that this strategy resulted in improved

Table 1. Observed Compliance of Healthcare Workers with Recommended Handwashing Practices in Intensive Care Units

Author	Year	Percent Compliance
Preston	1981	30%
Albert	1981	28%–41%
Donowitz	1987	30%
Graham	1990	32%
Dubbert	1990	81%
Pettinger	1991	51%
Doebbeling	1992	40%
Pittet	1999	36%

compliance of ICU personnel with recommended hand hygiene practices (54). This strategy warrants further evaluation as a means of improving hand hygiene in ICUs.

Several studies suggest that in ICUs where MRSA is endemic or epidemic, universal glove use may help control the spread of MRSA (13,42). This strategy requires that all health-care workers wear gloves when caring for all patients in the affected intensive care unit.

Other control measures that have been used in some ICUs where MRSA is endemic or epidemic include labeling patients charts and identifying known MRSA patients' at the time of readmission. Although screening patients for MRSA carriage at the time of admission to high-risk units has been shown to contribute to control of MRSA transmission in an ICU in Europe, this approach is used infrequently in United States. However, it warrants serious consideration in ICUs where MRSA is poorly controlled, particularly if the organism is prevalent in other wards of the same hospital, or in other healthcare facilities that transfer patients to the ICU (55).

CONCLUSION

There are no standard criteria for use of decolonization therapy in the ICUs. It has been recommended that hospitals consider administering intranasal mupirocin ointment to colonized high-risk patients during MRSA outbreaks in an effort to reduce the reservoir of the organism (9). No current data exist regarding how frequently this strategy is used in ICUs in United States, but it is less commonly used than in some European countries. Most experts agree that epidemiologically-implicated health-care workers with MRSA nasal carriage should be treated with an agent such as mupirocin ointment (56,57,58).

In summary, ongoing transmission of MRSA in ICUs leads to serious infections, prolonged length of stays and mortality among affected patients, excess hospital costs for which hospitals are seldom reimbursed, spread of the organism from the ICU to other wards, and increased use of vancomycin, which promotes emergence of organisms with reduced susceptibility to vancomycin. These factors should serve as an impetus for hospitals to continue their efforts to control the spread of MRSA.

REFERENCES

1. Fridkin S, Gaynes R. Antimicrobial Resistance in Intensive Care Units. Clinics in Chest Medicine 1999;20:303–316.
2. Thompson RL, Cabezudo I, Wenzel RP. Epidemiology of nosocomial infections caused by methicillin-resistant *Staphylococcus aureus*. Ann Intern Med 1982;97:309–317.
3. Archibald L, Phillips L, Monnet D, McGowan JE, Jr, Tenover F, Gaynes R. Antimicrobial resistance in isolates from inpatients and outpatients in the United States: Increasing importance of the intensive care unit. Clin Infect Dis 1997;24:211–215.
4. Gerberding JL, et al. Semiannual Report: Aggregated Data from the National Nosocomial Infections Surveillance (NNIS) System. NNIS SAR 1999; December 1999:1–34.
5. Pujol M, Pena C, Pallares R, Ariza J, Ayats J, Dominguez MA, Gudiol F. Nosocomial *Staphylococcus aureus* bacteremia among nasal carriers of methicillin-resistant and methicillin-susceptible strains. Am J Med 1996;100:509–516.
6. Arnow PM, Allyn PA, Nichols EM, Hill DL, Pezzlo M, Bartlett RH. Control of methicillin-resistant *Staphylococcus aureus* in a burn unit: role of nurse staffing. J Trauma 1982;22:954–959.

7. Haley RW, Cushion NB, Tenover FC, Bannerman TL, Dryer D, Ross J, Sanchez PJ, Siegel JD. Eradication of endemic methicillin-resistant *Staphylococcus aureus* infections from a neonatal intensive care unit. J Infect Dis 1995;171:614–624.
8. Boyce J. Methicillin-resistant *Staphylococcus aureus* and vancomycin-resistant enterococci in intensive care units. Current Opinion in Critical Care 1997;3:355–362.
9. Wenzel RP, Reagan D, Bertino J, Baron EJ, Arias K. Methicillin-resistant *Staphylococcus aureus* outbreak: A consensus panel's definition and management guidelines. Am J Infect Control 1998;26:102–110.
10. Saroglou G, Cromer M, Bisno AL. Methicillin-resistant *Staphylococcus aureus*: interstate spread of nosocomial infections with emergence of gentamicin-methicillin resistant strains. Infect Control 1980;1:81–89.
11. Locksley RM, Cohen ML, Quinn TC, Tompkins LS, Coyle MB, Kirihara JM, Counts GW. Multiply antibiotic-resistant *Staphylococcus aureus*: introduction, transmission, and evolution of nosocomial infection. Ann Intern Med 1982;97:317–324.
12. Peacock JE, Jr, Marsik FJ, Wenzel RP. Methicillin-resistant *Staphylococcus aureus*: introduction and spread within a hospital. Ann Intern Med 1980;93:526–532.
13. Hartstein AI, Denny MA, Morthland VH, LeMonte AM, Pfaller MA. Control of methicillin-resistant *Staphylococcus aureus* in a hospital and an intensive care unit. Infect Control Hosp Epidemiol 1995;16:405–411.
14. Craven DE, Reed C, Kollisch N, DeMaria A, Lichtenberg D, Shen K, McCabe WR. A large outbreak of infections caused by a strain of *Staphylococcus aureus* resistant to oxacillin and aminoglycosides. Am J Med 1981;71:53–58.
15. Gaynes R, Marosok R, Mowry-Hanley J, Laughlin C, Foley K, Friedman C, Kirsh M. Mediastinitis following coronary artery bypass surgery: A 3-year review. J Infect Dis 1991;163: 117–121.
16. Boyce JM, Opal SM, Potter-Bynoe G, Medeiros AA. Spread of methicillin-resistant *Staphylococcus aureus* in a hospital after exposure to a health care worker with chronic sinusitis. Clin Infect Dis 1993;17:496–504.
17. Sherertz RJ, Reagan DR, Hampton KD, Robertson KL, Streed SA, Hoen HM, Thomas R, Gwaltney JM, Jr. A cloud adult: The *Staphylococcus aureus*-virus interaction revisited. Ann Intern Med 1996;124:539–547.
18. Meier PA, Carter CD, Wallace SE, Hollis RJ, Pfaller MA, Herwaldt LA. Eradication of methicillin-resistant *Staphylococcus aureus* (MRSA) from the burn unit at a tertiary medical center. Infect Control Hosp Epidemiol 1996;17:798–802.
19. Rutala WA, Katz EBS, Sherertz RJ, Sarubbi FA, Jr. Environmental study of a methicillin-resistant *Staphylococcus aureus* epidemic in a burn unit. J Clin Microbiol 1983;18:683–688.
20. Boyce JM, Potter-Bynoe G, Chenevert C, King T. Environmental contamination due to methicillin-resistant *Staphylococcus aureus*: Possible infection control implications. Infect Control Hosp Epidemiol 1997;18:622–627.
21. Crossley K, Landesman B, Zaske D. An outbreak of infections caused by strains of *Staphylococcus aureus* resistant to methicillin and aminoglycosides. II Epidemiologic studies. J Infect Dis 1979;139:280–287.
22. Boyce JM, Landry M, Deetz TR, DuPont HL. Epidemiologic studies of an outbreak of nosocomial methicillin-resistant *Staphylococcus aureus* infections. Infect Control 1981;2:110–116.
23. Boyce JM, White RL, Causey WA, Lockwood WR. Burn units as a source of methicillin-resistant *Staphylococcus aureus* infections. JAMA 1983;249:2803–2807.
24. Linnemann CC, Jr, Mason M, Moore P, Korfhagen TR, Staneck JL. Methicillin-resistant *Staphylococcus aureus*: experience in a general hospital over four years. Am J Epidemiol 1982;115:941–950.
25. Crossley K, Loesch D, Landesman B, Mead K, Chern M, Strate R. An outbreak of infections caused by strains of *Staphylococcus aureus* resistant to methicillin and aminoglycosides. I. Clinical studies. J Infect Dis 1979;139:273–279.
26. Singh N, Paterson DL, Chang FY. Methicillin-Resistant *Staphylococcus aureus*: The Other Emerging Resistant Gram-Positive Coccus among Liver Transplant Recipients. Clin Infect Dis 2000;30: 322–327.
27. Myers JP, Linnemann CC, Jr. Bacteremia due to methicillin-resistant *Staphylococcus aureus*. J Infect Dis 1982;145:532–536.
28. Mest DR, Wong DH, Shimoda KJ, Mulligan ME, Wilson SE. Nasal colonization with methicillin-resistant *Staphylococcus aureus* on admission to the surgical intensive care unit increases the risk of infection. Anesth Analg 1994;78:644–650.

29. Sheridan RL, Weber J, Benjamin J, Pasternack MS, Tompkins RG. Control of methicillin-resistant *Staphylococcus aureus* in a pediatric burn unit. Am J Infect Control 1994;22:340–345.
30. Ribner BS, Landry MN, Kidd K, Peninger M, Riddick J. Outbreak of multiply resistant *Staphylococcus aureus* in a pediatric intensive care unit after consolidation with a surgical intensive care unit. Am J Infect Control 1989;17:244–249.
31. Holmbert SD, Solomon SL, Blake PA. Health and economic impacts of antimicrobial resistance. Rev Infect Dis 1987;9:1065–1078.
32. Everett ED, McNitt TR, Rahm AE, Jr, Stevens DL, Peterson HE. Epidemiologic investigation of methicillin-resistant *Staphylococcus aureus* in a burn unit. Melit Med 1978;143:165–167.
33. Reboli AC, John JF, Jr, Levkoff AH. Epidemic methicillin-gentamicin-resistant *Staphylococcus aureus* in a neonatal intensive care unit. Am J Dis Child 1989;143:34–39.
34. Rao N, Jacobs S, Joyce L. Cost-effective eradication of an outbreak of methicillin-resistant *Staphylococcus aureus* in a community teaching hospital. Infect Control Hosp Epidemiol 1988;9: 255–260.
35. Wakefield DS, Helms CM, Massanari RM, Mori M, Pfaller M. Cost of nosocomial infection: Relative contributions of laboratory, antibiotic, and per diem costs in serious *Staphylococcus aureus* infections. Am J Infect Control 1988;16:185–192.
36. Abramson MA, Sexton DJ. Nosocomial methicillin-resistant and methicillin-susceptible *Staphylococcus aureus* primary bacteremia: at what costs? Infect Control Hosp Epidemiol 1999;20:408–411.
37. Chaix C, Durand-Zaleski I, Alberti C. Control of Endemic Methicillin-Resistant *Staphylococcus Aureus*: A cost-benefit analysis in an intensive care unit. JAMA 1999;28:1745–1751.
38. Fridkin S, Edwards J, Pichette S, Pryor E, McGowan J, Tenover F, Culver D, Gaynes R. Determinants of Vancomycin Use in Adult Intensive Care Units in 41 United States Hospitals. Clin Infect Dis 1999;28:1119–1125.
39. Gerding DN. Is there a relationship between vancomycin-resistant enterococcal infection and *Clostridium difficile* infection? Clin Infect Dis 1997;25(suppl 2):206–210.
40. Smith TL, Pearson ML, Wilcox KR, Cruz C, Lancaster MV, Robinson-Dunn B, Tenover FC, Zervos MJ, Band JD, White E, Jarvis WR, Glycopeptide-Intermediate *Staphylococcus aureus* Working Group. Emergence of vancomycin resistance in *Staphylococcus aureus*. N Engl J Med 1999;340: 493–501.
41. Garner JS, Hospital Infection Control Practices Advisory Committee. Guideline for isolation precautions in hospitals. Infect Control Hosp Epidemiol 1996;17:53–80.
42. Maki DG, McCormick RD, Zilz MA, Stolz SM, Alvarado C. An MRSA outbreak in a SICU during universal precautions: new epidemiology for nosocomial MRSA: downside for universal precautions 1990 Program and abstracts of the 30th Interscience Conference on Antimicrobial Agents and Chemotherapy, Atlanta Abstr. #473
43. Jernigan JA, Titus MG, Groschel DHM, Getchell-White SI, Farr BM. Effectiveness of contact isolation during a hospital outbreak of methicillin-resistant *Staphylococcus aureus*. Am J Epidemiol 1996;143:496–504.
44. Preston GA, Larson EL, Stamm WE. The effect of private isolation rooms on patient care practices, colonization and infection in an intensive care unit. Am J Med 1981;70:641–645.
45. Albert RK, Condie F. Hand-washing patterns in medical intensive-care units. N Engl J Med 1981;304:1465–1466.
46. Donowitz LG. Handwashing technique in a pediatric intensive care unit. Am J Dis Child 1987;141:683–685.
47. Graham M. Frequency and duration of handwashing in an intensive care unit. Am J Infect Control 1990;18:77–80.
48. Dubbert PM, Dolce J, Richter W, Miller M, Chapman SW. Increasing ICU staff handwashing: Effects of education and group feedback. Infect Control Hosp Epidemiol 1990;11:191–193.
49. Pettinger A, Nettleman MD. Epidemiology of isolation precautions. Infect Control Hosp Epidemiol 1991;12:303–307.
50. Doebbeling BN, Stanley GL, Sheetz CT, Pfaller MA, Houston AK, Annis L, Li N, Wenzel RP. Comparative efficacy of alternative hand-washing agents in reducing nosocomial infections in intensive care units. N Engl J Med 1992;327:88–93.
51. Pittet D, Mourouga P, Perneger TV, Members of the Infection Control Program. Compliance with handwashing in a teaching hospital. Ann Intern Med 1999;130:126–130.
52. Kretzer EK, Larson EL. Behavioral interventions to improve infection control practices. Am J Infect Control 1998;26:245–253.

53. Voss A, Widmer AF. No time for handwashing!? Handwashing versus alcoholic rub: Can we afford 100% compliance? Infect Control Hosp Epidemiol 1997;18:205–208.
54. Bischoff WE, Reynolds TM, Sessler CN, Edmond MB, Wenzel RP, Bischoff WE, Reynolds TM, Sessler CN, Edmond MB, Wenzel RP. Handwashing compliance by health care workers: the impact of an education and patient awareness program and the introduction of a new hand disinfectant1998540Program and Abstracts of the 38th Annual ICAACAbstr #K-132.
55. Girou E, Pujade G, Legrand P, Cizeau F, Brun-Buisson C. Selective screening of carriers for control of methicillin-resistant *Staphylococcus aureus* (MRSA) in high-risk hospital areas with a high level of endemic MRSA. Clin Infect Dis 1998;27:543–550.
56. Mulligan ME, Murray-Leisure KA, Ribner BS, Standiford HC, John JJ, Korvick JA, Kauffman CA, Yu VL. Methicillin-resistant *Staphylococcus aureus*: A consensus review of the microbiology, pathogenesis, and epidemiology with implications for prevention and management. Am J Med 1993;94:313–328.
57. Boyce JM, Jackson MM, Pugliese G, Batt MD, Fleming D, Garner JS, Hartstein AI, Kauffman CA, Simmons M, Weinstein R, O'Boyle Williams C. Methicillin-resistant *Staphylococcus aureus* (MRSA): a briefing for acute care hospitals and nursing facilities. Infect Control Hosp Epidemiol 1994;15:105–115.
58. Herwaldt LA. Control of methicillin-resistant *Staphylococcus aureus* in the hospital setting. Am J Med 1999;106(Suppl 5A):11S–18S.

6. ACINETOBACTER: EPIDEMIOLOGY AND CONTROL

JAMES J. RAHAL, M.D. AND CARL URBAN, PH.D.

The New York Hospital Medical Center of Queens, Flushing, N.Y. 11355-5095, USA

MICROBIOLOGY

Microscopic examination of gram stained members of Acinetobacter may reveal several morphologies including short, plump rods, longer rods and coccoid forms depending on various parameters including the stage of cell growth and whether beta-lactam antibiotics are present. The cells may be in pairs and/or clusters, are frequently gram-variable, and occasionally exhibit large halos indicating the presence of a capsule. Biochemically, members of the genus Acinetobacter are nonfermenting strict aerobes that are oxidase negative and catalase positive. Growth at different temperatures and on MacConkey agar may vary, as do results of assimilation tests, even within a species of Acinetobacter (1). The API 20 NE® system (bioMérieux Vitek, Inc., Hazelwood, Mo., USA) is widely used for the identification of Acinetobacter species and consists of 8 conventional biochemical tests and 12 assimilation tests (2). Since phenotypic differences are sometimes observed within a species, genetic techniques including DNA-DNA hybridization and PCR must be used to definitively assign Acinetobacter isolates to a specific genomospecies (1).

Taxonomy and Related Clinical Disease

The genus Acinetobacter has evolved from the former "Mimeae Tribei" which consisted primarily of *Mima polymorpha*, *Herrelia vaginicola* and *Moraxella* species (3). During the 1960s studies of Mima and Herrelia identified their natural reservoir in

R.A. Weinstein and M.J.M. Bonten (eds.). INFECTION CONTROL IN THE ICU ENVIRONMENT.

humans as the oropharynx, vagina, other mucosal surfaces and moist skin (axilla, intertriginous areas). They were not found as part of the normal gastrointestinal flora (4–6). Many publications described acute urethritis, endocarditis, meningitis, and conjunctivitis due to Mima and Herrelia—community acquired infectious not currently associated with Acinetobacter (7–10). However, nosocomial outbreaks occurred in situations in which Acinetobacter are now isolated frequently; namely nosocomial pneumonia, burn infections, and catheter associated bacteremias (11). Reclassification has now included both Mima and Herrelia into the genus Acinetobacter, with the exception of oxidase negative isolates. *Mima polymorpha*, var. oxidans which caused most of the community acquired infections described above is now included among *Moraxella* species. Oxidase negative *Mima polymorpha* and *Herrelia vaginicola* first evolved to *Acinetobacter calcoaceticus* and *Acinetobacter anitratus*. Genetic methods have now identified at least 19 species of Acinetobacter with *A. calcoaceticus* and *A. anitratus* included as the *Acinetobacter calcoaceticus—baumannii* complex (12). Although this complex (usually referred to as *A. baumannii*) is most commonly associated with nosocomial infection, severe community acquired pneumonia occurs occasionally in patients with alcohol-induced liver disease, diabetes, chronic obstructive pulmonary disease, silicosis, and other host defense deficiencies. These pneumonias are often complicated by bacteremia, neutropenia, disseminated intravascular coagulation, shock and a high mortality (13).

Clinical and Molecular Epidemiology

Microbiologic and epidemiologic observations suggest that nosocomial invasive Acinetobacter strains, many of which are multiply antibiotic resistant, are derived from strains which exist as normal human microflora. Such resistant isolates appear to have evolved from exposure to antibiotics after patients are admitted to the hospital. However, Acinetobacter species are also commonly isolated from water, soil, food and sewage (12). It is therefore unclear whether nosocomial multi-resistant strains originate from human or environmental sources. In 1997 Seifert and colleagues used genotyping to compare colonizing Acinetobacter isolates from patients upon hospital admission with those recovered from healthy controls (14). They found more frequent colonization of patients than controls, but both groups harbored a variety of species other than A. baumannii, the cause of most nosocomial infections. A subsequent study by Berlan and coworker also indicates that normal skin flora is not the source of multi-resistant *A. baumannii* (15). Whether such multi-resistant strains are, in fact, complex genetic mutants of normal colonizing species or have evolved from other environmental sources remains to be determined. Regardless of the original source of nosocomial multi-resistant *A. baumannii*, most molecular epidemiologic studies of outbreaks have demonstrated dissemination of relatively few clones, often with predominance of a single clone (16–21). Molecular techniques most useful in characterizing the epidemiology of Acinetobacter outbreaks include protein profiles, multilocus enzyme electrophoresis, plasmid profiles, pulsed-field gel electrophoresis, ribotyping and polymerase chain reaction (22–24). The primarily clonal nature of nosocomial Acinetobacter infection contrasts with the molecular epidemiology of extended spectrum beta lactamase-producing Klebsiella and *E. coli*. High level antibiotic resistance in these enteric species is plasmid mediated and readily transferable among multiple intestinal clones. Although Acinetobacter is not an enteric genus, a few studies have demonstrated intestinal carriage of pathogenic clones in outbreak situations (25–27). However, plasmid mediated resistance transfer has been demonstrated relatively rarely, and not as yet in North American isolates. In the critical care environment, clonal multi-resistant isolates have been recovered frequently from inanimate objects. These include ventilatory equipment, laryngoscopes, air conditioners, and bedding (15–21). Thus, molecular and clinical epidemiologic findings implicate infection control deficiencies as the major cause of nosocomial outbreaks of multi-resistant acinetobacter infections.

Virulence

Because Acinetobacter species are found among normal human microflora, their isolation from sputum or wound cultures of hospitalized patients may represent either colonization or infection. The virulence of Acinetobacter has been questioned, and is most definitively addressed by examination of bacteremic cases. Recent published literature demonstrates an attributable mortality of 19–34% with a 20–25% incidence of shock or disseminated intravascular coagulation (28–30). Of interest is the relatively low mortality of intravascular catheter-associated bacteremia due to Acinetobacter. Thus, the majority of bacteremic deaths are related to pneumonia, indicating that Acinetobacter (usually *A. baumannii*) is an invasive pulmonary pathogen. Bacteremia due to infection of intravascular catheters may be caused by either *A. baumannii* or *A. lwoffii*, and is associated with a lower mortality than bacteremic pneumonia.

Control of Nosocomial Antibiotic-Resistant Infection: General Principles

Control of nosocomial antibiotic-resistant infection due to any invasive pathogen requires a multidisciplinary approach. A position paper by the Society for Healthcare Epidemiology of America and the Infectious Diseases Society of America has proposed specific methods to interdict the dissemination of resistant strains (31). These methods include procedures to monitor resistant organisms; characterize such isolates phenotypically and genotypically; maintain control of selected antibiotics; educate medical personnel to achieve cooperation; establish stable infection control methods; and measure outcomes. Flaherty and Weinstein have reviewed thoroughly procedures for control of endemic and epidemic antimicrobial resistance (32). For control of endemic antibiotic resistance, they have suggested unit-based microbiologic surveillance, reinforcement of routine asepsis (handwashing, etc.), barrier precautions for patients colonized or infected with resistant organisms, and antibiotic control. For episodes of epidemic resistance, clinical and molecular epidemiologic investigations should be conducted to detect common environmental sources or personnel carriers. This may require cultures of personnel and treatment of carriers if genetic linkage can be established between colonizing and outbreak strains. Reinforcement of housekeeping procedures for routine cleaning and disinfection is essential for control of environmental colonization. Cohorting of patients and/or personnel may also be considered as well as possible topical antimicrobial prophylaxis. Prompt and cooperative implementation of these measures should obviate the necessity for closure of specific units as the ultimate method of epidemic control.

Antibiotic control may, like infection control, be implemented to varying degrees of intensity, depending upon the level of endemic or epidemic antibiotic resistance. General guidelines for therapeutic and prophylactic use, supplemented by computer-based or other educational techniques may be sufficient for institutions at low risk for development of antibiotic resistance. In such situations, the presence of few demographic risk factors for antibiotic resistance may limit the necessity for restriction of specific agents or antibiotic classes. Such risk factors may include advanced age, complexity of disease, need for ventilatory assistance, immunosuppression, referral from long term care facilities and other patient characteristics which predispose to increased antibiotic utilization and reduced host defenses. As these risk factors increase, selective restriction of broad spectrum agents may be useful, particularly if surveillance demonstrates evolving endemic resistance. The more draconian approach of restricting an entire class of antibiotics, or rotation of antibiotics by class, may be necessary only when epidemic resistance to one or more classes may threaten to abrogate antibiotic efficacy against highly invasive pathogens (33). Such situations may occur throughout an institution or be limited to specific units. Thus, infection control and antibiotic restriction, both important measures, may vary in their relative contributions, depending upon knowledge of mechanisms of resistance and mechanisms of spread of specific pathogens.

Control of Nosocomial Acinetobacter Infection: U.S. Experience

Our experience with epidemic nosocomial imipenem-resistant acinetobacter infection in 1991 and 1992 provided further evidence for the critical role of infection control in the prevention of such outbreaks (21). During this period *A. baumannii* isolates demonstrated four antibiotic susceptibility patterns, designated as Groups 1–4. Group 1 was susceptible to most extended spectrum beta lactam agents, quinolones, trimethoprim-sulfamethoxazole, and aminoglycosides. Group 2 demonstrated resistance to all antibiotics routinely tested, including imipenem. Groups 3 and 4 were susceptible only to imipenem, or only to imipenem and amikacin, respectively. Restriction endonuclease study of representative isolates from each group showed that those isolates which were either imipenem-resistant, susceptible only to imipenem, or susceptible only to imipenem and amikacin (Groups 2–4) were highly associated genetically, and markedly different from those which were susceptible to most antibiotics (Group 1). Our findings suggested an outbreak due to a single clone (Group 2), or a few very closely related clones (Groups 2, 3 and 4). In these groups antibiotic susceptibility to imipenem and amikacin fluctuated, depending upon expression of chromosomal mechanisms, particularly those governing chromosomal AMP C beta lactamase production and antibiotic permeability. Resistance to ceftazidime, probably due to both decreased permeability and derepression of AMP C beta lactamase, was common to all three groups. We therefore strictly inforced contact isolation of all patients harboring organisms within groups 2, 3 and 4. Those patients with pulmonary infection or colonization by strains which were imipenem resistant (Group 2) were cared for with respiratory precautions. Patients in the Surgical Intensive Care Unit (SICU) harboring such strains were also cohorted geographically and by nursing care whenever possible. All Acinetobacter isolates were susceptible to polymyxin B, and many to sulbactam. Susceptibility to these agents is not tested routinely in our hospital, or in most others in the United States. We applied polymyxin B solution to colonized or infected wounds to further control multiresistant Acinetobacter during the outbreak.

Because the most serious infections within the outbreak occurred in the SICU, serial surveillance cultures were taken from inanimate objects and the hands of personnel in that unit. Early in the outbreak isolates belonging to all four groups were recovered, including multi-resistant isolates from laryngoscopes, hands of personnel, and the SICU environment. Cultures taken after institution of the above infection control measures yielded only highly susceptible isolates from Group 1. Since the end of this outbreak imipenem resistant Acinetobacter has not reappeared except for a rare individual isolate. However, strains susceptible to imipenem alone or imipenem and amikacin (Groups 3 and 4) have remained endemic, and strict contact isolation of colonized or infected patients continues. In this outbreak molecular epidemiologic study showed that isolates with different antibiotic susceptibility were genetically related. In contrast, other studies have demonstrated separate genotypes among strains with the same susceptibility pattern (18,19). Knowledge of the geographic distribution of major epidemic clones serves to orient infection control efforts in the most effective directions. Thus, molecular epidemiologic techniques have become essential to the control of nosocomial multi-resistant pathogens by focusing efforts against specific resistant clones. An outbreak of imipenem-resistant Acinetobacter in France was found to be due to two distinct epidemic strains by PFGE analysis. However, extensive environmental contamination necessitated temporary closure of intensive care units for disinfection and control of that outbreak (34).

In other U.S. experiences, Zuccotti and Currie have used pulsed-field gel electrophoresis to define two sequential outbreaks of acinetobacter infection by separate clones at a single institution (35). One was associated with horizontal transmission between patients with shared geographic and temporal hospital experiences. This clone was controlled by strictly inforced contact isolation. The second outbreak was associated with specific exposure to an intensive care unit environment. These authors also showed that the same risk factor predisposed to both colonizing and infecting isolates (36). However, infected patients were more likely to have been treated in an intensive care unit. Such findings suggest that colonization with virulent, multi-resistant Acinetobacter often precedes infection by the same strain. Several other U.S. experiences have demonstrated clonal outbreaks of acinetobacter infection associated with the intensive care unit setting, contaminated respirator equipment, prior broad spectrum antibiotic therapy (particularly late generation cephalosporins) and serious underlying disease (16,18,19). Inadequate decontamination of ventilator equipment and infrequent changing of gloves by personnel have been identified as the cause of these outbreaks. A pediatric outbreak of acinetobacter bacteremia has been associated with contaminated air conditioners with aerosolization of the organism (17). This and several other reports have noted a seasonal association of nosocomial acinetobacter infection with summer months (37–38). Prolonged survival in moisture as well as on dry surfaces may contribute to persistent environmental contamination by Acinetobacter (39).

In a molecular epidemiologic case control study, patients infected with *A. baumannii* had a higher mortality rate than colonized patients or those without acinetobacter colonization or infection (16). Thus, a sequential relationship appears to exist between colonization of wounds, burns or sputum, subsequent infection, and increased mortality due to multi-resistant Acinetobacter. Further studies are needed to determine whether early identification of colonization, isolation of colonized patients, and eradication of colonization by local antibacterial application to nasal, lower respiratory or gastrointestinal mucosa, or to wounds may enhance the effect of standard infection control procedures in aborting nosocomial outbreaks (21,40,41).

Antibiotic Therapy

The therapeutic challenge presented by acinetobacter infections exists primarily in hospitalized patients with underlying disease. Blood stream infections usually arise from pneumonia, infected intravascular catheters, and skin and soft tissue infections, implicating these as the most common sites of invasive infections due to Acinetobacter (28–30). Respiratory colonization is frequent, often creating difficulty in avoiding undertreatment of potentially fatal disease and overtreatment of non-invasive local bacterial overgrowth (42). A large literature and much controversy exists regarding the definition of nosocomial pneumonia, particularly ventilator-associated pneumonia. Bacterial criteria vary, and may be limited to repeated sputum or endotracheal cultures showing the same species, or require quantitative cultures of specimens from protected bronchial brushing or endobronchial lavage (43). At the other end of the diagnostic spectrum, clinical criteria may be used exclusively, abandoning respiratory cultures as non-reproducible and unreliable (44–45). Certainly, most investigators would regard bacteremia (documented by one or more positive blood cultures) as definitive evidence of respiratory infection when associated with recovery of the same organism from respiratory secretions, and/or compatible clinical or radiologic findings.

After concluding that acinetobacter pulmonary infection exists, the choice of antibiotic depends upon results of standard susceptibility testing. Highly susceptible isolates may be treated with one of several agents. Among the beta lactam-beta-lactamase inhibitor combinations, piperacillin-tazobactam is the most active. For optimal effect against nosocomial pneumonia, this agent should be given as 3.375 gm every four hours if creatinine clearance is above 70 ml/min. The addition of an aminoglycoside is necessary for efficacy against pseudomonas pneumonia, and is probably beneficial for other gram-negative pneumonias if susceptibility exists (46,47). The efficacy of ampicillin-sulbactam is due entirely to the antibacterial effect of sulbactam which is not available as a single agent in the United States (48). This combination should be reserved for use against multiply resistant strains which may retain susceptibility to sulbactam. Among the quinolones, ciprofloxacin remains the most active and least toxic drug against Acinetobacter. Again, a maximum dose (400 mg every 8 hours) should be used for patients with nosocomial pneumonia and normal renal function (49). Trimethoprim-sulfamethoxazole is a useful agent against susceptible strains, but also should be used in high doses for pulmonary infection (160 mg trimethoprim every 6–8 hours) with appropriate adjustment for renal dysfunction. Aminoglycosides given alone are widely considered to be inadequate therapy for gram-negative pneumonia, although the use of large initial doses or single daily dose therapy remains to be fully evaluated (50). Ceftriaxone, cefotaxime and ceftazidime are active against Acinetobacter but are susceptible to inactivation by amp C beta lactamase, particularly when derepressed mutants with high level enzyme production are selected by use of one of these agents. Thus, as is the case with serious infections due to Enterobacter, avoidance of cephalosporins may be prudent in institutions where resistance to ceftazidime has appeared in either Enterobacter, Serratia or Acinetobacter (51). Of interest is the finding that selection of resistant *Pseudomonas aeruginosa* is least likely in the presence of ceftazidime, as compared to other beta lactam agents (52). Thus, while carbapenem resistance in *Pseudomonas aeruginosa* has reached 20–40% in many institutions due to selection of mutants with altered outer membrane permeability, carbapenems remain the most active beta lactam antibiotics against multi-resistant Acinetobacter, with greatest activity provided by imipenem. Thus carbapenems, amikacin and ampicillin-sulbactam frequently are, to varying degrees, the only active agents against multi-resistant strains. As described earlier, evolution to resistance to all routinely tested antibiotics is an increasing phenomenon among such isolates. The polymyxins, not routinely evaluated in most institutions, remain an exception to the potential resistance of Acinetobacter to all antibiotics (21). In vitro studies have demonstrated synergy between polymyxin or colistin plus rifampin, polymyxin plus imipenem, and ampicillin-sulbactam plus rifampin against multiresistant Acinetobacter (53–55). Most of the tested strains exhibited susceptibility to polymyxins or ampicillin-sulbactam alone, intermediate susceptibility to imipenem, and variable susceptibility to rifampin.

A limited number of infections due to isolates resistant to imipenem have been treated successfully with colistin (colistimethate sodium or colistin sodium methane sulfonate), polymyxin B sulfate, ampicillin-sulbactam, and sulbactam alone (56–61). Systemic polymyxins have been effective in clearing bacteremia, and central nervous system infection has been cured by the addition of direct subarachroid installation. However, pneumonia has responded poorly due to inadequate penetration of these agents into pulmonary parenchyma. Similarly, sulbactam alone has been effective against mild to moderately severe infections, and remains to be tested in more serious situations. Anecdotal personal communications have suggested that triple therapy with imipenem, polymyxin B sulfate and rifampin has benefitted selected patients with serious infections due to isolates of Acinetobacter which were resistant to all agents except polymyxin B. Studies in a mouse model of multiresistant *A. baumannii* pneumonia suggest that combinations of rifampin with imipenem or ticarcillin-clavulanate–sulbactam have a beneficial effect on survival (62). The above findings indicate that combination therapy against serious acinetobacter infection should be studied prospectively with clinical and microbiologic follow up.

REFERENCES

1. Streckenberger PC, von Graevenitz A. Acinetobacter, Alcaligenes, Moraxella, Methylobacterium, and other nonfermentative gram-negative rods. In: Murray PR, ed. Manual of Clinical Microbiology 7th Edition, Washington, DC: 1999:539–560.
2. API 20 NE® Identification system for non-enteric gram-negative rods (1998) by BioMérieux Vitek Inc. Hazelwood, MO. pp 1–9.
3. Editorial. Bacteria of the tribe Mimeae. JAMA 1963;186:947.
4. Taplin D, Rebell G, Zaias N. The human skin as a source of Mima-Herrelia infections. JAMA 1963;186:166–168.
5. Grehn M, von Graevenitz A. Search for Acinetobacter calcoaceticus, subsp. anitratus: enrichment of fecal samples. J Clin Microbiol 1978;8:342–343.
6. Rosenthal S, Tager TB. Prevalence of gram-negative rods in the normal pharyngeal flora. Ann Intern Med 1975;83:355–357.
7. Kozub WR, Bucolo S, Sami AW, Chatman CE, Pribor HC. Gonorrhea-like urethritis due to Mima polymorpha var. oxidans. Arch Intern Med 1968;122:514–516.
8. Alami SY, Riley HD Jr. Infections caused by Mimeae, with special reference to Mima polymorpha: A review. Am J Med Sci 1966;252:537–544.
9. Shea DW, Phillips JH. Mimeae endocarditis; A clinical syndrome? Am J Med Sci 1966;252:201–205.
10. Hirsch SR, Koch ML. Herellea (Bacterium anitratum) endocarditis. JAMA 1964;187;148–150.
11. Daly AK, Postic B, Kass E.H. Infections due to organisms of the genus Herellea. Arch Intern Med 1962;110:580–591.
12. Berezin-Bergogne E, Towner KJ. Acinetobacter spp. as nosocomial pathogens: microbiological, clinical, and epidemiological features. Clin Microbiol Rev 1996;9:148–165.
13. Anstey NM, Currie BJ, Withnall KM. Community-acquired Acinetobacter pneumonia in the northern territory of Australia. Clin Infect Dis 1992;14:83–91.
14. Seifert H, Dijkshoorn L, Gerner-Smidt P, Pelzer N, Tjernberg I, Vaneechoutte M. Distribution of Acinetobacter species on human skin: comparison of phenotypic and genotypic identification methods. J Clin Microbiol 1997;35:2819–2825.
15. Berlau J, Aucken H, Malnick H, Pitt T. Distribution of Acinetobacter species on skin of healthy humans. Eur J Clin Microbiol Infect Dis 1999;18:179–183.
16. Sader HS, Mendes CF, Pignatari AC, Pfaller MA. Use of macrorestriction analysis to demonstrate interhospital spread of multiresistant Acinetobacter baumannii in Sao Paulo, Brazil. Clin Infect Dis 1996;23:631–634.
17. Scerpella EG, Wanger AR, Armitige L, Anderlini P, Ericsson CD. Nosocomial outbreak caused by a multiresistant clone of Acinetobacter baumannii: Results of the case-control and molecular epidemiologic investigations. Infect Control Hosp Epidemiol 1995;16:92–97.
18. McDonald LC, Walker M, Carson L, Arduino M, Aguero SM, Gomez P, McNeil P, Jarvis WR. Outbreak of Acinetobacter spp. bloodstream infections in a nursery associated with contaminated aerosols and air conditioners. Pediatr Infect Dis J. 1998;17:716–722.
19. Patterson JE, Vecchio J, Pantelick EL, Farrel P, Mazon D, Zervos MJ, Hierholzer WJ. Association of contaminated gloves with transmission of Acinetobacter calcoaceticus var. anitratus in an intensive care unit. Am J Med 1991;91:479–483.
20. Tankovic J, Legrand P, DeGatines G, Chemineau V, Brun-Buisson C, Duval J. Characterization of a hospital outbreak of imipenem-resistant Acinetobacter baumannii by phenotypic and genotypic typing methods. J Clin Microbiol 1994;32:2677–2681.
21. Go ES, Urban C, Burns J, Kreiswirth B, Eisner W, Mariano N, Mosinka-Snipas K, Rahal JJ. Clinical and molecular epidemiology of acinetobacter infections sensitive only to polymyxin B and sulbactam. Lancet 1994;344:1329–1332.

22. Seifert H, Schulze A, Baginski R, Pulverer G. Comparison of four different methods for epidemiologic typing of Acinetobacter baumannii. J Clin Microbiol 1994;32:1816–1819.
23. Seifert H, Gerner-Smidt P. Comparison of ribotyping and pulsed-field gel electrophoresis for molecular typing of Acinetobacter isolate. J Clin Microbiol 1995;33:1402–1407.
24. Snelling AM, Gerner-Smidt P, Hawkey PM, Heritage J, Parnell P, Porter C, Bodenham AR, Inglis T. Validation of use of whole-cell repetitive extragenic palindromic sequence-based PCR (REP-PCR) for typing strains belonging to the Acinetobacter calcoaceticus-Acinetobacter baumannii complex and application of the method to the investigation of a hospital outbreak. J Clin Microbiol 1996;34:1193–1202.
25. Timsit JF, Garrait V, Misset B, Goldstein FW, Renaud B. Carlet J. The digestive tract is a major site for Acinetobacter baumannii colonization in intensive care unit patients. J Infect Dis 1993;168:1336–1337.
26. Corbella X, Pujol M, Ayats J, Sendra M, Ardanuy C, Dominguez MA, Linares J, Ariza J, Gudiol F. Relevance of digestive tract colonization in the epidemiology of nosocomial infections due to multiresistant Acinetobacter baumannii. Clin Infect Dis 1996;23:329–334.
27. Lortholary O, Fagon JY, Hoi AB, Mahieu G, Gutmann L. Colonization by Acinetobacter baumannii in intensive-care-unit patients. Infect Control Hosp Epidemiol 1998;19:188–190.
28. Seifert H, Strate A, Pulverer G. Nosocomial bacteremia due to Acinetobacter baumannii. Clinical features, epidemiology, and predictors of mortality. Medicine 1995;74:340–349.
29. Tilley PAG, Roberts FJ. Bacteremia with acinetobacter species: risk factors and prognosis in different clinical settings. Clin Infect Dis. 1994;18:896–900.
30. Cisneros JM, Reyes MJ, Pachon J, Becerril B, Caballero FJ, Garcia-Garmendia, JL, Ortiz C, Cobacho AR. Bacteremia due to Acinetobacter baumannii: epidemiology, clinical findings and prognostic features. Clin Infect Dis 1996;22:1026–1032.
31. Shlaes DM, Gerding DN, John JF Jr, Craig WA, Bornstein DL, Duncan RA, Eckman MR, Farrer WE, Greene WH, Lorian V, Levy S, McGowan JE Jr, Paul SM, Ruskin J, Tenover FC, Watanakunakorn C. Society for Healthcare Epidemiology of America and Infectious Diseases Society of America Joint Committee on the Prevention of Antimicrobial Resistance: guidelines for the prevention of antimicrobial resistance in hospitals. Infect Control Hosp Epidemiol 1997;18:275–291.
32. Flaherty JP, Weinstein RA. Nosocomial infection caused by antibiotic-resistant organisms in the intensive care unit. Infect Control Hosp Epidemiol 1996;17:236–248.
33. Rahal JJ, Urban C, Horn D, Freeman K, Segal-Maurer S, Maurer J, Mariano N, Marks S, Burns JM, Dominick D, Lim M. Class restriction of cephalosporin use to control total cephalosporin resistance in nosocomial Klebsiella. JAMA 1998;280:1233–1237.
34. Tankovic J, Legrand P, DeGatines G, Chemineau V, Brun-Buisson C. Duval J. Characterization of a hospital outbreak of imipenem-resistant Acinetobacter baumannii by phenotypic and genotypic typing methods. J Clin Microbiol 1994;32:2677–2681.
35. Zuccotti G, Currie BP. Molecular epidemiology of multiple antibiotic resistant (MAR) Acinetobacter anitratus isolates at a single hospital. Society for Healthcare Epidemiology of America 1998. Washington, D.C. Abstract #59.
36. Zuccotti G, Currie BP. An investigation of the relationship of colonizing and infecting nosocomial Acinetobacter anitratus isolates. Society for Healthcare Epidemiology of America 1998. Washington, D.C. Abstract #56.
37. McDonald LC, Banerjee SN, Jarvis WR, NISS Hospital Infections Program. Seasonal variation of Acinetobacter spp. infections reported to the National Nosocomial Infection Surveillance (NNIS) system: 1987–1996. Society for Healthcare Epidemiology of America 1998. Washington, D.C. Abstract #55.
38. Christie C, Mazon D, Hierholzer W, Patterson JE. Molecular heterogeneity of Acinetobacter baumannii isolates during seasonal increase in prevalence. Infect Control Hosp Epidemiol 1995;16:590–594.
39. Jawad A, Seifert H, Snelling AM, Heritage J, Hawkey PM. Survival of Acinetobacter baumannii on dry surfaces: comparison of outbreak and sporadic isolates. J Clin Microbiol 1998;36:1938–1941.
40. Brun-Buisson C, Legrand P. Can topical and nonabsorbable antimicrobials prevent cross-transmission of resistant strains in ICUs? Infect Control Hosp Epidemiol 1994;15:447–455.
41. DíAmico Roberto, Pifferi S, Leonetti C, Torri V, Tinazzi A, Liberati A. Effectiveness of antibiotic prophylaxis in critically ill adult patients: systematic review of randomised controlled trials. Brit Med J 1998;316:1275–1285.
42. Greene JN. The microbiology of colonization, including techniques for assessing and measuring colonization. Infect Control Hosp Epidemiol 1996;17:114–118.

43. George DL, Falk PS, Wunderink RG, Leeper KV, Umberto Meduri G, Steere EL, Corbett CE, Mayhall CG. Epidemiology of ventilator-acquired pneumonia based on protected bronchoscopic sampling. Am J Respir Crit Care Med 1998;158:1839–1847.
44. Luna CM, Vujacich P, Niederman MS. Vay C, Gherardi C, Matera J, Jolly EC. Impact of BAL data on the therapy and outcome of ventilator-associated pneumonia. Chest 1997;111:676–685.
45. Sanchez-Nieto JM, Torres A, Garcia-Cordoba F, El-Ebiary M, Carrillo A, Ruiz J, Nunez ML, Niederman M. Impact of invasive and noninvasive quantitative culture sampling on outcome of ventilator-associated pneumonia. Am J Resp Crit Care Med 1998;157:371–376.
46. Joshi M, Bernstein J, Solomkin J, Wester BA, Juye O. Piperacillin/tazobactam plus tobramycin versus ceftazidime plus tobramycin for the treatment of patients with nosocomial lower respiratory tract infection. Piperacillin/ tazobactam nosocomial pneumoniae study group. J Antimicrob Chemother 1999;43:389–397.
47. Trouillet J-L, Chastre J, Vuagnat A, Joly-Guillou, M-L, Combaux D, Dombret M-C, Gibert C. Ventilator-associated pneumonia caused by potentially drug-resistant bacteria. AM J Respir Crit Care Med 1998;157:531–539.
48. Urban C, Go E, Mariano N, Rahal JJ. Interaction of sulbactam, clavulanic acid and tazobactam with penicillin-binding proteins of imipenem-resistant and susceptible Acinetobacter baumannii. FEMS Microbiol Letters 1995;125:193–198.
49. Lipman J, Scribante J, Gous AGS, Hon H, Tshukutsoane S, and The Baragwanath Ciprofloxacin Study Group. Pharmacokinetic profiles of high-dose intravenous ciprofloxacin in severe sepsis. Antimicrob Agents Chemother 1998;42:2235–2239.
50. Kashuba ADM, Nafziger AN, Drusano GL, Bertino JS. Optimizing aminoglycoside therapy for nosocomial pneumonia caused by gram-negative bacteria. Antimicrob Agents and Chemother 1999;43:623–629.
51. Anstey NM. Use of cefotaxime for treatment of acinetobacter infections. Clin Infect Dis 1992;15: 374–375.
52. Carmeli Y, Troillet N, Eliopoulos GM, Samore MH. Emergence of antibiotic-resistant Pseudomonas aeruginosa: comparison of risks associated with different antipseudomonal agents. Antimicrob Agents Chemother 1999;43:1379–1382.
53. Chini NX, Scully B, Della-Latta P. In-vitro synergy of polymyxin B with imipenem and other antimicrobial agents against Acinetobacter, Klebsiella and Pseudomonas species. 38th Interscience Conference on Antimicrobial Chemotherapy. Sept. 24–27, 1998, San Diego, CA. Abstract E56.
54. Hogg GM, Barr JG, Webb CH. In-vitro activity of the combination of colistin and rifampicin against multidrug-resistant strains of Acinetobacter baumannii. J Antimicrob Chemother 1998;41: 494–495.
55. Tascini C, Menichetti F, Bozza S, Del Favero A, Bistoni F. Evaluation of the activities of two-drug combination of rifampicin, polymyxin B and ampicillin/sulbactam against Acinetobacter baumannii. J Antimicrob Chemother 1998;42:270–271.
56. Wood CA, Reboli AC. Infections caused by imipenem-resistant Acinetobacter calcoaceticus biotype anitratus. J Infect dis 1993;168:1602–1603.
57. Urban C, Go E, Mariano N, Berger BJ, Avraham I, Rubin D, Rahal JJ. Effect of sulbactam on infections caused by imipenem-resistant Acinetobacter calcoaceticus biotype anitratus. J Infect Dis 1993;167:448–451.
58. Jimenez-Mejias ME, Pachon J, Becerril B,. Palomino-Nicas J, Rodriquez-Cobaco A, Revuelta M. Treatment of multidrug-resistant Acinetobacter baumannii meningitis with ampicillin/sulbactam. Clin Infect Dis 1997;24:932–935.
59. Corbella X, Ariza J, Ardanuy C, Vuelta M, Tubau F, Sora M, Pujol M, Gudiol F. Efficacy of sulbactam alone and in combination with ampicillin in nosocomial infections caused by multiresistant Acinetobacter baumannii. J Antimicrob Chemother 1998;42:793–802.
60. Levin AS, Barone AA, Penco J, Santos MV, Marinho IS, Arruda EAG, Manrique EI, Costa SF, Intravenous colistin as therapy for nosocomial infections caused by multidrug-resistant Pseudomonas aeruginosa and Acinetobacter baumannii. Clin Infect Dis 1999;28:1008–1011.
61. Fernandez-Viladrich P, Corbella X, Corral L, Tubau F, Mateu A. Successful treatment of ventriculitis due to carbapenem-resistant Acinetobacter baumannii with intraventricular colistin sulfomethate sodium. Clin Infect Dis 1999;28:916–917.
62. Wolff M, Joly-Guillou ML, Farinotti R, Carbon C. In-Vivo efficacies of combinations of *B*-lactams, *B*-lactamase inhibitors, and rifampin against Acinetobacter baumannii in a mouse pneumonia model. Antimicrob Agents Chemother 1999;43:1406–1411.

7. ACINETOBACTER: EPIDEMIOLOGY AND CONTROL

JAVIER ARIZA, M.D. AND XAVIER CORBELLA, M.D.

Infectious Disease Service, Hospital de Bellvitge, Barcelona, Spain

INTRODUCTION

Over the last 15 years *Acinetobacter baumannii* has emerged as an important nosocomial pathogen and outbreaks caused by these organisms have been progressively reported worldwide (1–13). *Acinetobacter* organisms are ubiquitous non-fermentative gram-negative coccobacilli belonging to the family of Moraxellaceae (14), which is widely distributed in nature and found in soil, water, foods and as a normal inhabitant of human skin (15,16). The genus has undergone confusing taxonomic changes over many years, making the comparison between historical and modern series difficult. Among the 19 genomic species currently recognized, three are the usually isolated in hospitalized populations: species 2 (*A. baumannii*), 3 and 13 (17–20). These three species are included in the so-called *A. calcoaceticus-A. baumannii* complex group, which establish a clear difference between those *Acinetobacter* species ubiquitous in nature and those found clinically (21–23).

Nowadays, *A. baumannii* isolates are almost exclusively hospital-acquired and rarely found in the community (24). Similarly to other nosocomial pathogens, *A. baumannii* commonly causes epidemic infections, which mainly occur in ICU settings. Several aspects of the hospital epidemiology still remain poorly known, although there is no doubt that both the surprising ability of *A. baumannii* to acquire antimicrobial multiresistance and its high capacity for survival on most environmental surfaces are determinant factors for their spread and persistance in hospitals. In fact, many contaminated objects in the hospital environment have been implicated as the main

R.A. Weinstein and M.J.M. Bonten (eds.). INFECTION CONTROL IN THE ICU ENVIRONMENT.

source of infections. The ability to control multiresistant *A. baumannii* epidemic infections has varied widely from one hospital to another, probably depending on several epidemiological differences. In some institutions, in which epidemic infections were circumscribed to a sole ICU ward, a common contaminated object (ventilators, humidifiers, mattresses, etc.) could be identified as the source of infection (25–29). In such cases, the implementation of isolation precautions and the revision of cleaning procedures usually resulted in a prompt eradication of the outbreak. In other hospitals, epidemic infections have become endemic, remaining the clinical and microbiological epidemiology of such endemic infections as yet obscure. Under these circumstances many investigations failed to identify a single environmental source of infection (2,8,9,12), and pointed toward patients as an additional potential reservoir (2,30,31).

Beginning in 1992, a sustained outbreak due to *A. baumannii* has been noted in our 1,000-bed institution in Barcelona, Spain, involving more than 1,900 patients (60–70% of them during ICU-stay). Currently, this organism constitutes one of the most common causes of nosocomial infection, originating about 20% of ICU infections (31% of the total infections of the respiratory tract, 17% of surgical wound, 12% of vascular catheter-related, 10% of urinary tract). Molecular typing procedures showed that endemic isolates pertained to five main clones (12). Although control measures were repeatedly reinforced during this time, only transitory decreases in the incidence rates of *A. baumannii* were observed following each reinforcement. Large outbreaks due to *A. baumannii* have been registered in other hospitals in Spain as well as in several European countries such as France, Germany, The Netherlands, and Denmark (2,9,13,20,31). A 6-month survey conducted by Bergogne-Berezin et al. (*Acinetobacter* study group) during 1995–96 in several hospitals from 7 countries (Belgium, France, Germany, Israel, South Africa, Spain, and United Kingdom), detected that 14% of large institutions had an incidence rate of *Acinetobacter sp.* infections ranging from 5 to >10% (32). Reported data from a multicenter study of surveillance of antibiotic resistance in European ICUs (June 1994–June 1995) including 7,308 patients from 18 hospitals in Belgium, 40 in France, 20 in Portugal, 30 in Spain, and 10 in Sweden (33). The study showed that *Acinetobacter spp* were 2% of isolates from Belgium, 10% from France, 6% from Portugal, 8% from Spain, and 3% from Sweden. Surveillance of nosocomial infections were also carried out in 30 Spanish ICUs, and included data from more than 7,000 patients. *Acinetobacter spp* was the etiologic agent of ventilator-associated pneumonia in 18% of cases in 1994, 10% in 1995 and 13% in 1996. Furthermore, these resistant organisms caused 7% of primary bacteremia in 1996 (34,35).

A. baumannii nosocomial infections are mainly related to the presence of invasive procedures and continuous manipulations or catheters such as intubation-associated respiratory tract infections, surgical wounds, urinary tract, and primary bacteremia. While *Acinetobacter spp* have been classically recognized to be of low virulence, some authors have reported high rates of mortality associated with nosocomial pneumonia or bacteremia due to *A. baumannii* (36–39). In our experience, morbidity and mortality due to *A. baumannii* is lower than that observed by other hospital-acquired gram-negative bacilli and many *A. baumannii* organisms isolated during admission often reflect colonization rather than infection. Only controlled investigations may determine the true virulence, although they are extremely difficult to do since the clinical relevance of isolates is uncertain, they are most often polymicrobial, most occur in severelly-ill ICU patients, and are usually associated with multiple invasive procedures.

EPIDEMIOLOGY

Numerous efforts have been conducted to clarify the epidemiology of *A. baumannii* hospital outbreaks. Results indicated that environmental contamination and colonized patients may act as the major epidemiological reservoirs for infection, and that inadequate prevention of cross-transmission is the main determinant for its spread and persistence.

Colonized Patients as Reservoirs

Since the genus *Acinetobacter* is known to be a normal inhabitant of human skin, several authors have postulated that, in addition to the contaminated environment, patients could be a major reservoir for hospital spread in endemic settings (2,5,8–11,30,31). In agreement with this thinking, our group and several other authors showed that not only the skin but also the pharynx, the respiratory tract, and the digestive tract of ICU patients may be colonized by *A. baumannii*, providing permanent carriage and a source for epidemic infections (2,30,40,41). Of relevance was the observation that *A. baumannii* may colonize the digestive tract, since these organisms are not considered to be inhabitants of the bowel in healthy humans (42). However, it is well-known that in severely-ill hospitalized patients, the normal digestive flora which provides intestinal colonization resistance can be modified (43), predisposing patients to acquire persistent colonization by exogenous nosocomial epidemic pathogens.

With the above observations in mind, several prospective studies showed high rates of patients' colonization during large outbreaks. In our experience, 66% of ICU patients were found to have axillar, pharyngeal, or rectal colonization by *A. baumannii* (44). Of concern was the surprising speed with which patients were colonized (77% during the first week of ICU stay), and these results agreed with those of other previous reports (8). Furthermore, at the time of initial detection, more than half of the patients had 2 or 3 concomitant positive body-sites, which hampered the identification of a hypothetical sequence of colonization. The probability of remaining free of colonization was less than 25% at 30 days of ICU admission.

When potential risk factors for *A. baumannii* acquisition have been evaluated, terms such as the severity of illness, length of ICU stay, previous days with invasive procedures and, almost uniformly, prior antibiotic administration were found to be the main predisposing conditions, like those reported for other hospital infections (7,13,31,36,39,45). However, when prospective screening for patients' colonization was done, we observed that the previous state of *A. baumannii* carrier was the major

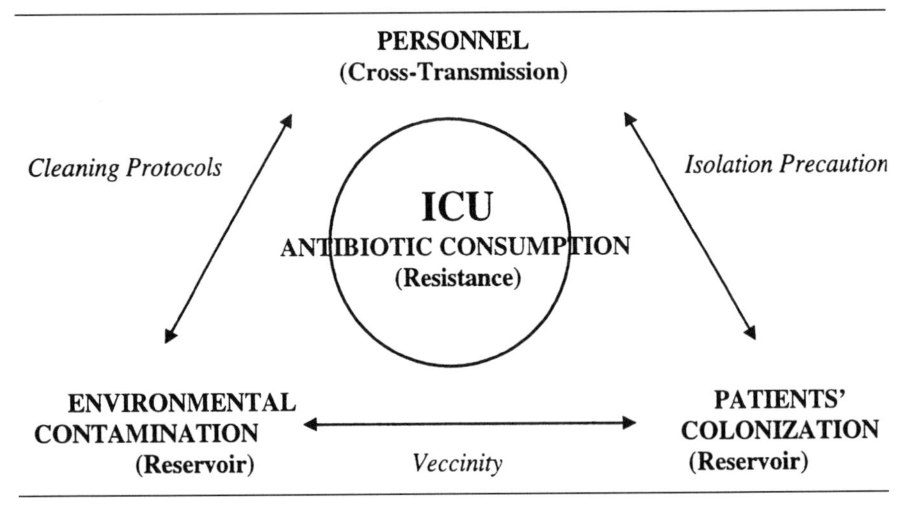

Figure 1. Epidemiology of *A. baumannii* hospital infections.

attribute for the subsequent development of infections, with regard to those classically associated factors. In fact, this previous carrier state may be detected in almost all patients who developed positive clinical samples, with a mean of 7 days between detection of body-site carriage and clinical colonization or infection.

Under the special circumstances noted in our ICUs, analysis selected those patients submitted to continuous manipulations such as those with polytrauma, or those who were admitted in an ICU ward with a high "tonnage" of colonized patients, to be at higher risk for body-site colonization. Thus, colonized patients may constitute an additional "animate" object of the ICU environment and a continuous reservoir for recontamination of the immediate environment and the hands of health-care-workers. In this way, patients may facillitate the maintainance of the epidemiological cycle of *A. baumannii* infections: environment—staff—patients—staff—environment (Figure 1).

Inanimate Environment Contamination as Reservoir

It is well-known that the ability of the genus *Acinetobacter* to persist on dry surfaces weighty contributes to the development and persistence of hospital outbreaks. This survival, which has been shown to be for more than two weeks (a time longer than that observed for other gram-negative rods), seems to be in part due to the intrinsic capacity of the organism to survive at different conditions of humidity, temperature, and pH (46–48).

Evaluation of environmental contamination rates in endemic/epidemic settings may differ widely depending on several factors, such as the magnitude of the outbreak at the time of sampling, the type of items cultured, and the technique used. In fact, the overall rates reported for authors ranged between 0% and 18% (10). Outbreaks affecting a small number of patients can show lower grades of contam-

Table 1. Positive environmental cultures for *A. baumannii* comparing mointened swabs versus moistened gauze pads*

	Swab	Gauze
Clean Room		
Monitor	1/5	1/5
BPG[1]	0/4	1/4
Lamp	0/6	0/6
Mattress	0/5	1/5
Persian	0/5	0/5
Unit		
Table	2/5	4/5
Cupboard	0/8	2/8
ECG[2]	0/3	1/3
Cart	2/4	4/4
Crane	0/3	2/3
Telephone	0/1	1/1
BGM[3]	0/1	1/1
TOTAL	5/50	18/50

*The proportion of colonized/infected *A. baumannii* patients admitted at the ICUs at the time to perform environmental cultures were 35% (16/46). [1]BPG = Blood Pressure Gauge, [2]ECG = Electrocardiograph, [3]BGM = Blood Glucose Meter.

ination than those which are large and sustained. In addition, the items placed in the immediate environment of a colonized patient may show higher contamination rates.

Microbiological techniques used for culturing surfaces may also play a role in such differences. Recommended techniques included Rodac impression agar plates and cotton tipped swabs moistened with Brain Heart Infusion Broth (BHIB). To improve the ability to detect environmental contamination, our group modified the swab-technique by using sterile gauzes rather than cotton applicator swabs (49). In a comparative study using both techniques, 50 different ICU items usually found to be negative by the swab-technique were selected for sampling (Table 1).

Cultures obtained by the gauze-technique showed higher rates of positivity than those by the swab-technique (36% vs 10%; $p < 0.05$). Results showed not only improved ability to detect contamination but, of major epidemiological relevance, several previously unrecognized environmental reservoirs by using the recommended swabs. These observations may indicate a possible underdetection of environmental contamination rates in several other outbreaks previously reported. Immediately following the study, we applied a continuous environmental surveillance program in our ICUs using the sterile gauze-technique. After an 18-month survey, 265 (42%) of a total of 629 items sampled were found to be contaminated. Isolates belonged to the same clones found in the clinical samples. Furthermore, the results demonstrated how some items pertaining to a free-bed patient's room (39%), some placed into ICU stores while waiting for patients (39%), some apparatus which daily moved from patient-to-patient (54%), some placed in the unit (45%) or some clothes worn by the personnel (43%) can remain contaminated after inadequate cleaning or completion of barrier measures.

Mode of Transmission: The Role of Health-Care-Workers

During *A. baumannii* hospital outbreaks, most authors pointed towards the inadequate compliance with handwashing and gloves removal by personnel as the main determinant factor for the dissemination of these infections. The relevance of ICU health-care-workers acting as transient carriers facilitating cross-contamination via the hands has been clearly supported by several studies which documented positive hand and glove cultures from staff members who had been caring for patients (3,26,50,51).

In contrast to what occurs in MRSA hospital outbreaks, in *A. baumannii* epidemics/endemics health-care-workers do not become permanent carriers. This fact was demonstrated in two different studies (18). In our experience, none of the 25 ICU personnel caring for colonized patients showed *A. baumannii* colonization, either axillar or on the hands, before and after an 8-hour day in the ICUs (52).

Some authors have also speculated that airbone spread is a possible mode of transmission since positive air samples have been found using environmental plates or by means of slit-samplers, ranging from 11 to 20% (5,53). These studies suggested that the morphology of *Acinetobacter* cells, similar in size and shape to staphylococci, might favour airborne spread (46). In any case, air contamination probably depends on the contamination of immediate inanimate surfaces, playing a secondary epidemiological role with regards to cross-transmission.

Antibiotic Cosumption

There are few doubts that antibiotic consumption plays a relevant role in the emergence of resistant organisms in ICUs. In addition to other attributes, the use of broad-spectrum antibiotics may by itself contribute to the selection of hospital populations and to the spread of antimicrobial resistance (54). It is well known that overuse of third-generation cephaloporins clearly predispose the appearance of infections due to *Enterococcus faecalis* or extended-spectrum betalactamases producing *Klebsiella pneumoniae* and vancomycin use may promote infections by vancomycin-resistant *Enterococcus faecium* (55–57). In these circumstances, specific antibiotic restriction-use usually contributes to controlling the outbreak.

In *A. baumannii* outbreaks, the role of antibiotic use is difficult to state. Over the past two decades, *A. baumannii* has exhibited one of the most alarming pattern towards antimicrobial resistance, which currently includes all commercially available antibiotics. Exposure to antibiotics may determine a selective advantage for those multiresistant clones over competing with more susceptible ones (6,8,58). In fact, antibiotic administration has uniformly been reported among the associated risk factors for developing nosocomial infections by the majority of authors (6,8,13,31).

Nowadays, most *A. baumannii* strains isolated in European hospitals are highly resistant to modern β-lactams, aminoglycosides, and fluoroquinolones. It is of great concern that resistance to carbapenems, the last recognized antibiotic alternative, has already emerged in Europe. Reported data from the European Surveillance study mentioned above showed carbapenem-resistant strains in 12% of *Acinetobacter* isolates in Belgium, 9% in France, 5% in Portugal, 16% in Spain, and 19% in Sweden (33). In our hospital, carbapenem resistance emerged and rapidly spread among *A. baumannii* population in 1997, after 5 years of sustained outbreak. Molecular typing showed that carbapenem resistance was due to the introduction of a new clone colonizing a patient moved from an ICU of another Spanish hospital (58). Now, in our ICUs, most strains are only sensitive to polymyxins.

Typing Methods

In contrast to other nosocomial pathogens, antibiogram may be of less value when identifying the emergence of *A. baumannii* epidemics. Multiresistance is inherent in most current strains isolated worldwide, and unrelated organisms may exhibite the same antibiogram. Furthermore, changes in susceptibility patterns may occur during sustained endemics (8,11,59).

Molecular typing methods such as pulsed-field gel electrophoresis (PFGE) and polymerase chain reaction (PCR) fingerprinting may contribute to a better epidemiological approach in emerging outbreaks, differentiating endemic from epidemic or sporadic infections. Studies often show that several clones may concur during uncontrolled epidemics or sustained endemics by *A. baumannii* (9,12). However, a complete correlation between susceptibility pattern and genotyping may be documented in such circumstances (44,60), facillitating the infection-control management of the outbreak. In any case, molecular typing seem to be required not only for a modern approach in large outbreaks, but in order to identify the sources and modes of transmission, and better outline the control strategies for spread prevention (61–63).

CONTROL MEASURES

Although standard infection-control measures may be the recommended basis for cointainment of infection for almost all nosocomial pathogens, the particular epidemiology of each organisms should lead physicians to specifically design the interventions to be applied. It has already been mentioned that emerging epidemics by *A. baumannii* limited to a sole ward may usually be erradicated after the identification of a common source of infection. Nevertheless, control of large and sustained outbreaks is much more difficult since a variety of potential sources may concur, making infection-control management a serious challenge. In fact, no well-defined recommendations has been esatblished yet in such outbreaks, and the sequence and priority with which control measures should be applied and the results that physicians could expect remain unknown (Table 2).

Reinforcement of Barrier Measures

Handwashing and isolation methods, including the use of protective gloves and gowns, remain as the cornerstone of control programs in *A. baumannii* outbreaks. Since body-site colonization precedes clinical samples (in our setting with a mean

Table 2. Recommended control measures in large endemics due to *A. baumannii*

1. Reinforcement of Barrier measures—Cross-transmission prevention
Prospective screening for colonized patients using body-site swabs
Cutaneous isolation of patients known to be colonized
Cohorting patients
Correct use of gloves and gowns
Use of cast off or frequent routine spare clothing
Correct handwashing compliance
Handwashing facilities into the rooms
Assignation of an infection-control nurse regarding compliance with measures
Attention to the use of medical apparatus moved patient-to-patient
Attention to movement of colonized patients througout the hospital
2. Revision of Cleaning Procedures—Environment Contamination Reduction
Revision of housekeeping practices
Revision of medical equipment decontamination procedures
Initial approach to potential environmental sources for infection
Implementation of a routine surveillance of environment contamination
Transitory closing of the ICUs for complete decontamination
Global redesign of the ICUs
3. Rational Use of Antibiotics—Reduction of Selective Advantage
Design of antibiotic alternatives for treatment of A. baumannii infections
Antibiotic rotation policies for empirical regimens
Transitory restriction use of specific antibiotics
4. Patient decontamination (?)—Reduction of Colonized Patients as Reservoirs
Selective intestinal decontamination
Concomitant digestive, pharyngeal, and cutaneous decontamination
5. Continuous Personnel Education—Compliance with Basic Control Measures
Educational programs for adequate cross-transmission prevention
Providing feedback of data referring to rates of contamination
Providing feedback of data referring to compliance with basic control measures

of 7 days) in most patients admitted to ICU wards, a surveillance program based on the identification of positive clinical samples could be too late to prevent cross-transmission and the spread of the outbreak. Therefore, in emerging outbreaks, continued prospective screening for colonized patients releying on body-site swabs seems to be mandatory as the initial approach and for early implementation of barrier measures. According to our results, the weekly practice of a single body-site swab (either cutaneous, phryngeal or rectal) missed fewer than a quarter of the total of colonized patients (44). From the cost-profit point of view, one should consider whether this miss rate is reasonable or whether in some special circunstances more accurate detection rates by means of a pharyngeal-rectal swab combination (which may detect about 90% of total colonized patients) might be more appropriate.

Unfortunately, appropriate compliance with barrier measures is not always carried out in a busy ICU (observational studies revealed adequate compliance in only 36–65% of observed opportunities), explaining in part the failure to control *A. baumannii* in endemic settings (64). Cohorting patients has been shown useful in *A. baumannii* outbreaks as well as other kind of hospital epidemics (8,9,65). However, in some *A. baumannii* settings, this accumulation of colonized patients could determine a "boomerang" effect, leading to higher rates of environment contamination in those wards if cleaning protocols and cross-transmission prevention are not effectively ensured. Special attention should be taken with all those medical apparatus such as electrocardiographs or x-rays that move daily patient-to-patient as well as when contaminated patients leave the ICU wards for diagnostic or therapeutic procedures. Furthermore, the fact that the microorganism may survive several days on clothes used by staff in ICU wards should be taken into account.

In settings with endemic infections with high rates of contamination, routine screening for new colonized patients may be controversial. Cost-effectiveness and the assumption of the ineluctable advance of increasing rates due to *A. baumannii* and other resistant organisms, may be offered by some ICU workers as an excuse for inaction and decreased compliance with barrier measures. The placing of hand-washing facilities in all ICU rooms, the use of cast off or the frequent routine spare clothing, and the assignation of an infection-control nurse at the ICUs providing continuous personnel education, and feedback of data regarding hand carriage and contamination rates might enhance the compliance with basic isolation precautions. Nevertheless, infection-control teams have the final responsibility in noting that it is possible to reduce cross-transmission, and in renewing efforts for maintain infection control programs.

Revision of Cleaning Procedures and Surveillance of Environmental Contamination

Routine environmental studies are recommended as a useful measure not only to detect the sources for the epidemics, but also to help physicians in detecting potentially unrecognized reservoirs of infection and in monitoring compliance with basic control measures. In this way, we believe that the use of moistened sterile gauze pads probably provides a more sensitive method for sampling and allows us to become aware of the real of environment contamination. Environmental air surveillance probably plays a more secondary role.

For careful environmental surveillance, items could be grouped as follows: group 1, those belonging to rooms free of patients cultured after terminal cleaning; group 2. those placed into an ICU storage room while waiting for new patients; group 3, those that are moved daily from patient-to-patient; and group 4, those placed inside the units and commonly shared by personel. Results of environmental surveillance focusing on those groups of items may identify which procedures are susceptible to improvement and can direct the efforts for appropriate compliance on the part of personnel responsible. Thus, groups 1, 2, and 3 indicate compliance with housekeeping and cleaning procedures, and group 4 mainly involves compliance with barrier measures and handwashing. Revision and reinforcement of cleaning protocols should be mandatory when results indicate extensive environmental contamination. Protocols should detail all housekeeping practices and medical equipment decontamination procedures and indicate periodicity as well as the personnel responsible for cleaning.

Sometimes only the transitory closure of the ICUs may assure complete decontamination (1,59). In our experience, in an ICU setting with high icidence rates of

A. baumannii, we repeatedly documented the inability of our cleaning procedures to provide systematic negative cultures in samples obtained from rooms free of patients after terminal cleaning. In contrast, all cultures carried out after the sequential closing, decontaminating, and painting of the ICU wards were found negative. However, efforts to decontaminate the ICUs may unfortunately fail if colonized patients are newly readmitted after decontamination. This troublesome practice may occur in those tertiary-care public institutions in which the high pressures on medical care and the high density of colonized patients usually determine the rapid recontamination of the ICUs. In endemic settings in which intensive surveillance fails to control the outbreak, other draconian measures such as the structural redesign of the ICUs may be required.

Rational Use of Antibiotics

Rational use of antibiotics is decisive in containing the development of bacterial multiresistance in ICUs. The main bases may be: 1/ adjusting their empirical use according to clinical criteria and based on microbiological data of in vitro antibotic susceptibility of the particular flora of each unit, 2/ using preferably narrow-spectrum antibiotics according to antibiogram results when the microorganism has been identified, and 3/ diversifying overall antibiotic consumption (54).

In outlining empirical schedules it may be very important to know the antibiogram of the *A. baumannii* clones prevailing in each ICU. Because of its low virulence, clinical judgment in the selection of the sort of patients who really need antibiotics is mandatory. Some infections may respond to the removal of foreign bodies, debridement, or topical therapy (66). Multiresistance could make the treatment of infections a challenge for physicians, prompting the use of unusual antibiotics such as sulbactam (8,67–69), as a rational alternative for treating in vitro susceptible strains. While strongly insuring strict compliance with basic control measures, antibiotic restriction programs may contribute to containing the spread of antibiotic resistance among *A. baumannii* population.

Selective Intestinal Decontamination

Since the demonstration of the digestive tract as an important reservoir for *A. baumannii* in ICU patients, some authors have proposed selective decontamination as a measure for control. These optimistic expectations have been challenged by two recent studies showing that selective digestive decontamination may not be an effective strategy in preventing *A. baumannii* infections such as nosocomial pneumonia (70,71). Possible reasons are the fact that such infections may be mainly exogenous in origin, either from the inanimate environment or from other concomitant colonized body-sites such as the skin or the respiratory tract. Both the environment and skin are not only contaminated due to the extension from digestive tract colonization (as occurs in other nosocomial gram-negative bacteria), and probably reflect a more natural habitat for *Acinetobacter sp.* Furthermore, the extremely narrow therapeutic margin shown by *A. baumannii* population worldwide now casts doubts on the real efficacy of digestive decontamination, since many strains are aminoglycoside resistant (a family of antibiotics usually included in decontamination schedules along with polymyxins).

Taking into account all these reflexions, we believe the risk of failure with using monotherapy and the potential selection of more resistant *A. baumannii* strains may be reasons discouraging selective intestinal decontamination in some settings. However, if it is considered, basic infection-control interventions such as strict compliance with cleaning procedures and cross-transmission prevention should be strongly insured, and decontamination should probably not be circumscribed to the digestive tract, but also to the skin and respiratory tract. Under such circumstances, its hypothetic role in contributing to decreasing secondary environment contamination and thus increasing the efficacy of other control measures is not known. As the organisms are associated with low-moderate morbidity, one should consider if attempts to prevent or eradicate *A. baumannii* infections by the implementation of body-site decontamination programs may be reasonable or not.

SUMMARY

Nosocomial outbreaks caused by *Acinetobacter baumannii* have been progressively reported worldwide, including many European countries. These infections are usually of low virulence and include those of the respiratory tract, surgical wounds, primary bacteremia and urinary tract, mainly involving ICU patients. Their treatment may be a challenge for the physicians, because of the surprising ability of the microorganism to acquire antimicrobial multiresistance. This characteristic along with its high capacity for survival on most environmental surfaces are determinant factors for their spread and persistance in hospitals. Environmental contamination of a wide variety of inanimate objetes in hospitals and patients' colonization in different body-sites such as the skin, pharynx and digestive tract, may act as the major epidemiological reservoirs for infection. Inadequate compliance with preventing cross-transmission (handwashing and gloves removal) by health-care-workers, as the main determinant factor for the hospital-wide dissemination. In such circumstances, exposure to antibiotics may provide a selective advantage for some multiresistant colonizing clones over competing with more susceptible ones. The apply of a modified environmental technique for sampling surfaces by using sterile gauzes probably provides the best results to detect unrecognized environmental reservoirs. Molecular typing are required for a modern approach in large outbreaks, often showing that several clones may concur during uncontrolled epidemics. Continued prospective screening for colonized patients releying on body-site swabs seems to be mandatory for early implementation of barrier measures. Handwashing and isolation methods, including the use of protective gloves and gowns, remain as the cornerstone of control programs. Revision and reinforcement of cleaning protocols should be mandatory when results indicate extensive environmental contamination. Cohorting patients may be necessary and sometimes only the transitory closure of the ICUs may assure complete decontamination.

REFERENCES

1. Sherertz RJ, Sullivan ML. An outbreak of infection with *Acinetobacter calcoaceticus* in burn patients: contamination of patients' mattresses. J Infect Dis 1985;151:252–258.
2. Gerner-Smidt P. Endemic occurrence of *Acinetobacter calcoaceticus* biovar *anitratus* in an intensive care unit. J Hosp Infect 1987;10:265–272.
3. Hartstein AI, Rashad AL, Liebler JM, Actis LA, Freeman J, Rourke JW, Stibolt TB, Tolmasky ME, Ellis GR, Crosa JH. Multiple intensive care unit outbreak of *Acinetobacter calcoaceticus* subspecies *anitratus* respiratory infection and colonization associated with contaminated, reusable ventilator circuits and resucitation bags. Am J Med 1988;85:624–631.
4. Sakata H, Fujita K, Maruyama S, Kakehashi H, Mori Y, Yoshioka H. *Acinetobacter calcoaceticus* biovar. *anitratus* septicaemia in a neonatal intensive care unit: epidemiology and control. J Hosp Infect 1989;14:15–22.
5. Crombach WHJ, Dijkshoorn L, van Noort-Klaassen M, Niessen J, van Knippenberg-Gordebeke G. Control of an epidemic spread of a multi-resistant strain of *Acinetobacter calcoaceticus* in a hospital. Intensive Care Med 1989;15:166–170.
6. Buisson Y, Tran van Nhieu G, Ginot L, Bouvet P, Shill H, Driot L, Meyran M. Nosocomial outbreaks due to amikacin-resistant tobramycin-sensitive *Acinetobacter* species: correlation with amikacin usage. J Hosp Infect 1990;15:83–93.
7. Bergogne-Berezin E, Joly-Guillou ML. Hospital infection with *Acinetobacter* spp.: an increasing problem. J Hosp Infect 1991;18(Suppl A):250–255.
8. Go ES, Urban C, Burns J, Kreiswirth B, Eisner W, Mariano N, Mosinka-Snipas K, Rahal JJ. Clinical and molecular epidemiology of *Acinetobacter* infections sensitive only to polymyxin B and sulbactam. Lancet 1994;344:1329–1332.
9. Seifert H, Boullion B, Schulze A, Pulverer G. Plasmid DNA profiles of *Acinetobacter baumannii*: clinical application in a complex endemic setting. Infect Control Hosp Epidemiol 1994;15:520–528.
10. Bergogne-Berezin E, Towner KJ. *Acinetobacter* spp. as nosocomial pathogens: microbiological, clinical, and epidemiological features. Clin Microbiol Rev 1996;9:148–165.
11. Fang FC, Madinger NE. Resistant nosocomial gram-negative bacillary pathogens: *Acinetobacter baumannii*, *Xanthomonas maltophilia*, and *Pseudomonas cepacia*. Current Topics in Infectious Diseases, pg 52–75.
12. Dominguez MA, Ayats J, Ardanuy C, Corbella X, Liñares J, Martin R. Evolution and molecular characterization of epidemic clones of multiresistant *Acinetobacter baumannii* (1992–97). Abstract K-124. 38th Interscience Conference on Antimicrobial Agents and Chemotherapy. San Diego, (USA), 1998.
13. Villers D, Espaze E, Coste-Burel M, Grauffret F, Nimin E, Nicolas F, Richet H. Nosocomial *Acinetobacter baumannii* infections: microbiological and clinical epidemiology. Ann Intern Med 1998;129:182–189.
14. Rossau R, van Landschoot A, Gillis M, De Levy J. Taxonomy of Moracellaceae fam. nov., a new bacterial family to accomodate the genera *Moraxella*, *Acinetobacter* and *Psychrobacter* and related organisms. Int J Syst Bacteriol 1991;41:310–319.
15. Baumann P. Isolation of *Acinetobacter* from soil and water. J Bacteriol 1968;96:39–42.
16. Taplin D, Rebell G, Zaias N. The human skin as a source of *Mima-Herellea* infections. J Am Med Assoc 1963;186:952–954.
17. Tjernberg I, Ursing J. Clinical starins of *Acinetobacter* classified by DNA-DNA hybridization. Acta Pathol Microbiol Immunol Scand 1989;97:595–605.
18. Joly-Guillou ML, Bergogne-Berezin E, Vieu JF. Epidemiology of *Acinetobacter* strains isolated from nosocomial infections in France. In: The biology of *Acinetobacter*. Towner KJ, Bergogne-Berezin E, Fewson CA. (Eds). Plenum Press, New York, 1991, pg 63–68.
19. Seifert H, Baginsky R, Schlze A, Pulverer G. Thre distribution of *Acinetobacter* species in clinical culture materials. Zentrabl Bakteriol 1993;279:544–552.
20. Dijkshoorn L, Aucken HM, Gerner-Smidt P, Kaufmann ME, Ursing J, Pitt TL. Correlation of typing methods for *Acinetobacter* isolates from hospital outbreaks. J Clin Microbiol 1993;31:702–705.
21. Bouvet PJM, Jeanjean S. Delineation of new proteolytic genospecies in the genus *Acinetobacter*. Res Microbiol 1989;140:291–299.
22. Gerner-Smidt P, Tjernberg I, Ursing J. Reliability of phemotypic tests for identification of *Acinetobacter* species. J Clin Microbiol 1991;29:277–282.
23. Gennari M, Lombardi P. Comparative characterization of *Acinetobacter* strains isolated from different foods and clinical sources. Zentrabl Bakteriol 1993;279:553–564.

24. Joly-Guillou ML, Brun Buisson C. Epidemiology of *Acinetobacter* spp.: Surveillance and management of outbreaks. In: *Acinetobacter*: Microbiology, Epidemiology, Infections, managemenet. Bergonge-Berezin E, Joly-Guillou ML, Towner KJ (eds). CRC Press Inc, Boca Raton Florida 1996, pg 73–75.
25. Smith PW, Masanari RM. Room humidifiers as the source of *Acinetobacter* infections. JAMA 1977;237:797.
26. Vandenbroucke CMJE, Kerver AJH, Rommes JH, Jansen R, den Dekker C, Verhoef J. Endemic *Acinetobacter anitratus* in a surgical intensive care unit: mechanical ventilators as reservoir. Eur J Clin Microbiol Infect Dis 1988;7:485–489.
27. Contant J, Kemeny E, Oxley C, Perry E, Garber G. Investigation of an outbreak of *Acinetobacter calcoaceticus* var. *anitratus* infections in an adult intensive care unit. Am J Infect Control 1990;18:288–291.
28. Cefai C, Richards J, Gould FK, McPeake P. An outbreak of *Acinetobacter* respiratory tract infection resulting from incomplete disinfection ventilatory equipment. J Hosp Infect 1990;15:177–182.
29. Weernink A, Severin WPJ, Tjernberg I, Dijkshoorn L. Pillows, an unexpected source of *Acinetobacter*. J Hosp Infect 1995;29:189–199.
30. Wise KA, Tosolini FA. Epidemiological surveillance of *Acinetobacter* species. J Hosp Infect 1990;16:319–329.
31. Mulin B, Talon D, Viel JF, Vincent C, Leprat R, Thouverez M, Michel-Briand Y. Risk factors for nosocomial colonization with multiresistant *Acinetobacter baumannii*. Eur J Clin Microbiol Infect Dis 1995;14:569–576.
32. Bergogne-Berezin E. *Acinetobacter*: a challenge to infection control. *Acinetobacter* 96. 4th International Symposium on the Biology of *Acinetobacter*. Eilat, Israel, 3–5 November 1996.
33. Hanberger H, García Rodríguez JA, Gobernado M, Goossens H, Nilsson LE, Struelens MJ, and the French and Portuguese ICU study groups. Antibiotic susceptibility among aerobic gram-negative bacilli in intensive care units in 5 European countries. JAMA 1999;281:67–71.
34. Palomar M, Alvárez Lerma F, de la Cal MA, Insausti J, Olaechea P and the ENVIN-UCI Study Group. ICU-acquired infections in Spain. Predominant pathogens. Intensive Care Med 1997:23(Suppl 1):123.
35. Palomar M, Alvárez Lerma F, de la Cal MA, Insausti J, Olaechea P and the ENVIN-UCI Study Group. Etiología y patrones de sensibilidad de las infecciones adquiridas en los Servicios de Medicina Intensiva. XXXII Congreso Nacional de la Sociedad Española de Medicina Intensiva y Unidades Coronarias (SEMIUC), 1997.
36. Lortholary O, Fagon JY, Buu-Hoi A, Slama MA, Pierre J, Giral PH, Rosenzweig R, Gutmann L, Safar M, Acar J. Nosocomial adquisition of multiresistant *Acinetobacter baumannii*: risk factors and prognosis. Clin Infect Dis 1995;20:790–796.
37. Cisneros JM, Reyes MJ, Pachon J, Becerril B, Caballero CJ, García-Garmendia JL, Ortiz C, Cobacho AR. Bacteremia due to *Acinetobacter baumannii*: epidemiology, clinical findings, and pronostic features. Clin Infect Dis 1996;22:1026–1032.
38. Fagon JY, Chastre J, Domart Y, Trouillet JL, Gibert C. Mortality due to ventilator-associated pneumonia or colonization with *Pseudomonas* or *Acinetobacter* species; assessment by quantitative culture of samples obtained by a protected specimen brush. Clin Infect Dis 1996;23:538–542.
39. Kaul R, burt JA, Cork L, Dedler H, García M, Kennedy C, Brunton J, Krajden M, Conly J. Investigation of a multiyear critical care unit outbreak due to relatively drug-sensitive *Acinetobacter baumannii*: risk factors and attributable mortality. J Infect Dis 1996;174:1279–1287.
40. Timsit JF, Garrait V, Misset B, Goldstein FW, Renaud B, Carlet J. The digestive tract is a major site for *Acinetobacter baumannii* colonization in intensive care unit patients. J Infect Dis 1993;168: 1336–1337.
41. Corbella X, Pujol M, Ayats J, Sendra M, Ardanuy C, Dominguez MA, Ariza J, Gudiol F. Relevance of digestive tract colonization in the epidemiology of multiresistant *Acinetobacter baumannii*. Clin Infect Dis 1996;23:329–334.
42. Grehn M, von Graevenitz A. Search of *Acinetobacter calcoaceticus* subsp. *anitratus*: enrichment of fecal samples. J Clin Microbiol 1978;8:342–343.
43. Brun-Buisson C, Legrand P. Can topical and nonabsorbable antimicrobials prevent cross-transmission of resistant strains in ICUs? Infect Control Hosp Epidemiol 1994;15:447–455.
44. Ayats J, Corbella X, Ardanuy C, Domínguez MA, Ricart A, Ariza J, Martin R, Liñares J. Epidemiological significance of cutaneous, pharyngeal, and digestive tract colonization by multiresistant *Acinetobacter baumannii* in ICU patients. J Hosp Infect 1997;37:287–295.
45. Seifert H, Strate A, Pulverer G. Nosocomial bacteremia due to *Acinetobacter baumannii*: Clinical features, epidemiology and predictros of mortality. Medicine 1995;74:340–349.

46. Getschell-White SI, Donowitz LG, Groschel DHM. The inanimate environment of an intensive care unit as a potential source of nosocomial bacteria: evidence for long survival of *Acinetobacter calcoaceticus*. Infect Control Hosp Epidemiol 1989;10:402–406.
47. Musa EK, Desai N, Casewell MW. The survival of *Acinetobacter calcoaceticus* inoculated on fingertips and on formica. J Hosp Infect 1990;15:219–227.
48. Wendt C, Dietze B, Ruden H. Survival of Acinetobacter species on dry surfaces. 3rd International Symposium Biology of Acinetobacter. Edinburgh, 1994.
49. Corbella X, Pujol M, Argerich MJ, Ayats J, Sendra M, Peña C, Ariza J. Environmental sampling of *Acinetobacter baumannii*: moistened swabs versus moistened sterile gauze pads. Infect Control Hosp Epidemiol 1999;20:458–460.
50. Buxton AE, Anderson RL, Werdegar D, Atlas E. Nosocomial respiratory tract infection and colonization with *Acinetobacter calcoaceticus*. Epidemiologic characteristics. Am J Med 1978;65:507–513.
51. Patterson JE, Vecchio J, Pantelick EL, Farrel P, Mazon D, Zervus MJ, Hierholzer WJ. Association of contaminated gloves with transmission of *Acinetobacter calcoaceticus* var. *anitratus* in an intensive care unit. Am J Med 1991;91:479–483.
52. Corbella X, Pujol M, Ayats J, Sendra M, Ardanuy C, Domínguez MA, Ariza J. Clinical epidemiology of a large and sustained hospital outbreak of infections due to multiresistant acinetobacter baumannii in Barcelona. *Acinetobacter* 96. 4th International Symposium on the Biology of *Acinetobacter*. Eilat, Israel, 3–5 November 1996.
53. Allen KD, Green HT. Hospital outbreak of multi-resistant *Acinetobacter anitratus*: an airborne mode of spread. J Hosp Infect 1987;9:110–119.
54. Gaynes R. Antibiotic resistance in ICUs: a multifaceted problem requiring a multifaceted solution. Inf Control Hosp Epidemiol 1995;16:328–330.
55. Pallarés R, Pujol M, Peña C, Ariza J, Martin R, Gudiol F. Cephalosporins as a risk factor for nosocomial *Enterococcus faecalis* bacteremia. A matched case-control study. Arch Intern Med 1993;153:1581–1586.
56. Peña C, Pujol M, Ardanuy C, Ricart A, Pallarés R, Liñares J, Ariza J, Gudiol F. Epidemiology and successful control of a large outbreak due to *Klebsiella pneumoniae* producing extended-spectrum β-lactamases. Antimicrob Agents Chemother 1998;42:53–58.
57. Bonten MJ, Hayden MK, Nathan C, van-Voorhisd, Matushek M, Slaughter S, Rice T, Weinstein RA. Epidemiology of colonization of patients and environment with vancomycin-resistant enterococci. Lancet 1996;348:1615–1619.
58. Corbella X, Montero A, Pujol M, Domínguez MA, Ayats J, Argerich MJ, Garrigosa F, Ariza J, Gudiol F. Emergence of Carbapenem Resistance during a Large Hospital Endemic by Multiresistant *Acinetobacter baumannii*: Epidemiology and Control Measures. 38th International Conference of Antimicrobial Agent and Chemotherapy (ICAAC), San Diego, CA, USA, 1998.
59. Tankovic J, Legrand P, de Gatines G, Chemineaud V, Brun-Buisson C, Duval J. Characterization of a hospital outbreak of imipenem resistant *Acinetobacter baumannii* by phenotypic and genotypic typing methods. J Clin Microbiol 1994;32:2677–2681.
60. Vila J, Amela M, Jimenez de Anta MT. Laboratory investigation of hospital outbreak caused by two different multiresistant *Acinetobacter calcoaceticus* subsp. *anitratus* strains. J Clin Microbiol 1989;27: 1086–1089.
61. Vila J, Marcos MA, Jimenez de Anta MT. A comparative study of different typing methods for epidemiological typing of *Acinetobacter calcoaceticus-A. baumannii* complex. J Med Microbiol 1996;44: 482–489.
62. Seifert H, Schulze A, Baginsky R, Pulverer G. Comparison of four different typing methods for epidemiological typing of *Acinetobacter baumannii*. J Clin Microbiol 1994;32:1816–1819.
63. Dijkshoorn L. Acinetobacter: Microbiology. In: *Acinetobacter*: Microbiology, Epidemiology, Infections, managemenet. Bergonge-Berezin E, Joly-Guillou ML, Towner KJ (eds). CRC Press Inc, Boca Raton Florida 1996, pg 41–64.
64. Wenzel RP, Edmon MB. Vancomycin-resistant *Staphylococcus aureus*: infection control considerations. Clin Infect Dis 1998;27:245–251.
65. French GL, Casewell MW, Roncoroni AJ, Knight S, Phillips I. A hospital outbreak of antibiotic resistant *Acinetobacter anitratus*: epidemiology and control. J Hosp Infect 1980;1:125–131.
66. Viladrich PF, Corbella X, Corral L, Tubau F, Mateu A. Successful treatment of carbapenem-resistant *Acinetobacter baumannii* ventriculitis with intraventricular colistin sulphomethate sodium. Clin Infect Dis 1999;28:916–917.
67. Urban C, Go E, Mariano N, Berger BJ, Rubin D, Rahal JJ. Effect of sulbactam on infections caused by imipenem-resistant Acinetobacter calcoaceticus biotype *anitratus*. J Infect Dis 1993;167:448–451.

68. Jiménez-Mejías ME, Pachón J, Becerril B, Palomino-Nicás J, Rodríguez-Cobacho A, Revuelta M. Treatment of multi-resistant *Acinetobacter baumannii* meningitis with ampicillin/sulbactam. Clin Infect Dis 1997;24:932–935.
69. Corbella X, Ariza J, Ardanuy C, Vuelta M, Tubau F, Sora M, Ariza J, Gudiol F. Efficacy of sulbactam alone and in association with ampicillin in nosocomial infections due to *Acinetobacter baumannii*. J Antimicrobial Chemother 1998;42:793–802.
70. Joly-Guillou ML, Wolff M, Decré D, Calvat S, Bergogne-Berezin E. Colonization and infection with *A. baumannii* in ICU patients receiving selective digestive decontamination: results of a case control and molecular epidemiologic investigations. 34th Interscience Conference on Antimicrobial Agents and Chemotherapy. Orlando (USA), 1994.
71. Lance-Sauders G, Hammond JMJ, Potgieter PD, Plum HA, Forder AA. Microbiological surveillance during selective decontamination of the digestive tract (SDD). J Antimicrobial Chemother 1994;34: 529–544.

8. FUNGAL INFECTIONS: THE ROLE OF PROPHYLACTIC AND EMPIRIC ANTIFUNGAL THERAPY IN ICU PATIENTS

PAUL O. GUBBINS, PHARM D.

University of Arkansas for Medical Sciences, Little Rock, AR 72205-7122

INTRODUCTION

In 1990 National Nosocomial Infection Surveillance (NISS) Program data heightened the awareness of nosocomial fungal infections in the U.S. During the 1980s nosocomial fungal infection rates doubled and *Candida* species (*Candida* sp.) emerged as the sixth most common nosocomial pathogen. Increases in fungal infection rates occurred regardless of hospital type or size and were primarily due to one genus, *Candida* sp, which caused nearly 80% of all nosocomial fungal infections (1,2).

More striking, the increases in nosocomial fungal infection rates occurred across all infection sites, especially in the bloodstream (1). By 1990, *Candida* sp. caused nearly 8% of all nosocomial bloodstream infections (BSI) (3,4). The rate of nosocomial candidemia had risen nearly 500% in large teaching hospitals, and 200% or more in small teaching hospitals and large nonteaching hospitals (3). Generally, these trends have continued throughout this decade (5). NNIS data from 1990 to 1996 show *Candida* sp. are the sixth most common nosocomial pathogen, and still cause nearly 9% of all nosocomial BSI (6). Other national surveillance programs confirm that *Candida* sp. are currently the fourth leading cause of BSI (7).

The importance of preventing nosocomial fungal infections has become clear, particularly on oncology wards and bone marrow transplant (BMT) units. In these settings measures used to prevent invasive mycoses include antifungal prophylaxis, controlled environments and other extensive infection control practices. In the U.S., the importance of preventing nosocomial fungal infections in the intensive care units

R.A. Weinstein and M.J.M. Bonten (eds.). INFECTION CONTROL IN THE ICU ENVIRONMENT.

(ICU) is widely recognized, but effective preventative measures in this setting are still evolving as our understanding of these infections improves. Antifungal prophylaxis in the BMT setting has recently been reviewed and will not be addressed in this chapter (8). This chapter will examine the role of prophylaxis and empiric antifungal therapy in the ICU setting. Specifically, the epidemiology and risk factors of invasive mycoses in the ICU environment will be reviewed and the role of antifungal prophylaxis and empiric therapy in this setting will be addressed.

FUNGAL INFECTIONS IN THE ICU

Epidemiology

Generally, fungal infections are more prevalent in the ICU setting than on the general medical wards (5,7,9). For at least two decades the epidemiological trends for fungal infections in the ICU have mirrored the hospital-wide trends described above. In the 1980s, nationwide, the nosocomial fungal infection rate per 1,000 discharges rose 124% among patients on surgical services. Moreover, between 1986 and 1990, subspecialties with the highest fungal infection rates were burn/trauma, cardiac and general surgery services (1).

These trends have also continued throughout this decade (5,9–15). In the U.S., fungal infections in the ICU setting occur most often in the bloodstream and urinary tract. Between 1986 and 1995 the proportion of urinary tract infections (UTI) in the ICU caused by fungi increased 33% (12). During that period, fungi also caused approximately 10% of all BSI in the ICU setting (12). Fungal infection rates at specific sites vary depending on the type of ICU. At a large teaching hospital during a 7-year period, 50% of all nosocomial fungal BSI occurred in the SICU and haematology unit. In contrast, at that center, abdominal fungal infections occurred primarily in the BMT and haematology unit and 33% of all nosocomial catheter-related fungal UTIs occurred in the SICU and medical intensive care unit (MICU) (5). In contrast, at another institution, surgical wounds and urine were the most common infection sites during a two-year SICU surveillance (13).

National surveillances also show infection sites vary by ICU type. According to NNIS data from 1986 to 1995, overall, catheter-related UTIs have been the most common nosocomial fungal infection in the ICU setting (12,14). In the U.S., between 1992 and 1997, fungi caused approximately 40% of all UTIs in the MICU setting (15). However, in the National Epidemiology of Mycoses Survey (NEMIS), a 2-year (1993–95) study of fungal infections in the SICU and neonatal ICU (NICU) settings of six different medical centers, BSI was the most common nosocomial fungal infection (10,11). According to this surveillance, fungal infections of sterile body fluids and wounds, though prevalent, were much less common. NEMIS data also indicate *Candida* sp. caused nearly 10 BSI per 1,000 admissions in the SICU setting and approximately 12 BSI per 1,000 admissions in the NICU (11). Clearly, patients in the SICU and NICU are among those at greatest risk for developing nosocomial fungal infections.

Fungal Pathogens in the ICU

Numerous *Candida* sp. exist, however, less than 20 have been associated with human infections. For at least 20 years *Candida* sp. have been the most prominent fungal pathogens in the ICU. During the 1980s, *Candida* sp. caused 10% of all BSI, 25% of all UTIs and were the fourth most commonly isolated pathogen in the ICU setting (1,2,14). According to NNIS data these trends have continued throughout the 1990s. Between 1990 and 1995, *Candida* sp. accounted for 20% of all isolates from catheter-associated UTIs and approximately 11% of all catheter-associated BSI in the ICU (12). From 1992 to 1997, *Candida* sp. accounted for 31% of all isolates from UTIs and 11% of all catheter-associated BSI, in the MICU (15).

In the ICU setting, *Candida albicans* (*C. albicans*) is the primary fungal pathogen (10,11,15). Among all ICU pathogens, *C. albicans* is the second most common pathogen of nosocomial catheter-associated UTIs, superseded only by *Escherichia coli* (12). Between 1992 and 1997, *C. albicans* was the most common cause of UTIs in the MICU setting (15). Moreover, *C. albicans* is the fourth most common pathogen of BSI in the ICU setting, superseded only by coagulase-negative staphylococci, *Staphylococcus aureus*, and enterococci. (12,15).

Approximately 43% of *Candida* sp. in the SICU and NICU setting are non-*albicans Candida* sp. (10,11). In the NEMIS study *Candida glabrata* (*C. glabrata*) and *Candida parapsilosis* (*C. parapsilosis*) were the most common non-*albicans Candida* sp. in the SICU and NICU settings (10,11). In the U.S., *C. glabrata* is among the ten most common causes of nosocomial BSI and UTIs in the MICU setting (15). *Candida krusei* (*C. krusei*) and *Candida tropicalis* (*C. tropicalis*) are less prevalent non-*albicans Candida* sp. (10,11). In the NEMIS study approximately 3% of *Candida* isolates were not speciated, other notable species such as *Candida lusitaniae* (*C. lusitaniae*) likely cause infections in the ICU as well (10,11).

Within specific ICU settings there is substantial variation in the species causing nosocomial fungal infections. For example, fungal infections in the SICU and MICU are typically caused by a variety *Candida* sp. in contrast, in the NICU, they are primarily caused by two species, *C. albicans* and *C. parapsilosis* (10,11,15). Though such distributions may be somewhat influenced by local clusters of infections, others have noted a high prevalence of these two species in the NICU (16–21). Species distribution and susceptibility to antifungal agents also varies geographically (10,11,22–24). In an ongoing national surveillance of nosocomial BSI in 49 hospitals across the U.S., most isolates (69%) came from the eastern U.S. Overall, the majority (53%) of the isolates were *C. albicans*, however, in the eastern U.S., 51% of the BSI were caused by non-*albicans Candida* species. In contrast, in the western U.S., only 36% of the BSI were caused by non-*albicans Candida* sp. (7,22,23). The overall susceptibility patterns of the *Candida* sp. in this surveillance were similar to previous observations, however, regional differences in susceptibility to fluconazole, itraconazole and 5-FC were noted for *C. albicans*. Regional differences in susceptibility to itraconazole were also noted among non-*albicans Candida* sp. (22,23).

DEFINING THE ROLE OF PROPHYLAXIS OR EMPIRIC ANTIFUNGAL THERAPY IN THE ICU

Clinical manifestations of fungal infections in critically ill patients are often nonspecific. Moreover, limited microbiological resources, especially in smaller institutions, can make isolation and identification of certain fungal pathogens difficult (25,26). As a result, in the U.S., the indication for prophylactic or empiric antifungal therapy in the ICU often hinges on ability to identify patients at risk for systemic mycosis. Therefore to define the role of prophylactic and empiric antifungal therapy in ICU patients, the origin, risks and outcomes of fungal infections in the ICU must be understood.

Etiology of Fungal Infections in the ICU

C. albicans, *C. glabrata*, *C. tropicalis*, *C. lusitaniae* and perhaps *C. krusei* are commensals of the gastrointestinal (GI) tract. BSI caused by these species likely arise endogenously from the GI tract (27,28,29). Prior to infection, patients are colonized at multiple body sites, over time, with a unique strain (22,29–34). In the ICU setting, depending on the body site, patients can be colonized for prolonged intervals prior to developing infection (32). When infection develops, the genotype of the colonizing and infecting strains are often identical (32). Exogenous transmission of *C. albicans* has been reported in the NICU setting, but is uncommon in other ICU settings (20,21,30,32,35,36). In contrast, exogenous transmission of the non-*albicans Candida* sp. in the ICU setting, through indirect contact with other patients or the ICU environment, is fairly common (23,34,37). *C. parapsilosis* is unlike other non-*albicans Candida* sp.; it is not a known human commensal and colonization does not precede infection (30,38). Rather, *C. parapsilosis* infections arise exogenously, through indirect contact with the ICU environment or other patients (38,39). Healthcare workers may be a primary reservoir for exogenous transmission of *Candida* sp. in the ICU. In one study 58% of ICU healthcare workers carried *Candida* sp. on their hands. *C. parapsilosis* was isolated from 52% of these healthcare workers' hands (40).

Prognosis of Fungal Infections in the ICU

In the ICU fungal infections, particularly *Candida* BSI, are difficult to detect. It is usually not possible to distinguish bacterial and fungal BSI on the basis of symptoms. *Candida* sp. are cleared from the blood very efficiently by several organs; not surprisingly, blood cultures can be negative in approximately 50% of patients with hematogenously disseminated candidiasis (41,42).

Difficulty in establishing a diagnosis likely contributes to the relatively poor prognosis associated with *Candida* BSI in the U.S. Among critically ill patients, regardless of etiology, the attributable mortality of nosocomial BSI is 35% (43). In the U.S., BSI due to *Candida* sp. alone produce comparable mortality rates. At some centers the *Candida* sp. BSI mortality rates are the highest among any type of BSI (44). The crude mortality rate associated with *Candida* BSI hospital-wide and in the ICU setting, is roughly 35–69%, and the attributable mortality is 38% (44,45). Moreover, *Candida* sp. are the only pathogens that have been identified as an independent predictor of mortality (44). In addition, candidemia adds approximately one month to the length of hospital stay of surviving patients (46).

In the ICU setting, systemic fungal infections are common, difficult to diagnosis, and carry a poor prognosis. Therefore, the ability to identify patients at risk for fungal infections is crucial to defining the indication for prophylactic or empirical antifungal use in this setting.

Risk Factors for Fungal Infections in the ICU

Risk factors for *Candida* BSI are well described (Table 1). Several, including broad-spectrum antimicrobial use, colonization with *Candida* sp., indwelling vascular catheters, and hemodialysis have been identified as independent risk factors for *Candida* BSI (44). Many of the risk factors are not unique to the ICU setting, but in this environment, most are unavoidable. Therefore, clinicians should understand with each risk factor, the odds of the patient developing infection multiplies.

As discussed above, often colonization with *Candida* sp. is a prerequisite to developing infection. Although the importance of colonization is widely recognized, the ability to predict the likelihood a colonized site will progress to infection is disputed. One study suggests that in SICU patients no single site of colonization is better than any given site in predicting the subsequent development of infection (13). In another study, the interval between a positive culture from a colonized site and the blood was shorter when the likelihood of isolating identical colonizing and infecting strains was high (32). Investigators noted that patients colonized with *Candida* sp. at common infection sites (i.e. urine or on a catheter tip) developed BSI more quickly than patients colonized at other less common infection sites (i.e. respiratory tract) (32). Other investigators have also suggested colonization of the urinary tract (e.g. candiduria) is a harbinger of disseminated candidiasis in the ICU setting (47). However, several studies have shown progression of infection from a urinary source to the bloodstream rarely occurs. Instead, candiduria may reflect a previously undetected BSI (48).

Studies have demonstrated that in the GI tract, at a threshold inoculum size, *Candida* sp. can translocate to the bloodstream (41,49). Many epidemiologic studies have identified antibiotic use as a risk for *Candida* BSI. Therefore, as a consequence

Table 1. Commonly Identified Risk Factors for Candida BSI in the U.S.

Broad-spectrum Antibiotic Use*	Multiple Blood Transfusions
Candida Colonization*	Length of ICU Stay
Hemodialysis*	Diabetes Mellitus
Presence of Hickman Catheter*	Corticosteroid Therapy
Neutropenia	Immunosuppressive Therapy
Prolonged Central Venous Catheter Use	Total Parenteral Nutrition (TPN)
Mechanical Ventilation	Presence of Urinary Catheter

*Identified as independent risk factors by multivariate analysis

of antibiotic-induced changes in endogenous microflora, the threshold *Candida* inoculum size is apparently achieved often. In U.S. hospitals, broad-spectrum antibiotic use is ubiquitous in the ICU environment. Patients in the ICU account for less than 20% of hospital admissions, yet broad-spectrum antibiotic use in this setting is significantly higher than in the non-ICU setting (50,51). Researchers in the U.S. determined the number of antibiotics given and the total number of days of antibiotic therapy were significant risk factors for *Candida* BSI by univariate analysis (44). Others have identified the number of antibiotics given as a predictor of mortality in candidemic patients using univariate methods (52). However in a multivariate analysis the duration of antibiotic therapy was not a significant risk or predictor, rather only the number of antibiotics as a predictor of developing *Candida* BSI was identified as significant (44,52).

For ICU patients the risk of developing *Candida* infections associated with central venous access is likely not limited to the Hickman catheter. Other catheter types have been identified by univariate methods, as significant predictors of *Candida* infections. Since *Candida* infections, particularly those due to *C. parapsilosis*, can develop from exogenous origins, central venous access can be an important source of these infections.

ANTIFUNGAL USE IN THE ICU SETTING

Despite increased awareness of risks factors, ICU fungal infection rates in the U.S. have not decreased. Given the incidence, the difficulty in diagnosing, and the poor prognosis of invasive mycoses in the ICU, preventative measures in this setting are clearly needed. Fungal infections in the ICU arise endogenously, and in some cases, by a complex cycling of pathogens between patients, the ICU environment, and healthcare workers or other patients. Therefore ideally, measures to prevent invasive mycosis should include both traditional infection control methods (handwashing, gloving, etc), and pharmacologic intervention.

Indications for Prophylactic or Empiric Therapy

In the U.S., all ICU settings should have traditional infection control measures in place. However, there is no consensus regarding prophylactic or empiric antifungal use in the ICU. Prophylactic and empiric antifungal therapy are not the same. Prophylactic therapy is the initiation of antifungal therapy in anticipation of infection developing (i.e., the absence of any symptoms or other evidence of infection). Empiric therapy is the initiation of antifungal therapy upon the first clinical suspicion of infection (i.e., in the presence of a clinical manifestation of infection in a patient at risk). Unlike patients in the BMT unit, not all patients in the ICU setting are at risk of developing invasive mycoses and in need preventative pharmacologic therapy. Therefore, prophylactic antifungal therapy in the ICU setting is hard to justify.

From the epidemiological data summarised above, ICU patients at high risk of developing invasive mycoses can be identified. Because fungal infections in these patients are common, difficult to diagnose, and associated with significant morbidity or mortality, clinicians cannot delay therapy until cultures become positive. Therefore, empiric therapy can be justified in these high risk patients, in whom a poor outcome is likely if treatment is not provided in a timely fashion.

Options for Empiric Therapy

In the U.S. options for empiric therapy are limited to amphotericin B, fluconazole, or itraconazole. Moreover, empiric therapy in the ICU setting has not been studied in a multi-center, controlled fashion; therefore, the optimal antifungal agent for empiric use is unclear. Nevertheless, the trends described above and the poor prognosis associated with infection, have fuelled widespread use of antifungals, particularly fluconazole in ICU patients in the absence of an established source of fungal infection. Data from one center indicate fluconazole is frequently used in ICU patients presumed to be at risk for yeast infections (5). At that center, after fluconazole was available in the U.S., the use of amphotericin B decreased slightly, however, the proportion of patients treated with antifungals who received amphotericin B declined markedly. Between 1990 and 1995 one University Hospital reported nearly a 16-fold increase in fluconazole use in the SICU, while during the same period admissions to the SICU rose 26% but the number of SICU beds remained constant (53).

For many years, amphotericin B was the lone option for the treatment of invasive mycoses in the ICU. However, clinicians have been reluctant to use this agent as empiric therapy because of the risk of nephrotoxicity. Consequently, the initiation of empiric amphotericin B therapy was often delayed. In addition, the effective preventative dose of amphotericin B is unknown. Data in patients who are not critically ill show that low dose amphotericin B is well tolerated (54). A retrospective study in general surgical patients with at least one blood culture positive for *Candida* sp. demonstrated that treatment with ≥210 mg of amphotericin B was associated with a significant protective effect (55). This study did not address the empiric use of amphotericin B in critically ill patients; therefore the efficacy of low dose amphotericin B for empiric therapy is unclear.

Lipid formulations of amphotericin B have lowered the risk of nephrotoxicity associated with amphotericin B, however, in the U.S. there are no data regarding the empiric use of the lipid amphotericin B formulations in the ICU setting. The results of a recent empiric therapy study in febrile neutropenic patients should not be extrapolated to the ICU setting. The study compared liposomal amphotericin B to amphotericin B, and showed no difference in the primary efficacy endpoints, fever resolution and 7 day survival (56). Moreover, a subgroup analysis revealed the liposomal formulation lowered the incidence of proven breakthrough infections (56). However, overall there was no difference between the agents to prevent all breakthrough infections, proven or otherwise. In this study, the liposomal formulation was less nephrotoxic, and it was associated with significantly less infusion related adverse effects (56). Even so, there was no difference between the agents in the premature discontinuation due to toxicity or lack of efficacy. According to this study more than 100 patients would have to be treated to prevent 1 infection (56).

Therefore, the liposomal formulation may be suitable for the neutropenic BMT population where the length of therapy may be longer and the risk of deadly non-*Candida* infections is higher than in the general ICU setting. Given the cost of the lipid amphotericin B formulations in the U.S., and concerns raised above, these formulations are likely not a cost effective means to prevent invasive mycoses in the ICU setting.

Fluconazole is safe, well tolerated and available orally or intravenously. In addition, the pharmacokinetic profile of fluconazole, particularly its oral availability, is well suited for the ICU setting. Several small studies in this setting have demonstrated the oral availability of fluconazole is maintained (i.e. 77–97%), even when administered through a nasogastric or feeding tube in surgical or trauma patients in the ICU (57,58). Given the disparity between the costs and infectious risks associated with i.v administration, this could be a cost-effective way to give fluconazole to these types of patients.

Fluconazole has been studied in high-risk non-surgical groups such as BMT recipients and neutropenic cancer patients as prophylaxis, not empiric therapy. The studies showed prophylactic fluconazole reduces the colonization with, and the number of infections due to, *C. albicans* (9). However the impact of fluconazole prophylaxis on morbidity and mortality in these populations is unclear (9). Moreover, the optimum dose is also unclear (9). Nonetheless, although in the U.S. clinicians may use fluconazole prophylactically in the ICU, there are no large trials assessing the efficacy of prophylactic or empiric fluconazole use in this setting.

The use of itraconazole in the ICU was limited by difficulty administering the capsule through feeding and NG tubes. However, the advent of an oral solution in the U.S. enables this drug to be more widely used in the ICU. The marketing of an i.v. itraconazole formulation may further increase its use in this setting in the future. Nonetheless in the U.S. there are no data regarding the empiric or prophylactic use of itraconazole in the ICU setting. Furthermore, despite more convenient dosage forms, the use itraconazole in the ICU may still be limited by a significant drug-drug interaction profile with agents commonly used in the ICU.

Effects of Empiric Therapy on the Etiology of *Candida* Infections

In the U.S. a concern surrounding prophylactic or empiric antifungal use in the ICU setting, particularly with the azoles, is a perceived shift in the etiology of *Candida* infections, and the selection of less susceptible *Candida* sp. (59). Since the mid-1990s many reports have suggested a shift in pathogen distribution may be occurring (5,9,22,23,53,60,61). During a 7-year period at a large teaching hospital, the prevalence of fungal infections caused by *C. albicans* dwindled while infections caused by *C. glabrata*, the second most prominent *Candida* sp., increased substantially (5). In a 4-year, multicenter, prospective observational study of *Candida* BSI, the prevalence of non-*albicans Candida* sp. continually increased at all centers and by the end of the study period, 53% of candidemias were caused by non-*albicans Candida* sp. Moreover, for the first time, *C. glabrata* supplanted *C. tropicalis* as the primary non-*albicans Candida* sp. causing candidemia (60). A nationwide surveillance made comparable findings (23).

Similar trends have been noted in the ICU setting. In a 5-year two-center, surveillance of fungal infections in the SICU setting, the prevalence of infections caused by *C. albicans* declined slightly at both institutions but a modest increase in the prevalence of infections due to *C. glabrata* was noted at only one center (53).

These data are compelling, yet national data derived from BSI isolates of *Candida* sp. obtained between 1992 and 1998, from 50 U.S. medical centers indicate the frequency of BSI caused by *Candida* sp. in general, has remained relatively stable (62). Although collectively there was no increase in infections due to non-*albicans Candida* sp., this study did note a significant increase in the incidence of *C. glabrata* BSI isolates (62). In the U.S., shifts in the etiology of *Candida* infections in the ICU setting may be occurring locally, however, nationally many of these shifts may be obscured by the species variation geographically and within specific ICUs. Accordingly, the consistent finding that *C. glabrata* infections are increasing in prevalence, locally and nationally is troubling.

The selection of non-*albicans Candida* sp. has been attributed to prophylactic use of fluconazole in BMT recipients (63,64). Outside of the BMT setting a possible association between azole use and the emergence of non-*albicans Candida* sp., particularly *C. glabrata*, and *Candida krusei* (*C. krusei*) has been noted (5,10,23,53,60,61,65). A large study in cancer patients noted a sharp decline in hematogenous candidiasis corresponding to the introduction of fluconazole prophylaxis at that institution. The decline resulted from a reduction in infections due to *C. albicans* and *C. tropicalis*, species typically sensitive to fluconazole, and an increased incidence of infections due to *C. krusei* and *C. glabrata*, species typically resistant to fluconazole (65). This suggests the selective pressure exerted by the empiric or prophylactic use of azoles within the ICU setting has contributed to the emergence of non-*albicans Candida* sp., specifically *C. glabrata*. However, in the U.S. there are conflicting data.

At a large teaching hospital shifts in pathogen distribution observed during a 7-year period occurred in conjunction with increased azole use. However, there was no correlation between the use of any individual antifungal agent within a particular ICU and the shifts in fungal etiology specific to that unit (5). Another university hospital has noted similar increases in the incidence of *C. glabrata* infections in the SICU setting that correspond to marked increases in fluconazole use (53). However, another university reported no increase in infections due to non-*albicans Candida* sp. in the SICU setting despite increased fluconazole use (53). Similarly, the stable overall trends and the slight increase in *C. glabrata* infections noted in the national analysis of BSI isolates of *Candida* sp. from 50 U.S. medical centers, occurred with widespread fluconazole use (62). A definitive link between azole use and the rising prominence of non-*albicans Candida* sp. is lacking. However, a growing body of evidence suggests the emergence of certain species, such as *C. glabrata*, in the ICU setting, may be somewhat related to selective pressures exerted by the use of the azoles (5,53,62).

CONCLUSIONS

In summary, in the U.S. fungal infections in the ICU setting have continued to increase throughout the decade. *Candida* sp. continue to be the predominant fungal pathogen in this setting. In the ICU, systemic fungal infections due to these species can be deadly and costly. Risk factors that predict the development of infection are well known. But their recognition alone has not improved the outcome of infections. In the at-risk ICU patient, it is now recognized that failure to treat in a timely fashion will likely lead to a poor outcome. Consequently in these patients empiric antifungal therapy can be justified. Unfortunately, in the U.S., controlled trials addressing empiric antifungal therapy in the ICU have not yet been performed. Therefore, the choice of therapy hinges on the epidemiology of infection, and the clinical setting.

REFERENCES

1. Beck-Sagué CM, Jarvis WR. National Nosocomial Infection Surveillance System. Secular trends in the epidemiology of nosocomial fungal infections in the United States. 1980–1990. J Infect Dis 1993;167:1247–1251.
2. Jarvis WR, Martone WJ. Predominant pathogens in hospital infections. J Antimicrob Chemother 1991;28:15–19.
3. Banerjee SN, Emori TG, Culver DH, Gaynes RP, Jarvis WR, Horan T, Edwards JR, Tolson J, Henderson T, Martone WJ. Secular trends in nosocomial primary bloodstream infections in the United States, 1980–1989. Am J Med 1991;91(Suppl 3B):86S–89S.
4. Schaberg DA, Culver DH, Gaynes RP. Major trends in the microbial etiology of nosocomial infection. Am J Med 1991;91(Suppl 3B):72S–75S.
5. Berrouane YF, Herwaldt LA, Pfaller MA. Trends in antifungal use and epidemiology of nosocomial yeast infections in a university hospital. J Clin Microiol 1999;37:531–537.
6. The National Nosocomial Infections Surveillance System. National Nosocomial Infections Surveillance (NNIS) Report, data summary from October 1986–April 1996, issued May 1996. Am J Infect Control 1996;24:380–388.
7. Edmond MB, Wallace SE, McClish DK, Pfaller MA, Jones RN, Wenzel RP. Nosocomial bloodstream infections in United States hospitals: a three-year analysis. Clin Infect Dis 1999;29:239–244.
8. Gubbins PO, Bowman JL, Penzak SR. Antifungal prophylaxis to prevent invasive mycoses among bone marrow transplant recipients. Pharmacother 1998;18:549–564.
9. Wenzel RP. Nosocomial candidemia: Risk factors and attributable mortality. Clin Infect Dis 1995;20:1531–1534.
10. Pfaller MA, Messer SA, Houston A, Rangel-Frausto MS, Wilbin T, Blumberg HM, Edwards JE, Jarvis W, Martin MA, Neu HC, Saiman L, Patterson JE, Dibb JC, Roldan CM, Rinaldi MG, Wenzel RP. National epidemiology of mycoses survey: A multicenter study of strain variation and antifungal susceptibility among isolates of Candida species. Diagn Microbiol Infect Dis 1998;31: 289–296.
11. Rangel-Frausto MS, Wiblin T, Blumberg HM, Saiman L, Patterson J, Rinaldi M, Pfaller M, Edwards JE, Jarvis W, Dawson J, Wenzel RP. National epidemiology of mycosis survey (NEMIS): Variations in rates of bloodstream infections due to Candida species in seven surgical intensive care units and six neonatal intensive care units. Clin Infect Dis 1999;29:253–258.
12. Fridkin SK, Welbel SF, Weinstein RA. Magnitude and prevention of nosocomial infections in the intensive care unit. Infect Dis Clin N Amer 1997;11:479–496.
13. Cornwell EE, Belzberg H, Berne TV, Dougherty WR, Morales IR, Asensio J, Demetriades D. The pattern of fungal infections in critically ill surgical patients. Am Surg 1995;61:847–850.
14. Jarvis WR, Edwards JR, Culver DH. Nosocomial infection rates in adult and pediatric intensive care units in the United States. Am J Med 1991;91(Suppl 3B):185S–191S.
15. Richards MJ, Edwards JR, Culver DH, Gaynes RP. Nosocomial infections in medical intensive care units in the United States. Crit Care Med 1999;27:887–892.

16. Whitehouse JD, Everts RJ, Hader SL, Goldberg RN, Kirkland KB. Epidemiology of Candida colonization in a neonatal intensive care unit: A prospective surveillance study. [Abstract M1] In: Program and Abstracts of the 9th Annual Scientific Meeting of the Society for Healthcare Epidemiology of America, April 18, 1999, San Francisco, CA.
17. Cordero L, Sananes M, Ayers LW. Bloodstream infections in a neonatal intensive-care unit: 12 years' experience with an antibiotic control program. Infect Control Hosp Epidemiol 1999;20:242–246.
18. Khatib R, Thirumoorthi MC, Riederer KM, Strum L, Oney LA, Baran J. Clustering of *Candida* infections in the neonatal intensive care unit: Concurrent emergence of multiple strains simulating intermittent outbreak. Pediatr Infect Dis J 1998;17:130–134.
19. el-Mohandes AE, Johnson-Robbins L, Keiser JF, Simmons SJ, Aure MV. Incidence of *Candida parapsilosis* colonization in an intensive care nursery population and its association with invasive fungal disease. Pediatr Infect Dis J 1994;13:520–524.
20. Reef SE, Lasker BA, Butcher DS, McNeil MM, Pruitt R, Keyserling H, Jarvis WR. Nonperinatal nosocomial transmission of Candida albicans in a neonatal intensive care unit: Prospective study. J Clin Micro 1998;36:1255–1259.
21. Reagan DR, Pfaller MA, Hollis RJ, Wenzel RP. Evidence of nosocomial spread of Candida albicans causing bloodstream infection in a neonatal intensive care unit. Diagn Microbiol Infect Dis 1995;21:191–194.
22. Pfaller MA, Jones RN, Messer A, Edmond MB, Wenzel RP. National surveillance of nosocomial blood stream infection due to Candida albicans: Frequency of occurrence and antifungal susceptibility in the SCOPE Program. Diagn Microbiol Infect Dis 1998;31:327–332.
23. Pfaller MA, Jones RN, Messer A, Edmond MB, Wenzel RP. National surveillance of nosocomial blood stream infection due to species of Candida other than Candida albicans: Frequency of occurrence and antifungal susceptibility in the SCOPE Program. Diagn Microbiol Infect Dis 1998;30:121–129.
24. Pfaller MA, Lockhart SR, Pujol C, Swails-Wenger JA, Messer SA, Edmond MB, Jones RN, Wenzel RP, Soll DR. Hospital Specificity, region specificity, and fluconazole resistance of Candida albicans bloodstream isloates. J Clin Microbiol 1998;36:1518–1529.
25. Vincent JL, Anaissie E, Bruining H, Demajo W, El-Ebiary M, Haber J, Hiramatsu Y, Nitenberg G, Nystrom PO, Pittet D, Rogers T, Sandven P, Sganga G, Schaller MD, Solomkin J. Epidemiology, diagnosis and treatment of systemic Candida infection in surgical patients under intensive care. Intensive Care Med 1998;24:206–216.
26. Jarvis WR. Epidemiology of nosocomial fungal infections, with emphasis on Candida species. Clin Infect Dis 1995;20:1526–1530.
27. Odds FC. Candida and candidosis: A review and bibliography. 2nd ed. London: Balliere Tindall; 1988.
28. Cole GT, Halawa AA, Anaissie EJ. The role of the gastrointestinal tract in hematogenous candidiasis: From the laboratory to the beside. Clin Infect Dis 1996;22(Suppl 2):S73–S88.
29. Pfaller MA. Nosocomial candidiasis: Emerging species, reservoirs and modes of transmission. Clin Infect Dis 1996;22(Suppl 2):S89–S94.
30. Pfaller MA, Rhine-Chalberg J, Barry AL, Rex JH. Strain variation and antifungal susceptibility among bloodstream isolates of Candida species from 21 different medical institutions. Clin Infect Dis 1995;21:1507–1509.
31. Pfaller MA. Epidemiology and control of fungal infections. Clin Infect Dis 1994;19(Suppl 1):S8–S13.
32. Voss A, Hollis RJ, Pfaller MA, Wenzel RP, Doebbeling BN. Investigation of the sequence of colonization and candidemia in nonneutropenic patients. J Clin Microbiol 1994;32:975–980.
33. Wingard JR. Importance of Candida species other than C. albicans as pathogens in oncology patients. Clin Infect Dis 1995;20:115–125.
34. Sanchez V, Vazquez JA, Barth-Jones D, Dembry L, Sobel JD, Zervos MJ. Epidemiology of nosocomial acquisition of *Candida lusitaniae* J Clin Microbiol 1992;30:3005–3008.
35. Vazquez JA, Sanchez V, Dmuchowski C, Dembry LM, Sobel JD, Zervos MJ. Nosocomial acquisition of Candida albicans: An epidemiologic study. J Infect Dis 1993;168:195–201.
36. Voss A, Pfaller MA, Hollis RJ, Rhine-Chalberg J, Doebbeling BN. Investigation of Candida albicans transmission in a surgical intensive care unit by using genomic DNA typing methods. J Clin Microbiol 1995;33:576–580.
37. Vazquez JA, Dembry LM, Sanchez V, Vazquez MA, Sobel JD, Dmuchowski C, Zervos MJ. Noscomial *Candida glabrata* colonization: An epidemiologic study. J Clin Microbiol 1998;36:421–426.
38. Diekema DJ, Messer SA, Hollis RJ, Wenzel RP, Pfaller MA. An outbreak of *Candida parapsilosis* prosthetic valve endocarditis. Diagn Microbiol Infect Dis 1997;29:147–153.

39. Waggoner-Fountain LA, Whit Walker M, Hollis RJ, Pfaller MA, Ferguson JE, Wenzel RP, Donowitz LG. Vertical and horizontal transmission of unique *Candida* sp. to premature newborns. Clin Infect Dis 1996;22:803–808.
40. Strausbaugh LJ, Sewell DL, Ward TT, Pfaller MA, Heiztman T, Tjoelker R. High frequency of yeast carriage on hands of hospital personnel. J Clin Microbiol 1994;32:2299–2300.
41. Stone HH, Kolb LD, Currie CA, Geheber CE, Cuzzell JZ. Candida sepsis: pathogenesis and principles of treatments. Ann Surg 1974;179:697–711.
42. Dean DA, Burchard KW. Fungal infection in surgical patients. Am J Surg 1996;171:374–382.
43. Pittet D, Tarara D, Wenzel RP. Nosocomial bloodstream infections in critically ill patients: Excess length of stay, extra costs, and attributable mortality. JAMA 1994;271:1598–1601.
44. Wey SB, Mori M, Pfaller MA, Woolson RF, Wenzel RP. Risk factors for hospital-acquired candidemia: A matched case-control study. Arch Intern Med 1989;149:2349–2353.
45. Pittet D, Li Ning, Woolson RF, Wenzel RP. Microbiological factors influencing the outcome of nosocomial bloodstream infections: A 6-year validated, population-based model. Clin Infect Dis 1997;24: 1068–1078.
46. Wey SB, Motomi M, Pfaller MA, Woolson RF, Wenzel RP. Hospital-acquired candidemia: the attributable mortality and excess length of stay. Arch Intern Med 1988;148:2642–2645.
47. Nassoura Z, Ivatury RR, Simon RJ, Jabbour N, Stahl WM. Candiduria as an early marker of disseminated infection in critically ill surgical patients: The role of fluconazole therapy. J Trauma 1993;35:290–294.
48. Gubbins PO, McConnell SA, Penzak SR. Management of funguria. Am J Health-Sys Pharm 1999;56: 1929–1935.
49. Krause W, Matheis H, Wulf K. Fungaemia and funguria after oral administration of Candida albicans. Lancet 1969;1:598–599.
50. Weinstein RA. Epidemiology and control of nosocomial infections in adult intensive care units. Am J Med 1991;91(Suppl 3B):179S–184S.
51. Fridkin SK, Steward CD, Edwards JR, Pryor ER, McGowan JE, Archibald LK, Gaynes RP, Tenover FC. Surveillance of antimicrobial use and antimicrobial resistance in United States hospitals: Project ICARE Phase 2. Clin Infect Dis 1999;29:245–252.
52. Fraser VJ, Jone M, Dunkel J, Storfer S, Medoff G, Dunagan WC. Candidemia in a tertiary care hospital: Epidemiology, risk factors, and predictors of mortality. Clin Infect Dis 1992;15:414–421.
53. Gleason TG, May AK, Caparelli D, Farr O, Sawyer RG. Emerging evidence of selection of fluconazole-tolerant fungi in surgical intensive care units. Arch Surg 1997;132:1197–1201.
54. Pathak A, Pien FD, Carvalho L. Amphotericin B use in a community hospital with special emphasis on side effects. Clin Infect Dis 1998;26:334–338.
55. Tang E, Tang G, Berne TV. Prognostic indicators in fungemia of the surgical patient. Arch Surg 1993;128:759–763.
56. Walsh TJ, Finberg RW, Arndt C, Hiemenz J, Schwartz C, Bodesteiner D, Papps P, Seibel N, Greenberg RN, Dummer S, Schuster M, Holcenberg JS. Liposomal amphotericin B for empirical therapy in patients with persistent fever and neutropenia. N Engl J Med 1999;340:764–771.
57. Rosemurgy AS, Markowsky S, Goode SE, Plastino K, Kearney RE. Bioavailability of fluconazole in surgical intensive care patients. J Trauma 1995;39:445–447.
58. Nicolau DP, Crowe H, Nightingale CH, Quintiliani R. Bioavailability of fluconazole administered via a feeding tube in intensive care unit patients. J Antimicrob Chemother 1995;36:395–401.
59. Safran DB, Dawson E. The effect of prophylactic treatment with fluconazole on yeast isolates in a surgical trauma intensive care unit. Arch Surg 1997;132:11184–11188.
60. Nguyen MH, Peacock JE, Morris AJ, Tanner DC, Nguyen ML, Snydman DR, Wagener MM, Rinaldi MG, Yu VL. The changing face of candidemia: Emergence of non-Candida albicans species and antifungal resistance. Am J Med 1996;100:617–623.
61. Price MF, LaRocco MT, Gentry LO. Fluconazole susceptibilities of Candida species and distribution of species recovered from blood cultures over a 5-year period. Antimicrob Agents Chemother 1994;38:1422–1424.
62. Pfaller MA, Messer SA, Hollis RJ, Jones RN, Doern GV, Brandt ME, Hajjeh RA. Trends in species distribution and susceptibility to fluconazole among blood stream isolates of Candida species in the United States. Diagn Microbiol Infect Dis 1999;33:217–222.
63. Wingard JR, Merz WG, Rinaldi MG, Johnson TR, Karp JE, Saral R. Increase in Candida krusei infection among patients with bone marrow transplantation and neutropenia treated prophylactically with fluconazole. N Engl J Med 1991;325:1274–1277.

64. Wingard JR, Merz WG, Rinaldi MG, Miller CB, Karp JE, Saral R. Association of *Torulopsis glabrata* infections with fluconazole prophylaxis in neutropenic bone marrow transplant patients. Antimicrob Agents Chemother 1993;37:1847–1849.
65. Abi-Said D, Anaissie E, Uzun O, Raad I, Pinzcowski H, Vartivarian S. The epidemiology of hematogenous candidiasis by different Candida species. Clin Infect Dis 1997;24:1122–1128.

9. FUNGAL INFECTIONS: THE ROLE OF PROPHYLAXIS AND EMPIRIC THERAPY IN ICU PATIENTS

JACQUES F.G.M. MEIS AND PAUL E. VERWEIJ

University Medical Center St. Radboud, Nijmegen, The Netherlands

INTRODUCTION

It has been shown in the last decade that the incidence of nosocomial fungal infections is increasing both in the USA (1) and in European hospitals (2,3). In the ICU setting *Candida* species are the most common cause of invasive fungal infections. The increase in nosocomial invasive candidosis parallels the advance made in the medical and surgical supportive care towards survival of critically ill patients, which would previously have died of severe illness. One of the most important risk factors for development of invasive fungal infections in these debilitated patients is the enormous increase in appropriate or in-appropriate use of broad spectrum antibiotics. Carefully considered presumptive treatment of infectious diseases in the ICU prior to establishment of a diagnosis is a common and proper practice of medicine. However ill-considered use of antibiotics can lead to a spiraling empiricism of antibiotic therapy incurring unnecessary risk of side effects and ultimately fungal infections (4). Their modulation of the bacterial flora induces an overgrowth of gastrointestinal *Candida* colonization which is a major first step in the development of invasive candidosis. It is an important task for the ICU physician to prevent development of invasive fungal infections because of its high attributable mortality. Appropriate use of broad spectrum antibiotics, strict hygienic measures and preemptive treatment with antimycotics in a certain subset of ICU patients with identified risk factors should prove essential to decrease the number of patients with invasive fungal disease. Neutropenic patients and transplant recipients is a distinct group with regard

R.A. Weinstein and M.J.M. Bonten (eds.). INFECTION CONTROL IN THE ICU ENVIRONMENT.

to the use of prophylactic and empirical antifungal treatment and will not be discussed in this chapter.

EPIDEMIOLOGY

The incidence of hospital-acquired *Candida* infections has increased steadily since the 1970s. This is probably the combined result of increasing numbers of patients rendered susceptible to mycoses by modern medical intervention and the growing clinical awareness of the significance of *Candida* species as nosocomial pathogens (5). Surveys in the USA have shown the culture of *Candida* species from the blood at a rate of 5 to 10 per 10,000 admissions, representing up to 15% of all bloodstream infections (6). *Candida* is now among the top four most isolated microorganisms from blood cultures (7). Comparison of the rate of bloodstream infection in 1994 between the USA and Europe shows a rate of 0.98 episodes of candidemia per 10,000 patient days at the university of Iowa (8) and 0.72 in the Netherlands (2). The rates of candidemia in Dutch university hospitals showed the same increasing trend as in the USA but on a lower scale. It has been suggested that one of the explanations for this difference might be the restricted antibiotic policy enforced in the hospitals and the community. Crude mortality of candidemia is 60%, which is higher than most bacteremias (9,10). When accounting for the mortality due to the underlying disease there is still an attributable mortality of up to 40% (10) for blood stream infection with *Candida*. *Candida albicans* is the most commonly encountered pathogenic species with *C. glabrata*, *C. parapsilosis*, *C. tropicalis* and *C. krusei* responsible for the remaining infections. However there is now evidence for a decrease in the relative prevalence of *C. albicans* as the other species are reported more frequently. In the USA SCOPE survey for noscocomial bloodstream infections it appeared that 50% of *Candida* isolates were non-*albicans* species (11). These species tend to have decreased susceptibility to antifungal agents in vitro (12). Similar trends have been reported from Europe with a less pronounced shift although this is not clear cut since the prevalence of various species of *Candida* isolated from bloodstream infection may vary between countries, between institutions and even between patient groups. There is a better correlation between the emergence of resistant *Candida* species and the use of prophylactic antifungals. In neutropenic patients, *C. krusei* and *C. glabrata* emerge under prophylactic regimens of fluconazole as compared with placebo (13) or polyenes (14). The emergence of fluconazole resistance among *C. albicans* is found mainly in the AIDS population (15).

Risk factors for candidemia include colonization with *Candida*, central venous access devices, renal dysfunction and haemodialysis and the number of antibiotic classes to which the patient has been exposed (16–18). Patients with these risk factors are most commonly found in surgical ICUs (gastrointestinal and pancreatic surgery), medical ICUs and neonatal ICUs. Whether candidemia is a risk factor for mortality in ICUs is still a matter of debate. Increasing age, multi-organ failure (19) and failure to remove vascular catheters despite persisting candidemia (20) appear to be independent risk factors for mortality from fungal infection.

DIAGNOSIS

Candidosis is the major nosocomial fungal infection in European ICU's as determined in the EPIC study (21,22). The clinical presentation of invasive candidosis in ICU patients is very variable and non-specific with pyrexia and/or persistent leukocytosis during antibiotic treatment. The patient may develop a septic shock or remain hemodynamically stable. Muscular tenderness, cutaneous petechial microabscesses and, in non-neutropenic patients, an unilateral endophthalmitis may develop. There is a high correlation between the occurrence of eye-lesions and disseminated infection. Ophthalmologic examination is a true bedside diagnostic test for invasive candidosis with endophthalmitis occurring in previous studies in up to 37% of patients with systemic infection (23). In earlier studies of surgical patients receiving parenteral hyperalimentation, *Candida* endophthalmitis was detected in 15% of patients (24). These high figures might be related to the high treatment barrier with the toxic amphotericin B desoxycholate in the 1970ties and the existence of the concept of benign candidemia (25). A recent study from Europe with 180 episodes of candidemia, which were treated with antifungals, showed that only 3 patients developed delayed complications due to the fungemia (26). *Candida* is commonly cultured from sputum and lower respiratory tract secretions obtained during bronchoscopy, particularly after antibiotic treatment. Despite these common findings bronchogenic spread and resulting invasive disease is rare. In a recent autopsy-controlled study of lung histology in 38 patients with persistently positive *Candida* cultures from bronchial secretions only 1 patient appeared to have local invasive disease (27). Pulmonary candidosis as complication of hematogenous spread occurs more frequently but is still rare (28). Histologically proven *Candida* pneumonia was discovered at autopsy in only 8 of 106 candidemic patients (17). The diagnosis of *Candida* pneumonia is, without histology, impossible to establish due to the common isolation of *Candida* species from bronchial secretions which is not diagnostic. Unfortunately most patients, in which the diagnosis might be possible, are too critically ill to undergo a lung biopsy. The isolation of *Candida* from wounds or drainage sites in patient receiving antibiotics is more a sign of mere colonization than invasion, except in patients with severe burns. *Candida* peritonitis can be found in non-surgical patients undergoing peritoneal dialysis especially continuous ambulatory peritoneal dialysis (29). It is in seriously ill surgical ICU patients where isolation of *Candida* after abdominal surgery presents a diagnostic and therapeutic controversy (30). Several investigators have concluded that *Candida*, alone or as part of a polymicrobial peritoneal infection, can cause peritonitis, intra-abdominal abscess formation and subsequent candidemia (31–33). Candiduria is an even more difficult problem with regard to judgement of bladder colonization in the presence of a catheter, bladder infection or kidney involvement. Clinical judgement should determine whether the yeast found in the urine is a result of hematogenous dissemination, ascending infection or insignificant colonization (34). Patients under antibiotic treatment with a catheter without a history of diabetes, genitourinary abnormalities, renal transplantation and no fever in the presence of asymptomatic candiduria need no treatment

(34–36). However there is suggestive evidence that significant candiduria in critically ill ICU patient represents a significant indicator of disseminated disease (37). Molecular typing of *Candida* bloodculture isolates compared with colonizing strains from the gastrointestinal tract and urine demonstrated that the urine was the source of most candidemic episodes (38).

Because in an ICU environment many patients are at least colonized, the diagnosis of invasive candidosis for most patients is by the detection of *Candida* in the blood. Unfortunately routine bloodculture volumes are generally very insensitive to detect infection (39). In an autopsy controlled study a disappointing 43% of patients subsequently proved to have a tissue-proven invasive candidosis had positive blood cultures with the lysis centrifugation culture technique (40). *Candida* is much more often cultured from other sites than blood such as urine wounds, sputum, and bronchial secretions. The importance of a positive culture form these sites is variable and depends on the critical illness of the ICU patient. Most patients who develop a disseminated candidosis have had previous positive cultures from one or more sites. It appears that the more *Candida* culture positive sites are present the more risk exists for disseminated disease (41).

Because of the difficulty in establishing the diagnosis of invasive candidosis with certainty a variety of non-cultural methods are under investigation such as serology and molecular PCR based techniques. In certain European countries antibody detection has an important role in the management of non-neutropenic ICU patients. However a large prospective study from a German centre concluded that antibody detection was of no clinical use to guide the clinical management of patients (42). The detection of mannan, a major cell-wall polysaccharide antigen, which is released into the blood of patients with invasive candidosis have been the focus of many studies. A recent study from Europe showed that the presence of mannan in serum is inversely related to the presence of anti-mannan antibody (43). Circulating mannan alone could be detected in the serum of 40% of ICU patients with proven invasive candidosis and antibody in 53% of patients. However when the results of both tests were combined a sensitivity of 80% was achieved. The specificity of both tests combined was 93%. This EIA recently became commercially available (Platelia Candida, Sanofi Diagnostics Pasteur, Marne La Cocquet, France). Although limited data are available from patients with only gastrointestinal colonization, combination of antibody and antigen testing is an interesting new approach to the serodiagnosis of invasive candidosis.

The detection of microbial DNA by PCR is one of the most powerful tools for the early diagnosis of human pathogens. Several animal studies have shown that PCR on blood is more sensitive than culture for detecting candidemia (44). A higher sensitivity was also found for clinical specimens from patients with candidemia and those with histologically confirmed invasive candidosis (45). A very important finding is that *Candida* PCR of blood is negative in most patients with only gastrointestinal *Candida* colonization, including heavily colonized HIV patients (46,47). In addition to the detection of invasive candidosis, PCR can be used for monitoring of the response to antifungal therapy (47,48).

PREVENTION

Most invasive fungal infections with *Candida* are caused by endogenous organisms via translocation of the intact or damaged gastrointestinal tract or by spread from other body sites. However, horizontal transmission of *Candida* between patients followed by overgrowth in the oropharynx and gut has been described which reinforces the importance of infection control measures. Eradication of oropharyngeal and intestinal *Candida* carriage of patients in an outbreak situation with oral amphotericin B has been suggested to be of key importance to control an outbreak (49). Transmission by handcarriage of *Candida* between patients via staff is well recognized (50) and proven by molecular typing (51). Unfortunately hand-washing compliance of health care workers is disappointing, especially in the busy ICU environment (52). An approach to better compliance with hand-hygiene could be the uniformal use of alcohol-based hand disinfection (53).

PROPHYLAXIS

Before considering antifungal prophylaxis it is extremely important to eliminate the possibility of cross-infections between patients via the hands of healthcare workers. Neglection of principles of general hygienic care will frustrate all other, mostly expensive, strategies to reduce the risk of developing a fungal infection in the ICU. Oral and gastrointestinal colonization of patients in the ICU is a common finding and it seems reasonable to decrease or eliminate these fungi to preempt the development of a fungal infection. A recent small prophylaxis trial comparing 400 mg fluconazole (23 patients) with placebo (20 patients) in patients with abdominal surgery demonstrated that the infection rate and the colonization rate was lower in the treatment group (54). However at this moment in time antifungal prophylaxis for all ICU patients irrespective of individual risk factors has never been validated in controlled trials and is therefore not an option in the ICU. Furthermore widespread use of absorbable antifungals in the ICU would promote development of the inevitable resistance to azoles and selection of non-*Candida albicans* species which are difficult to treat (12,55). Because *Candida* inhabits the gastrointestinal tract of ICU patients, especially following broad-spectrum antibiotics, there is always a risk of endogenous infection. Although it is tempting to eliminate yeasts with topical oral amphotericin B in selective gut decontamination regimens, it has never been shown to decrease the incidence of fungal infection (56).

EMPIRIC TREATMENT

The rationale for empiric antifungal treatment is to treat the individual patient with a high risk of invasive candidosis at the earliest possible stage. Empirical therapy is perceived as an appropriate intervention in neutropenic patients with persistent fever of 3–7 days duration, despite appropriate broad-spectrum antibacterial therapy, no obvious source of the fever and no clue of a viral or bacterial infection. In the USA empiric treatment is started generally earlier (at 3 days of fever) and in more patients (80%) than in Europe (7 days and 30% of patients). Incorporating the results of surveillance cultures (qualitative and quantitative) could guide the selection of patients for preemptive treatment as has been proposed for neutropenic patients (57). This approach would be an attractive strategy for ICU patients. Individual patients with risk factors for developing candidosis (16) and with heavy and persistent colonization (41) are treated premptively in order to prevent the fungus from becoming invasive. However the studies supporting this management strategy are still scarce (58). A lack of response to antibacterial agents in the ICU patient, in the absence of fungal colonization, is not a sufficient indication for starting treatment with antifungal drugs. The exact determination of the *Candida* species involved in the infection is necessary to guide treatment. An uncomplicated proven or probable *Candida* infection can be treated with 400 to 800 mg/day of fluconazole for 14 days and, when possible, intravascular lines should be removed to shorten the duration of fungemia (59–62).

REFERENCES

1. Beck-Sague CM, Jarvis WR. Secular trends in the epidemiology of nosocomial fungal infections in the United States, 1980–1990. J Infect Dis 1993;167:1247–1251.
2. Voss A, Kluytmans JAJW, Koeleman JGM, et al. Occurrence of yeast bloodstream infections in Dutch university hospitals between 1987 and 1995. Eur J Clin Microbiol Infect Dis 1996;15:909–912.
3. Bruun B, Westh H, Stenderup J. Fungemia: an increasing problem in a Danish university hospital 1989 to 1994. Clin Microbiol Infect 1995;1:124–126.
4. Kim JH, Gallis HA. Observations on spiraling empiricism: its causes, allure, and perils, with particular reference to antibiotic therapy. Am J Med 1989;87:201–206.
5. Edwards JE. Invasive *Candida* infections. N Engl J Med 1991;324:1060–1062.
7. Pfaller M, Wenzel R. Impact of the changing epidemiology of fungal infections in the 1990s. Eur J Clin Microbiol Infect Dis 1992;11:287–291.
7. Wright WL, Wenzel RP. Nosocomial Candida. Epidemiology, transmission, and prevention. Infect Dis Clin North Am 1997;11:411–425.
8. Berrouane YF, Herwaldt LA, Pfaller MA. Trends in antifungal use and epidemiology of nosocomial yeast infections in a university hospital. J Clin Microbiol 1999;37:531–537.
9. Wenzel RP. Nosocomial candidemia: risk factors and attributable mortality. Clin Infect Dis 1995;20: 1531–1534.
10. Wey SB, Mori M, Pfaller MA, Woolson RF, Wenzel RP. Hospital-acquired candidemia. The attributable mortality and excess lenght of stay. Arch Intern Med 1988;148:2642–2645.
11. Pfaller MA, Jones R, Messer S, Edmond M, Wenzel RP. National surveillance of nosocomial bloodstream infections due to species of *Candida* other than *Candida albicans*: frequency of occurrence and antifungal susceptibility in the SCOPE program. Diagn Microbiol Infect Dis 1998;30:121–129.
12. Collin B, Clancy CJ, Hong Nguyen M. Antifungal resistance in non-*albicans Candida* species. Drug Res Update 1999;2:9–14.
13. Chandrasekar PH, Gatny CM. The effect of fluconazole prophylaxis on fungal colonization in neutropenic cancer patients. J Antimicrob Chemother 1994;33:309–318.
14. Akiyama H, Mori S, Tanikawa S, Sakamaki H, Onozawa Y. Fluconazole versus oral amphotericin B in preventing fungal infection in chemotherapy-induced neutropenic patients with haematological malignancies. Mycoses 1993;36:373–378.
15. Ruhnke M, Eigler A, Tennagen I, Geiseler B, Engelmann E, Trautmann M. Emergence of fluconazole-resistant strains of *Candida albicans* in patients with recurrent oropharyngeal candidosis and human immunodeficiency virus infection. Antimicrob Agents Chemother 1994;32: 2092–2098.
16. Wey SB, Mori M, Pfaller MA, Woolson RF, Wenzel RP. Risk factors for hospital-acquired candidemia. A matched case-control study. Arch Intern Med 1989;149:2349–2353.
17. Fraser VJ, Jones M, Dunkel J, et al. Candidemia in a tertiary care hospital: epidemiology, risk factors and predictors of mortality. Clin Infect Dis 1992;15:414–421.

18. Bross J, Talbot GT, Maislin G, et al. Riskfactors for nosocomial candidemia: a case-controlled study in adults without leukemia. Am J Med 1989;87:614–620.
19. Voss A, Le Noble JLML, Verduyn Lunel FM, Foudraine NA, Meis JFGM. Candidaemia in intensive care units: risk factors for mortality. Infection 1997;25:8–11.
20. Hong Nguyen M, Peacock JE, Tanner DC, et al. Therapeutic approaches in patients with candidemia. Arch Intern Med 1995;155:2429–2435.
21. Vincent JL, Bihari DJ, Suter PM, et al. The prevalence of nosocomial infection in intensive care units in Europe. Results of the European prevalence of infection in intensive care (EPIC) study. JAMA 1995;274:639–644.
22. Spencer RC. Predominant pathogens found in the European Prevalence of Infection in Intensive Care Study. Eur J Clin Microbiol Infect Dis 1996;15:281–285.
23. Menezes AV, Sigesmund DA, Demajo WA, Devenyi RG. Mortality of hospitalized patients with *Candida* endophthalmitis. Arch Intern Med 1994;154:2093–2097.
24. Henderson DK, Edwards JE, Montgomerie JZ. Hematogenous *Candida* endophthalmitis in patients receiving parenteral hyperalimentation fluids. J Infect Dis 1981;143:655–661.
25. Ellis CA, Spivack ML. The significance of candidemia. Ann Intern Med 1967;67:511–513.
26. Oude Lashof AML, Donnelly JP, Meis JFGM, Vander Meer JWM, Kullberg BJ. Duration of antifungal treatment and development of delayed complications in patients with candidemia. submitted.
27. Rello J, Esandi ME, Diaz E, Mariscal D, Gallego M, Valles J. The role of *Candida* species isolated from bronchoscopic samples in nonneutropenic patients. Chest 1998;114:146–149.
28. Haron E, Vartivarian S, Anaissie E, Dekmezian R, Bodey G. Primary *Candida* pneumonia. Medicine 1993;72:137–142.
29. Eisenberg ES, Leviton I, Soeiro R. Fungal peritonitis in patients receiving peritoneal dialysis: experience with 11 patients and review of the literature. Rev Infect Dis 1986;8:309–321.
30. Rudledge R, Mandel SR, Wild RE. *Candida* species. Insignificant contamination or pathogenic species. Am Surg 1986;52:299–302.
31. Marsh PK, Tally FP, Kellum J, et al. *Candida* infections in surgical patients. Ann Surg 1983;198:42–47.
32. Solomkin JS, Flohr AB, Quie PG, et al. The role of *Candida* in intraperitoneal infections. Surgery 1980;88:524–530.
33. Calandra T, Bille J, Schneider R, Mosimann F, Francioli P. Clinical significance of *Candida* isolated from peritoneum in surgical patients. Lancet 1989;ii:1437–1440.
34. Fisher JF, Newman CL, Sobel JD. Yeast in the urine: solutions for a budding problem. Clin Infect Dis 1995;20:183–189.
35. Leu H-S, Huang C-T. Clearance of funguria with short-course antifungal regimens: a prospective, randomized, controlled study. Clin Infect Dis 1995;20:1152–1157.
36. Ang BSP, Telenti A, King B, Steckelberg JM, Wilson WR. Candidemia from a urinary tract source: microbiological aspects and clinical significance. Clin Infect Dis 1993;17:662–666.
37. Nassoura Z, Ivatury RR, Simon RJ, et al. Candiduria as an early marker of disseminated infection in critically ill surgical patients: the role of fluconazole therapy. J Trauma 1993;35:290–294.
38. Voss A, Hollis RJ, Pfaller MA, et al. Investigation of the sequence of colonization and candidemia in nonneutropenic patients. J Clin Microbiol 1994;32:975–980.
39. Geha DJ, Roberts DT. Laboratory detection of fungemia. Clin Lab Med 1994;14:83–97.
40. Berenguer J, Buck M, Witebsky, Stock F, Pizzo PA, Walsh TJ. Lysis centrifugation blood cultures in the detection of tissue-proven invasive candidiasis: disseminated versus single organ infection. Diag Microbiol Infect Dis 1993;17:103–109.
41. Pittet D, Monod M, Sutter PM, Frenk E, Auckenthaler R. *Candida* colonization and subsequent infections in critically ill surgical patients. Ann Surg 1994;220:751–758.
42. Petri MG, Konig J, Moecke HP, et al. Epidemiology of invasive mycosis in ICU patients: a prospective multicenter study in 435 non-neutropenic patients. Intensive Care Med 1997;23:317–325.
43. Sendid B, Tabouret M, Poirot JL, Mathieu D, Fruit J, Poulain D. New enzyme immunoassays for sensitive detection of circulating *Candida albicans* mannan and antimannan antibodies: useful combined test for diagnosis of systemic candidiasis. J Clin Microbiol 1999;37:1510–1517.
44. Van Deventer AJ, Goessens WH, Van Belkum A, Van Vliet HJ, Van Etten EW, Verbrugh HA. Improved detection of *Candida albicans* by PCR in blood of neutropenic mice with systemic candidiasis. J Clin Microbiol 1995;33:625–628.
45. Flahaut M, Sanglard D, Monod M, Bille J, Rossier M. Rapid detection of *Candida albicans* in clinical samples by DNA amplification of common regions from *C. albicans*-secreted aspartic proteinase genes. J Clin Microbiol 1998;36:395–401.

46. Burnie JP, Golbang N, Matthews RC. Semiquantitative polymerase chain reaction enzyme immunoassay for diagnosis of disseminated candidiasis. Eur J Clin Microbiol Infect Dis 1997;16:346–350.
47. Chryssanthou E, Klingspor L, Tollemar J, et al. PCR and other non-culture methods for diagnosis of invasive *Candida* infections in allogeneic bone marrow and solid organ transplant recipients. Mycoses 1999;42:239–247.
48. Van Deventer AJ, Goessens WH, Van Belkum A, Van Etten EW, Van Vliet HJ, Verbrugh HA. PCR monitoring of response to liposomal amphotericin B treatment of systemic candidiasis in neutropenic mice. J Clin Microbiol 1996;34:25–28.
49. Van Saene HKF, Damjanovic V, Piser B, Petros AJ. Fungal infections in ICU. J Hosp Infect 1999;41: 337–340.
50. Burnie JP. *Candida* and hands. J Hosp Infect 1986;8:1–4.
51. Voss A, Pfaller MA, Hollis RJ, Rhine Chalberg J, Doebbeling BN. Investigation of *Candida albicans* transmission in a surgical intensive care unit cluster by using genomic DNA typing methods. J Clin Microbiol 1995;33:576–580.
52. Pittet D, Mourouga P, Perneger TV. Compliance with handwashing in a teaching hospital. Ann Intern Med 1999;130:126–130.
53. Pittet D. Why is it impossible to achieve full compliance with hand hygiene practices in the ICU? 37th Annual Meeting of IDSA; Philadelphia, 1999.
54. Eggimann P, Francioli P, Bille J, et al. Fluconazole prophylaxis prevents intraabdominal candidiasis in high-risk surgical patients. Crit Care Med 1999;27:1066–1072.
55. Martins M, Rex JH. Resistance to antifungal agents in the critical care setting: problems and perspectives. New Horizons 1996;4:338–344.
56. Bonten MJM, Weinstein RA. Selective decontamination of the digestive tract: a measure whose time has passed? Curr Opin Infect Dis 1996;9:270–275.
57. Guiot HF, Fibbe WE, van 't Wout JW. Risk factors for fungal infection in patients with malignant hematologic disorders: implications for empirical therapy and prophylaxis. Clin Infect Dis 1994;18:525–532.
58. British Society for Antimicrobial Chemotherapy Working Party. Management of deep *Candida* infection in surgical and intensive care unit patients. Intensive Care Med 1994;20:522–528.
59. Rex JH, Bennett JE, Sugar AM, et al. A randomized trial comparing fluconazole and amphotericin B for the treatment of candidemia in patients without neutropenia. N Engl J Med 1994;331: 1325–1330.
60. Demajo WA, Guimond JG, Rotstein C, et al. Guidelines for the management of nosocomial *Candida* infections in non-neutropenic intensive care patients. Can J Infect Dis 1997;8(suppl B):3b–9b.
61. Vincent JL, Anaissie E, Bruining H, et al. Epidemiology, diagnosis and treatment of systemic *Candida* infection in surgical patients under intensive care. Intensive Care Med 1998;24:206–216.
62. Edwards JE, et al. International conference for the development of a consensus on the management and prevention of severe candidal infections. Clin Infect Dis 1997;25:43–59.

10. NEWER APPROACHES TO PREVENTING VASCULAR CATHETER-RELATED SEPSIS

RABIH O. DAROUICHE, M.D.

Baylor College of Medicine and Veterans Affairs Medical Center, Houston, TX 77030 USA

INTRODUCTION

Despite our enhanced understanding of the pathogenesis and risk factors predisposing to infection of vascular catheters, bloodstream infection remains the most common serious complication of such intravascular devices. Most nosocomial cases of bloodstream infection are associated with the use of intravascular devices, which account for at least 200,000 such cases each year in the U.S. (1,2). The contribution of vascular catheters to sepsis is particularly prominent in the intensive care unit (ICU) setting where, for instance, patients with indwelling intravascular devices have substantially higher rates of bloodstream infection than those without such devices (3). Although ICU patients may require the insertion of different types of intravascular catheters, including peripheral arterial catheters, pulmonary artery catheters, peripheral venous catheters, and central venous catheters, the latter account for most cases of catheter-related bloodstream infection. The mortality attributable to catheter-related bloodstream infection in ICU patients approaches 25%, and patients who survive such an infection are hospitalized for a mean of 6.5 days longer than those who do not develop such an infection (4). The management of catheter-related bloodstream infections can be very expensive as it reportedly costs an additional mean of $29,000 to treat one such episode in ICU patients (4).

The life-threatening medical complications and tremendous financial burden associated with infections of vascular catheters have prompted a keen interest in preventing such infections. Although dozens of approaches have been suggested based

R.A. Weinstein and M.J.M. Bonten (eds.). INFECTION CONTROL IN THE ICU ENVIRONMENT.

on theoretical reasons and/or in vitro data to possess the potential for reducing the rate of catheter-related infection in human subjects, only a few have been examined in the clinical arena. The purpose of this chapter is not to provide an exhaustive review of all approaches that have been suggested to be potentially protective, but rather to critically assess the role of only those approaches that have been reported in clinical trials to reduce the rates of catheter-related bloodstream infection and/or catheter colonization. To better appreciate the scientific reasoning for the efficacy, or lack thereof, of various preventive approaches, this chapter will also provide a brief review of the pathogenesis and microbiology of infections associated with vascular catheters.

PATHOGENESIS AND MICROBIOLOGY

Infection of vascular catheters, like other medical devices, centers around the formation of a layer of biofilm around the indwelling catheter. The biofilm is composed of factors derived from both the infecting organism (for instance, the fibroglycocalyx present on the surface of coagulase-negative staphylococci) and the host (platelets and other tissue ligands, such as fibronectin, fibrinogen and fibrin that variably adhere to well described receptors on the surface of certain organisms, including the staphylococci and *Candida* organisms) (5). The resulting biofilm layer is conducive not only to bacterial adherence, but also to the survival of adherent organisms because it can act as a barrier that protects embedded organisms from host immune defenses including phagocytosis and opsonization (6,7), and can impair the penetration (8,9) and/or activity (10,11) of antibiotics against the slowly-growing, biofilm-embedded organisms.

Organisms that colonize the vascular catheter may originate from a number of potential sources, including the skin at the catheter insertion site, a contaminated catheter hub, a distant site of infection resulting in hematogenous seeding of the catheter, use of an infected infusate, etc. The two former sources cause the vast majority of cases of catheter-related infection and will be further discussed below.

The skin at the catheter insertion site is, by far, the most common source for organisms colonizing short-term (mean duration, <7–10 days) central venous catheters (12). Bacteria residing on the skin at the catheter insertion site colonize the external surface of the catheter then proceed to migrate along the subcutaneous segment into the distal intravascular segment, ultimately resulting in catheter-related bloodstream infection. A high concentration of bacteria colonizing the skin around the insertion site of catheters used for total parenteral nutrition has been correlated with a higher likelihood for catheter colonization and catheter-related sepsis (13). This relationship between the intensity of bacterial contamination of the skin and likelihood of developing catheter-related infection is further supported by finding that measures that promote bacterial growth at the catheter insertion site, such as using heavily contaminated disinfectants (14) or applying an occlusive transparent plastic dressing (15) may increase the risk of catheter-related infection; in contrast, measures that decrease bacterial growth at the catheter insertion site, such as topical application of antimicrobial agents (16) may decrease the risk of catheter colonization.

The catheter hub is usually contaminated by organisms that originate from the hands of medical personnel, then migrate along the internal surface of the catheter into the intravascular segment causing catheter-related bloodstream infection (17). The impact of hub contamination on luminal colonization of vascular catheters was supported by scanning electron microscopy studies which showed more biofilm formation along the internal surfaces than the external surfaces of catheters that had remained in place >10 days, but comparable formation of biofilm along the internal and external surfaces of the catheters that remained in place <10 days (18). Although there exists some controversy in the literature as to the source of most cases of catheter-related infection (i.e., organisms originating from the patient's skin vs. the contaminated hub), that controversy may be clarified, at least in part, by differences in the durations of catheters studied by various investigators (12,17). In general, it is reasonable to conclude that although the patient's skin is the major source of organisms causing infection of at least the short-term central venous catheters, a longer duration of catheter placement is associated with more extensive manipulation of the catheter hub resulting in hub contamination and eventually catheter-related infection.

The microbiology of infections associated with vascular catheters is a direct reflection of the pathogenesis of such infections. Because either the patient's skin around the catheter insertion site or the medical personnel hands' skin provides the source of bacteria responsible for most episodes of catheter-related infection, at least two-thirds of such cases are caused by staphylococcal organisms (coagulase-negative staphylococci and *Staphylococcus aureus)* (1,2,5,12,13,16,19). Other skin organisms that less commonly cause vascular catheter-related infection include Gram-positive bacilli, such as *Corynebacterium* (especially *C. jeikeium* sp.) and *Bacillus* species. Although enterococci rarely cause infections associated with vascular catheters, the increasing frequency of vascular catheter-related bloodstream infections due to vancomycin-resistant enterococci (VRE) has been worrisome. The contribution of Gram-negative bacilli and *Candida* species to catheter-related infection is probably more prominent with long-term than with short-term vascular catheters. Most Gram-negative bacilli that cause vascular catheter-related infection are hospital-acquired (such as *Acinetobacter* species, *Stenotrophomonas maltophilia, Pseudomonas* species, etc.) rather than enteric organisms (such as *Escherichia coli* and *Klebsiella pneumoniae*). Although *Candida albicans* still causes most cases of fungal infections of vascular catheters, *C. parapsilosis* has a particularly high predilection for causing infections of vascular catheters. Rapid-growing mycobacteria rarely cause vascular catheter-related infections in the general population, but can be occasional causative pathogens in immunocompromised patients.

PREVENTION

The ultimate evidence of clinical protection provided by a particular preventive approach is its ability to significantly reduce the rate of catheter-related bloodstream infection in prospective, randomized clinical trials. Because of the relatively low rate of catheter-related bloodstream infection in patients assigned to the control group

Table 1. Approaches for Prevention of vascular Catheter-Related Infection

(1) Approaches that reduce catheter colonization but not bloodstream infection
(a) Bed-side dipping of catheters in antibiotic solutions
(b) Topical polyantibiotic regimen (polymyxin-neomycin-bacitracin)
(2) Approaches with controversial clinical efficacy
(a) Routine guidewire-assisted exchange of catheters
(b) Antimicrobial-anticoagulant catheter flush
(c) Silver-chelated subcutaneous cuff
(d) Tunneling of catheters
(3) Approaches with proven clinical efficacy
(a) Skilled infusion therapy team
(b) Maximal sterile barriers
(c) Antiseptic catheter hub
(d) Catheters coated with chlorhexidine and silver-sulfadiazine
(e) Catheters coated with minocycline and rifampin

(range, 4–8%), studies comprising less than several hundred patients may not have enough statistical power to examine differences in the rates of catheter-related bloodstream infection. Although colonization of the catheter is a prelude to bloodstream infection, a significant reduction in the rate of catheter colonization is simply not adequate, in and of itself, to conclude that a particular approach is clinically protective. Based on the results of prospective, randomized clinical trials, the various preventive approaches can be divided into the following three categories (Table 1).

(1) Approaches that Reduce Catheter Colonization but not Bloodstream Infection

This category includes approaches that have been reported in prospective, randomized clinical trials to cause a significant reduction in the rate of catheter colonization, but have not been demonstrated to reduce the rate of catheter-related bloodstream infection.

(a) Bed-Side Dipping of Catheters in Antibiotic Solutions

This approach utilizes catheters that are pretreated with positively-charged surfactants (such as tridodecyl methyl ammonium chloride: TDMAC), which bind to negatively charged antibiotics (such as cephalosporins and glycopeptides). A prospective, randomized study showed that short-term central vascular catheters (venous or arterial) that were pretreated with TDMAC and dipped at the bedside in a solution of cefazolin were almost 7-fold less likely to be colonized than undipped catheters (2.1% vs. 13.6%, $P = 0.04$) (20). This dramatic decrease in the rate of catheter colonization may be explained by the possibility that although cefazolin is most active against methicillin-susceptible Gram-positive organisms, the high concentrations of this antibiotic on the surface of a freshly dipped catheter may provide some antimicrobial activity in vivo against some other organisms as well. Another group of investigators reported that bed-side immersion of central venous catheters in a solution of vancomycin just prior to catheter inser-tion was associated with about 22% reduction in the rate of catheter colonization (defined in that study as any level of bacterial growth by roll-plate cultures of the catheter tip), as compared with unimmeresed catheters (62% vs. 80%, P = 0.01) (21). However, neither study (20,21) reported the impact of dipping catheters in an antibiotic solution on the occurrence of catheter-related bloodstream infection. Other potential disadvantages that limit the utility of this approach include: 1) the impractical and time-consuming practice of preparing antibiotic solutions and dipping catheters in antibiotic solutions, particularly in the ICU setting; 2) the unknown dynamics of leaching of antibiotics off the dipped catheter; and 3) the preventive use of antibiotics such as cefazolin and vancomycin that are considered as drugs of choice for treatment of established catheter-related infection.

(b) Topical Polyantibiotic Regimen (Polymyxin-Neomycim-Bacitracin)

The purpose of this approach is to lower the microbial burden on the skin around the catheter insertion site. The efficacy of this approach was examined in a prospective, randomized, three-arm clinical trial that compared the topical application of polymyxin-neomycin-bacitracin to 1% povidone-iodine and to no ointment (negative control) (22). Although the triple antibiotic regimen was associated with significantly (P = 0.02) lower rates of catheter colonization (2.2%) than 1% povidone-iodine (3.6%) or no ointment (6.5%), it was associated with higher likelihood of colonization with *Candida*. More importantly, the rates of catheter-related bloodstream infection were similar (0.7%) in the three groups of patients.

(2) Approaches with Controversial Clinical Efficacy

This category is composed of approaches that have been reported in ≥1 prospective, randomized clinical trials to cause a significant reduction in the rate of catheter-related bloodstream infection, but the clinical efficacy of these approaches was not demonstrated in other trial(s).

(a) Routine Guidewire-Assisted Exchange of Catheters

There are both potential advantages and disadvantages for routine guidewire-assisted exchange of central venous catheters. On one hand, routine exchange of a catheter may be desirable because a shorter duration of catheter placement is associated with a lower risk of catheter-related infection, and guidewire-assisted exchange of a catheter is associated with a lower risk of mechanical complications (such as pneumothorax) than insertion of a new central venous catheter via a fresh stick. On the other hand, there is a potential concern that organisms already colonizing a pre-existing central venous catheter may be transferred over the guidewire to the newly inserted catheter. The results of earlier clinical trials had suggested that routine exchange of CVC can reduce the risk of catheter-related infections (23,24). However, two more recent prospective, randomized clinical trials failed to demonstrate any protection from regularly scheduled exchange of central venous catheters every three days over a guidewire vs. replacing the catheter only when clinically indicated (25,26). In fact, one of those clinical trials (25) showed that routine exchange of catheters over a guidewire was associated with a tendency for a higher rate of catheter-related bloodstream infection than replacement of catheters only when clinically indicated (mean duration of placement, 7 days). Because catheters that remain in place for longer periods of time may have higher risk of catheter-related infection, frequent (for instance, every 3 or 7 days) guidewire-assisted exchange of catheters may not necessarily be more risk-prone than clinically indicated replacement of catheters that remain in place for weeks. In patients in whom guidewire-assisted exchange of catheters is clinically desirable because of, for example, bleeding tendency, it may be reasonable to do that provided that the removed catheter is cultured. No further action would be indicated if cultures of the removed catheter are sterile; however, if the removed catheter is colonized (which occurs in the minority of instances), the newly exchanged catheter should be removed and another catheter inserted via a fresh venous stick, preferably on the contralateral side.

(b) Antimicrobial-Anticoagulant Catheter Flush

Because of the relationship between infection and thrombosis of vascular catheters, flushing catheters with a combination of antimicrobial-anticoagulant agents may seem reasonable. An earlier prospective, randomized study in immunocompromised children showed that flushing the lumen of long-term (median duration of placement, 247 days) central venous catheters with a solution of vancomycin-heparin significantly reduced the rate of catheter-related bloodstream infection due to luminal colonization by vancomycin-susceptible organisms, as compared with flushing catheters with heparin alone (0% vs. 21%, P = 0.04) (27). Although that same study (27) also showed that the use of vancomycin-heparin catheter flush was associated with a 4-fold reduction (5% vs. 21%) in the rate of catheter-related bloodstream infection due to luminal colonization by vancomycin-susceptible organisms, the differences were not statistically significant. Additionally, a more recent prospective, randomized study in pediatric patients who had cancer and/or were receiving total parenteral nutrition showed that flushing the lumen of long-term (median duration of placement, 137 days) central venous catheters with a solution of vancomycin-heparin did not reduce the rate of catheter-related bloodstream infection/1000 catheter-days due to luminal colonization by vancomycin-susceptible organisms, as compared with flushing catheters with heparin alone (1.4% vs. 0.6%, P = 0.25) (28). What made the catheter flush combination of vancomycin-heparin even less desirable was the finding in that later study (28) that catheters flushed with the combination of vancomycin-heparin were associated with a significant 4-fold increase in the rate of catheter-related bloodstream infection/1000 catheter-days due to luminal colonization by vancomycin-resistant organisms, as compared with flushing catheters with heparin alone (2.3% vs. 0.53%, P = 0.03). Because vancomycin is active only against Gram-positive bacteria and is the only drug approved in the U.S. for therapy of infections caused by methicillin-resistant staphylococci, flushing the lumen of catheters with vancomycin-containing solutions (as is bed-side dipping of catheters in vancomycin solution) is generally not recommended. Although flush solutions are primarily intended for use with long-term central venous catheters whose hub are likely to become contaminated with excessive manipulation, this approach does not provide protection against catheter-related infection that evolves due to bacterial colonization of the external surface of the catheter.

(c) Silver-Chelated Subcutaneous Cuff

Prospective, randomized clinical trials in critically ill patients showed that short-term (mean duration of placement, 9 days) untunneled central venous catheters affixed with a silver-chelated subcutaneous cuff reduce the incidences of catheter colonization by 3-folds (9.1% vs. 28.9%, P = 0.002) and catheter-related bloodstream infection by almost 4-folds (1% vs. 3.7%, P = 0.12), as compared with uncuffed catheters (12,29). However, long-term (median duration of placement, 145 days) tunneled Hickman catheters affixed with a silver-chelated subcutaneous cuff were as likely as control tunneled catheters affixed with a standard cuff to cause bloodstream infection (36% vs. 32%) (30). The results of all pertinent studies combined suggest that the mechanical barrier provided by a standard cuff may be more important than the antimicrobial activity provided by chelating the cuff with silver. The short-lived antimicrobial activity of the silver-chelated subcutaneous cuff (does not exceed 1 week because of the biodegradable nature of the collagen cuff) and its restricted ability to impair bacterial migration only along the external surface of the catheter may help explain why this approach is unlikely to be clinically beneficial when applied to long-term central venous catheters that may get infected secondary to bacterial migration along the internal surface following contamination of the catheter hub.

(d) Tunneling of Catheters

Subcutaneous tunneling of catheters is thought to retard the migration of organisms via the subcutaneous segment of the catheter, thereby possibly reducing the likelihhod of bacterial colonization of the intravascular segment resulting in bloodstream infection. Prospective, randomized studies showed that tunneled short-term (mean duration of placement, 8 days) internal jugular venous catheters were 3-fold less likely than untunneled catheters to cause bloodstream infection (rates of catheter-related bloodstream infection/100 catheter-days of 0.4 vs. 1.3, P = 0.02) (31). Although the same group of investigators found that tunneling of short-term (mean duration of placement, 8 days) femoral venous catheters were also associated with a 3-fold reduction in the rate of catheter-related bloodstream infection/100 catheter-days (0.073 vs. 0.23), the differences were not statistically significant (P = 0.18) (32). Furthermore, a recent meta-analysis of the results of five clinical trials showed that tunneling of short-term subclavian catheters does not significantly reduce the rate of catheter-related spsis, as compared with untunneled catheters (33). The practice of tunneling of short-term central venous catheters is, however, less common, at least in the U.S., than tunneling of long-term catheters inserted into the subclavian veins. Tunneling of long-term catheters has not been proven in prospective, randomized clinical trials to significantly reduce the rate of catheter-related bloodstream infection (34–36). For instance, although tunneled long-term (mean duration, 116 days) subclavian central venous catheters were less likley than untunneled catheters to cause bloodstream infection (2% vs. 5%) in immunocompromised patients, the differences were not statistically significant (34). Despite the lack of definite proof of clinical efficacy, the insertion of tunneled subclavian catheters in patients who require long-term vascular access is considered a standard of care in a large number of U.S. medical centers, including the author's.

(3) Approaches with Proven Clinical Efficacy

This category comprises approaches that have been demonstrated in all prospective, randomized clinical trials to significantly reduce the rate of catheter-related bloodstream infection. This category does not include approaches that had been shown in a single prospective, randomized clinical trial to protect against catheter-related bloodstream infection. For instance, cutaneous disinfection of the site of catheter insertion with 2% aqueous chlorhexidine was associated with about 5-fold reduction in the rate of catheter-related bloodstream infection, as compared with 10% povidone-iodine or 70% alcohol (16). Because 2% aqueous chlorhexidine is not commercially available in the US (where 2% or 4% alcoholic solutions of chlorhexidine are often used), the clinical efficacy of this particular antiseptic preparation was not assessed in other studies.

(a) Skilled Infusion Therapy Team

The institution of an experienced infusion therapy team for the insertion and maintenance of catheters can significantly decrease the rate of catheter-related infection and reduce the cost of health care (37–39). Establishing such a skilled team is particularly beneficial in medical centers that care for a large population of high-risk patients or have unacceptably high rates of catheter-related bloodstream infection.

(b) Maximal Sterile Barriers

Because catheters may become contaminated at the time of insertion, this approach is designed to help prevent field contamination at the time of catheter insertion in an attempt to prevent the eventual outcome of catheter-related infection. When compared to the previously routine aseptic practice that consisted only of wearing sterile gloves and using a small sterile drape, the use of maximal sterile barriers (including sterile gloves, a mask, a gown, and a cap, and using a large sterile drape) at the time of inserting central venous catheters has been demonstrated in prospective, randomized clinical trials to protect infection of central venous

(40) and pulmonary artery catheters (41). As with the institution of skilled infusion therapy team, the use of maximal sterile barriers can very well be a cost-saving measure.

(c) Antiseptic Catheter Hub

This hub model allows for passage of the needle through an antiseptic chamber that contains iodinated alcohol. The attachment of this antiseptic catheter hub to central venous catheters with a mean duration of placement of two weeks was shown in a prospective, randomized clinical trial to reduce the rate of catheter-related sepsis by 4-fold (42). Although quite novel, the antiseptic catheter hub is limited by its ability to protect only against organisms migrating through the hub along the internal surface of the catheter and, therefore, provides no antimicrobial activity against skin organisms that migrate along the external surface of the catheter.

(d) Catheters Coated with Chlorhexidine and Silver-Sulfadiazine

The external surfaces of such catheters are coated with the combination of chlorhexidine and silver sulfadiazine in an attempt to reduce the rate of catheter-related sepsis emanating from bacterial colonization of the external catheter surface. Although such a coated catheter is frequently referred to as the "antiseptic-coated catheter", this catheter contains the antibiotic sulfadiazine. When compared with uncoated catheters in a prospective, randomized clinical trial, polyurethane short-term (mean duration of placement, 1 week) catheters coated with chlorhexidine and silver sulfadiazine were shown to be 2-fold less likely to become colonized (13.5% vs. 24.1%, $P = 0.005$) and at least 4-fold less likely to cause bloodstream infection (1% vs. 4.6%, $P = 0.03$) (19). Although several other clinical trials (43,44) could not demonstrate the clinical efficacy of short-term catheters coated with chlorhexidine and silver sulfadiazine, none of those studies had adequate statistical power to examine differences in the rates of catheter-related bloodstream infection (that is why the author did not assign this preventive approach to the category of "approaches with controversial clinical efficacy"). Furthermore, a recent meta-analysis of the results of 12 clinical trials showed that short-term catheters coated with chlorhexidine and silver sulfadiazine reduce the rate of catheter-related bloodstream infection by 44% (45). Short-term catheters coated with the combination of chlorhexidine and silver sulfadiazine were also recently reported to reduce the cost of health care in patients at hish risk for developing catheter-related infection (46). However, the antimicrobial durability of catheters coated with chlorhexidine and silver sulfadiazine appears short-lived because a prospective, randomized large clinical trial demonstrated that longer-term catheters (mean duration of placement, 20 days) coated with this same combination of agents were not effective in reducing the rate of catheter-related bloodstream infection (47).

(e) Catheters Coated with Minocycline and Rifampin

Unlike the former catheters which are coated with chlorhexidine and silver sulfadiazine only on the external surfaces, catheters coated with the combination of minocycline and rifampin provide antimicrobial activity along both the external and internal surfaces. In contrast to vancomycin which is active only against Gram-positive bacteria, the presence of this unique combination of antibiotics in high local concentrations on the surfaces of the catheter provides broad-spectrum antimicrobial activity against Gram-positive bacteria, Gram-negative bacteria, and even *Candida* (48). What also makes this combination of antibiotics suitable for use in the prevention of catheter-related infection is that minocycline and rifampin, unlike vancomycin, are not considered as drugs of choice for therapy of established infections. Short-term (mean duration of placement, 6 days) polyurethane central venous catheters coated with minocycline and rifampin were demonstrated in a prospective, randomized, multi-center clinical trial to be 3-fold less likely than uncoated catheters to be colonized (8% vs. 26%, $P < 0.001$) and to prevent the occurrence of catheter-related bloodstream infection (0% vs. 5%, $P < 0.01$) (2).

A recently completed prospective, randomized, multi-center clinical trial demonstrated that short-term (mean duration of placement, 1 week) polyurethane central venous coated with minocycline and rifampin were 3-fold less likely to be colonized than catheters coated with chlorhexidine and silver sulfadiazine (7.9% vs. 22.8%, $P < 0.001$) and 12-fold less likely to cause bloodstream infection (0.3% vs. 3.4%, $P < 0.002$) (1). Several observations could help explain the superior clinical protection provided by catheters coated with minocycline and rifampin vs. catheters coated with chlorhexidine and silver sulfadiazine. First, the combination of minocycline and rifampin is simply more active than the combination of chlorhexidine and silver sulfadiazine against most potential pathogens, particularly the staphylococci. Second, rifampin retains its antimicrobial activity against bacteria embedded within the biofilm (49), whereas the ability of chlorhexidine and silver sulfadiazine to retain their antimicrobial activities in such an environment is unknown. Third, catheters coated with minocycline and rifampin had longer durability of antimicrobial activity (as assessed by zones of inhibition) than catheters coated with chlorhexidine and silver sulfadiazine. Finally, catheters coated with minocycline and rifampin have the potential to protect against bacterial colonization of both the external and internal surfaces, whereas catheters coated with with chlorhexidine and silver sulfadiazine provided antimicrobial activity only along the external surface.

The results of clinical trials showed a very low likelihood for developing antibiotic resistance in patients who had received short-term central venous catheters coated with minocycline and rifampin (1,2). The differences in the mechanisms of action of the two coating agents (minocycline inhibits protein synthesis, whereas rifampin inhibits DNA-dependent RNA polymerase) may serve to prevent emergence of bacterial resistance to either agent in the clinical scenario of catheter infection where the relatively low ratio of the concentration of infecting bacteria to concentrations of antibiotics on the surface of the coated catheter does not inherently favor development of resistance. Furthermore, the lack of detectable systemic antibiotic levels in the serum of patients who receive catheters coated with minocycline and rifampin makes it unlikely for these coating agents to cause antibiotic resistance among bacterial strains residing at sites distant from the catheter. Finally, scanning electron microscopy studies of central venous catheters removed from patients demonstrated that catheters coated with minocycline and rifampin are significantly less likely than uncoated catheters to display ultrastuctural bacterial colonization of the biofilm surrounding the catheters (50). Such a finding is particularly important in light of the recent reports of clinical infections by several staphylococcal strains (both *S. aureus* and *S. epidermidis*) with intermediate susceptibilities to vancomycin, the majority of which have been associated with indwelling vascular or peritoneal catheters (51–53). Because vanocomycin use in the ICU is heavily determined by the existing rates of catheter-related bloodstream infection (54), it is also possible that the likely reduction in the administration of vancomycin for the treatment of suspected or documented catheter-related infection due to the use of antimicrobial-coated catheters may help reduce the incidence of vancomycin resistance.

The use of antiinfective catheters should complement rather than replace aseptic procedures for insertion and maintenance of vascular catheters. So far, the clinical efficacy of antimicrobial-coated central venous catheters has been demonstrated only in patients at high risk for developing catheter-related infection (ICU patients, immunocompromised subjects, patients receiving total parenteral nutrition, etc.). It is probably neither necessary nor beneficial to use antimicrobial-coated central venous catheters in patients who are anticipated to have the catheter in place for just a couple of days (for instance, patients embarking on an elective procedure) and in those at low risk for developing catheter-related infection. There are ongoing clinical trials to assess the clinical efficacy of long-term, antimicrobial-coated central venous catheters.

Conflict-of-interest statement: Impregnation of catheters with minocycline and rifampin is described in two patents that are co-owned by Baylor College of Medicine, Houston, Texas. Both patents were licensed by Cook Critical Care, Bloomington, Indiana, with some royalty rights to Baylor College of Medicine. The author, an employee of Baylor College of Medicine, is a co-inventor of the two patents and receives a percentage of the royalties according to the official policy of the academic institution. Dr. Darouiche has no other financial links (such as equity interest, stock ownership, consultancies, and service on company board) with Cook Critical Care or other catheter-manufacturing companies that might constitute a potential conflict of interest.

REFERENCES

1. Darouiche RO, Raad II, Heard SO, et al. A comparison of two antimicrobial-impregnated central venous catheters. *N Eng J Med.* 1999;340:1–8.
2. Raad I, Darouiche R, Dupuis J, et al. Central venous catheters coated with minocycline and rifampin for the prevention of catheter-related colonization and bloodstream infections: a randomized, double-blind trial. *Ann Intern Med.* 1997;127:267–274.

3. Jarvis WR, Edwards JR, Culver DH, et al. Nosocomial infection rates in adult and pediatric intensive care units in the United States. *Am J Med*. 1991;91(Suppl.):185S–191S.
4. Pittet D, Tarara D, Wenzel RP. Nosocomial bloodstream infection in critically ill patients: Excess length of stay, extra costs, and attributable mortality. *JAMA*. 1994;271:1598–1601.
5. Raad II, Bodey GP. Infectious complications of indwelling vascular catheters. *Clin Infect Dis*. 1992;15: 197–210.
6. Costerton JW, Stewart PS, Greenberg EP. Bacterial biofilms: a common cause of persistent infections. *Science*. 1999;284:1318–1322.
7. Jensen ET, Kharazmi A, Lam K, Costerton JW, Hoiby N. Human polymorphonuclear leukocyte response to Pseudomonas aeruginosa grown in biofilms. *Infect. Immun*. 1990;58:2383–2385.
8. Hoyle BD, Alcantara J, Costerton JW. *Pseudomonas aeruginosa* biofilm as a diffusion barrier to piperacillin. *Antimicrob Agents Chemother*. 1992;36:2054–2056.
9. Kumon H, Tomochika K, Matunaga T, Ogawa M, Ohmori H. A sandwich cup method for the penetration assay of antimicrobial agents through *Pseudomonas* exopolysaccharides. *Microbiol Immunol*. 1994;38:615–619.
10. Stewart PS. Biofilm accumulation model that predicts antibiotic resistance of *Pseudomonas aeruginosa* biofilms. *Antimicrob Agents Chemother*. 1994;38:1052–1058.
11. Darouiche RO, Dhir A, Miller AJ, Landon GC, Raad II, Musher DM. Vancomycin penetration into biofilm covering infected prostheses and effect on bacteria. *J Infect Dis*. 1994;170:720–723.
12. Maki DG, Cobb L, Garman JK, Shapiro JM, Ringer M, Helgerson RB. An attachable silver-impregnated cuff for prevention of infection with central venous catheters: a prospective randomized multicenter trial. *Am J Med*. 1988;85:307–314.
13. Bjornson HS, Colley R, Bower RH, Duty VP, Schwartz-Fulton JT, Fisher JE. Association between microorganism growth at the catheter insertion site and colonization of the catheter in patients receiving total parenteral nutrition. *Surgery*. 1982;192:720–726.
14. Frank MJ, Schaffner W. Contaminated aqueous benzalkonium chloride. An unnecessary hospital infection hazard. *JAMA*. 1976;236:2418–2419.
15. Conly JM, Grieves K, Peters B. A prospective, randomized study comparing transparent and dry gauze dressings for central venous catheters. *J Infect Dis*. 1989;159:310–318.
16. Maki DG, Ringer M, Alvarado CJ. Prospective randomized trial of povidone-iodine, alcohol, and chlorhexidine for prevention of infection associated with central venous and arterial catheters. *Lancet*. 1991;338:339–343.
17. Sitges-Serra A, Hernandez R, Maestro S, Pi-Suner T, Garces JM, Segura M. Prevention of catheter sepsis: the hub. *Nutrition*. 1997;13(suppl.):30S–35S.
18. Raad I, Costerton JW, Sabharwal U, Sacilowski M, Anaissie E, Bodey GP. Ultrastructural analysis of indwelling vascular catheters: a quantitative relationship between luminal colonization and duration of placement. *J Infect Dis*. 1993;168:400–407.
19. Maki DG, Stolz SM, Wheeler S, Mermel LA. Prevention of central venous catheter-related bloodstream infection by use of an antiseptic-impregnated catheter: a randomized, controlled study. *Ann Intern Med*. 1997;127:257–266.
20. Kamal GD, Pfaller MA, Rempe LE, Jebson PJR. Reduced intravascular catheter infection by antibiotic bonding. *JAMA*. 1991;265:2364–2368.
21. Thornton J, Todd NJ, Webster NR. Central venous line sepsis in the intensive care unit: a study comparing antibiotic coated catheters with plain catheters. *Anesthesia*. 1996;51:1018–1020.
22. Maki DG, Band JD. A comparative study of polyantibiotic and iodophor ointments in prevention of vascular catheter-related infection. *Am J Med*. 1981;70:739–744.
23. Bozetti F, Terno G, Bonfanti G, et al. Prevention and treatment of central venous catheter sepsis by exchange via a guidewire: a prospective controlled trial. *Ann Surg*. 1983;198:48–52.
24. Gregory JA, Schiller WR. Subclavian catheter changes every third day in high risk patients. *Am Surg*. 1985;51:534–536.
25. Cobb DK, High KP, Sawyer RG, et al. A controlled trial of scheduled replacement of central venous and pulmonary-artery catheters. *N Engl J Med*. 1992;327:1062–1068.
26. Powell C, Kudsk KA, Kulich Pamandelbaum JA, Fabri PJ. Effect of frequent guidewire exchanges on triple lumen catheter sepsis. *JPEN Parenter Enteral Nutr*. 1988;12:464–465.
27. Schwartz C, Henrickson KJ, Roghmann K, Powell K. Prevention of bacteremia attributed to luminal colonization of tunneled central venous catheters with vancomycin-susceptible organisms. *J Clin Oncol*. 1990;8:591–597.

28. Rackoff WR, Weiman M, Jakobowski D, et al. A randomized, controlled trial of the efficacy of a heparin and vancomycin solution in preventing central venous catheter infections in children. *J Pediatr.* 1995;127:147–151.
29. Flowers RH III, Schwenzer KJ, Kopel RF, Fisch MJ, Tucker SI, Farr BM. Efficacy of an attachable subcutaneous cuff for the prevention of intravascular catheter-related infection. A randomized, controlled trial. *JAMA.* 1989;261:878–883.
30. Groeger JS, Lucas AB, Coit D, et al. A prospective, randomized evaluation of the effect of silver impregnated subcutaneous cuffs for preventing tunneled chronic venous access catheter infections in cancer patients. *Ann Surg.* 1993;218:206–210.
31. Timsit JF, Sebille V, Farkas JC, et al. Effect of subcutaneous tunneling on internal jugular catheter-related sepsis in critically ill patients: A prospective randomized multicenter study. *JAMA.* 1996;276: 1416–1420.
32. Timsit JF, Bruneel F, Cheval C, et al. Use of tunneled femoral catheters to prevent catheter-related infection: A randomized, controlled trial. *Ann Intern Med.* 1999;130:729–735.
33. Randolph AG, Cook DJ, Gonzales CA, Brun-Buisson C. Tunneling of short-term central venous catheters to prevent catheter-related infection: a meta-analysis of randomized, controlled trials. *Crit Care Med.* 1998;26:1452–1457.
34. Andrivet P, Bacquer A, Ngoc CV, et al. Lack of clinical benefit from subcutaneous tunnel insertion of central venous catheters in immunocompromised patients. *Clin Infect Dis.* 1994;18:199–206.
35. Von Meyenfeldt MMF, Stapert J, de Jong PCM, et al. TPN catheter sepsis: lack of effect of subcutaneous tunneling of PVC catheters on sepsis rate. *JPEN J Parent Enter Nutr.* 1980;4:514–517.
36. Moran KT, McEntee G, Jones B, et al. To tunnel or not to tunnel catheters for parenteral nutrition. *Ann R Coll Surg.* 1987;69:235–236.
37. Nelson DB, Kien CL, Mohr B, et al. Dressing changes by specialized personnel reduce infection rates in patients receiving central venous parenteral nutrition. *JPEN J Parenter Enteral Nutr.* 1986;10: 220–222.
38. Faubion WC, Wesley JR, Khalidi N, Silva J. Total parenteral nutrition catheter sepsis: impact of the team approach. *JPEN J Parenter Enteral Nutr.* 1986;10:642–645.
39. Tomford JW, Hershey CO, McLaren CE, Porter DK, Cohen DI. Intravenous therapy team and peripheral venous catheter-associated complications. A prospective controlled study. *Arch Intern Med.* 1984;144:1191–1194.
40. Raad II, Hohn DC, Gilbreath BJ, et al. Prevention of central venous catheter-related infections by using maximal sterile barrier precautions during insertion. *Infect Control Hosp Epidemiol.* 1994;15:231–238.
41. Mermel LA, McCormick RD, Springman SR, Maki DG. The pathogenesis and epidemiology of catheter-related infection with pulmonary artery Swan-Ganz catheters: a prospective study utilizing molecular subtyping. *Am J Med.* 1991;91(suppl. 3B):197S–205S.
42. Segura M, Alvarez-Lerma F, Tellado JM, et al. Advances in surgical technique: a clinical trial on the prevention of catheter-related sepsis using a new hub model. *Ann Surg.* 1996;223:363–369.
43. Heard SO, Wagle M, Vijayakumar E, et al. The influence of triple-lumen central venous catheters coated with chlorhexidine/silversulfadiazine on the incidence of catheter-related bacteremia: a randomized, controlled clinical trial. *Arch Intern Med.* 1998;158;81–87.
44. Ciresi D, Albrecht RM, Volkers PA, Scholten DJ. Failure of an antiseptic bonding to prevent central venous catheter-related infection and sepsis. *Am Surg.* 1996;62:641–646.
45. Veenstra DL, Saint S, Saha S, Lumley T, Sullivan SD. Efficacy of antiseptic-impregnated central venous catheters in preventing catheter-related bloodstream infection. *JAMA.* 1999;281:261–267.
46. Veenstra DL, Saint S, Sullivan SD. Cost-effectiveness of antiseptic-impregnated central venous catheters for the prevention of catheter-related bloodstream infection. *JAMA.* 1999;282:554–560.
47. Logghe C, Van Ossel C, D'Hoore W, Ezzedine H, Wauters G, Haxhe JJ. Evaluation of chlorhexidine and silver-sulfadiazine impregnated central venous catheters for the prevention of bloodstream infection in leukemic patients: a randomized controlled trial. *J Hosp Infect.* 1997;37:145–156.
48. Raad I, Darouiche R, Hachem R, Mansouri M, Bodey GP. The broad spectrum activity and efficacy of catheters coated with minocycline and rifampin. *J Infect Dis.* 1996;173:418–424.
49. Widmer AF, Frei R, Rajacic Z, Zimmerli W. Correlation between in vivo and in vitro efficacy of antimicrobial agents against foreign body infections. *J Infect Dis.* 1990;162:96–102.
50. Raad II, Darouiche RO, Hachem R, et al. Antimicrobial durability and rare ultrastructural colonization of indwelling central catheters coated with minocycline and rifampin. *Crit Care Med.* 1998;26:219–224.

51. Garrett DO, Jochimsen E, Murfitt K, et al. The emergence of decreased susceptibility to vancomycin in *Staphylococcus epidermidis*. *Infect Contr Hosp Epidemiol.* 1999;20:167–170.
52. Fridkin SK, Edwards JR, Pichette SC, at al. Determinants of vancomycin use in adult intensive care units in 41 United States Hospitals. *Clin Infect Dis.* 1999;28:1119–1125.
53. Sieradzki K, Roberts RB, Haber SW, Tomasz A. The development of vancomycin resistance in a patient with methicillin-resistant *Staphylococcus aureus* infection. *N Engl J Med.* 1999;340:517–523.
54. Smith TL, Pearson ML, Wilcox KR, et al. Emergece of vancomycin resistance in *Staphylococcus aureus*. *N Engl J Med* 1999;340:493–501.

11. NEWER APPROACHES TO PREVENTING INTRAVASCULAR DEVICE-RELATED BLOODSTREAM INFECTIONS

J. A. J. W. KLUYTMANS

Ignatius Hospital Breda., Department of Clinical Microbiology, PO Box 90158, 4800 RK Breda, The Netherlands, e-mail: jkluytmans@ignatius.nl

INTRODUCTION

Nosocomial bloodstream infections are frequent and serious complications of modern medicine. Each infection accounts for an estimated $6000 increase in hospital costs (1). In the ICU the incremental costs were calculated at $40,000 per survivor (2). Moreover the case fatality rate has been high, over 20% in two recent studies (2,3). Prevention of nosocomial bloodstream infections is therefore important. Prevention should be aimed at the primary source of the infection. When bloodstream infections are secondary to a source of infection elsewhere in the body, prevention should be aimed at this source and is beyond the scope of this chapter. This chapter focuses on the prevention of bloodstream infections due to intravascular devices.

Reliable access to the vascular system has become an essential feature of modern medical care. More than 60% of patients admitted to European hospitals received infusion therapy in a multicenter study (4). Recently, a Pan-European prevalence survey was performed by the European Study Group of Nosocomial Infections (ESGNI) (5). In the 112 participating hospitals more than 3,500,000 patients were admitted in 1997. Blood cultures were performed on nearly a quarter of all admitted patients and 14.4% of all blood cultures taken were positive. By extrapolation this results in 3.5 bacteremic episodes per 100 admissions. In the participating hospitals nearly 125,000 bacteremic episodes occurred in 1997. It was also found that intra-vascular catheters were the most important risk factor for nosocomial

R.A. Weinstein and M.J.M. Bonten (eds.). INFECTION CONTROL IN THE ICU ENVIRONMENT.

bacteremia. In Germany a large survey reported a prevalence of nosocomial primary bloodstream infections of 0.3%. The incidence density per 1000 intravascular device days was 0.3 for peripheral lines and 0.8 for central lines (6). For future studies it is important to incorporate the number of catheter days in the denominator for intravascular device-related infection-rates. In that way more reliable comparisons can be made.

Although the vast majority of intravascular catheters used are peripheral lines, bloodstream infections are mainly caused by central lines. These infections are largely preventable by adhering to simple and practical guidelines. Several guidelines have been published. The CDC-guideline for prevention of intravascular device-related infections has been updated in 1996 (7). No European guideline has been published so far. Some countries have their own guidelines, e.g. in The Netherlands there is a national guideline for the prevention of infection caused by intravascular devices. These guidelines are largely comparable to the CDC-guideline although local variations remain present. For the near future it is likely and desirable that a world standard is developed. No studies have been performed so far to compare the handling and procedures associated with intravascular devices between different countries.

PATHOGENESIS

There are four major sites where intravascular catheter-related bloodstream infections can arise. First, the insertion site is a major port of entrance. Pathogens can quickly migrate from the skin at the insertion site to the catheter tip along the outer surface of the catheter (8,9). At the catheter tip micro-organisms are incorporated in a bio-film consisting of a thick matrix of glycocalix. This so-called slime layer provides an ideal microclimate for bacteria and fungi to adhere and grow out. The slime layer protects the micro-organisms from the host defence mechanisms and from the activity of antibiotics. The second port of entry is colonisation of the hub. Catheter hubs are a common cause of intravascular catheter-related bloodstream infections (10,11). These two portals of entry are the most frequent causes of intravascular catheter-related bloodstream infections. The relative importance of the insertion site versus the hub may vary in different institutions due to differences in local care during insertion, different duration of catheterization, different types of catheter material and differences in care of the hub. Two other possible mechanisms, which are by far less frequent in modern settings, are hematogenous seeding from a remote focus of infection and contamination of the infusate. The latter used to be a frequent cause in earlier days when manufacturing of parental medication was less sophisticated. However, currently this problem should be under control.

MICROBIOLOGY

The microbiology of intravascular device-related infections is predominated by gram-positive bacteria. Especially, coagulase negative staphylococci (CNS) play an important role. This is not surprising, since most pathogens causing intravascular device related infections arise from the skin. In a recent German study (6), CNS accounted for 34.2% of all episodes and S. aureus for 15.8%. Gram-negative micro-organisms had a prevalence of 42.7% and yeast's were found in a small minority of cases (2.6%). An Italian survey (12) found CNS in 55.4%, S. aureus in 12.3% and other gram-positives in 12.3%. Gram-negative micro-organisms were encountered in 7.6% and yeast's in 12.3%. In cancer patients, a Belgian survey found only gram-positive micro-organisms in 32 episodes (13). A compilation of data from several surveys shows that generally, gram-positive micro-organisms are responsible for 70% of all episodes, gram-negatives for 20% and yeast for 10% or less (14).

DEFINITIONS

The term intravascular device-related infection is preferred above catheter-related bacteremia to include those infections caused by fungi. If a survey includes only a subset of devices or a subset of causative organisms it can be named accordingly, e.g. central venous catheter-related infection or intravascular device-related candidemia. For surveillance and comparison of infection rates it is essential to use uniform criteria. Besides the definitions themselves, this also implies the methods of gathering clinical data and the microbiological methods used. Many criteria have been developed and used. In Europe both national and European criteria have been developed (15). In a consensus meeting in 1998, the ESGNI proposed to use the CDC-criteria (16), for surveillance of nosocomial bloodstream infections. These criteria are currently being updated and are used widely. There is certainly some criticism on various aspects of these criteria, but to be able to compare data from different surveys it is important to come to a world standard. For more profound investigations into the subject of intravascular device-related infection, the CDC-criteria lack specificity and detail. For example, if one wants to know whether an infection is hub-related or insertion site-related the CDC-criteria offer no clue. For these purposes, Mermel has recently proposed a set of definitions (17). This proposal is highly accurate but requires elaborate laboratory techniques. Both semi-quantitaive (18) and quantitative (19–21) methods can be used to culture catheter segments. To prove concordance between strains cultured from different sites, fingerprinting of chromosomal DNA is mandatory, e.g. by pulsed field gel electrophoresis (22–23). The lack of standardisation of culturing techniques remains an important cause of bias between different surveys, and therefore is an important subject for consensus.

PREVENTION

Antibiotic Prophylaxis During Insertion

The few studies, which dealt with this issue, have resulted in conflicting results. Only for long-term catheters in institutions with high infection rates, a moderate reduction in early intravascular device-related infection was observed (24–26). This combined with the risk of widespread resistance associated with such extensive use of prophylactic antibiotics makes that this practice is not recommended (27).

Site of Insertion

The internal jugular vein is associated with a higher catheter colonisation rate and a higher intravascular catheter-related bloodstream infection rate than the subclavian vein (28–30). This is probably caused by an increased bacterial colonisation density at the internal jugular insertion site and by a more difficult immobilisation of the catheter at this site. On the other hand, insertion in the subclavian vein is associated with an increased risk for non-infectious complications, e.g. pneumothorax. The infectious risks of the femoral veins as insertion site remain controversial (28,29,31). Probably it is not higher than the internal jugular vein. When a short duration of catheterization is anticipated the jugular vein may be preferred because of its low mechanical complication rate.

Precautions During Insertion

During insertion of peripheral lines, wearing of sterile gloves is not recommended. Compared with central lines, peripheral lines have a low risk of infection. Several studies have examined the effect of maximal barrier precautions during insertion of central lines. This included wearing of a mask, a cap, a sterile gown, sterile gloves and a large sterile drape. All studies showed a significant reduction in the intravascular catheter-related bloodstream infection rate (32–34). The importance of the level of care during insertion and during follow-up has also been shown by several investigations looking at the effect of a specialised IV-team. Such teams were highly cost-effective in several studies (35). Still, many physicians do not take maximal barrier precautions during insertion and IV-teams have hardly been instituted.

Skin Antisepsis

The importance of the agent used for skin antisepsis of the insertion site was demonstrated in a large study by Maki et al. (36). They found that 2% aqueous chlorhexidine was associated with a significant lower intravascular catheter-related bloodstream infection rate than povidone-iodine 10% or alcohol 70%. Other studies evaluated the effect of adding alcohol to either iodine or chlorhexidine. Both combinations were superior to povidone-iodine alone. In Europe alcoholic combinations with either chlorhexidine or povidone-iodine have been used for decades and are the recommended disinfectants.

Topical Antimicrobial Ointments

Although the use of antibiotic ointments at the insertion site seems an attractive strategy from a theoretical point of view, there have been few well-designed studies performed to date. Polyantibiotic ointments were associated with a moderate effect on bacterial colonisation rates. Moreover, they were associated with increased Candida infection rates. Mupirocin ointment was associated with a lower catheter colonisation rate in several studies. No significant effect on the intravascular catheter-related bloodstream infection rate has been demonstrated. Interpretation of these results should be done with great caution. Colonisation as an outcome measure is a difficult item with antimicrobial ointments because they interfere with the reliability of culture results from the catheter tip. In view of these findings and the potential risk of resistance with this application of antibiotics it is currently not recommended (35). The most interesting studies in this field were done with skin antiseptics, i.e. povidone-iodine ointment. One study found no effect (37) while the other found a fourfold reduction (38). This strategy aimed at the insertion site is attractive and warrants more extensive investigations.

Dressings

The use of sterile gauze for dressing of the catheter insertion site is more and more replaced by transparent polyurethane dressings. The advantages of transparent dressings are that they permit continuous inspection of the insertion site, they secure the device reliable and are more comfortable to the patient. Moreover, they save time to hospital personnel. On the other hand they are more expensive and it is uncertain what the effect of occlusion of the skin surrounding the insertion site is on the cutaneous microflora. On peripheral catheters a number of studies have been performed. There is some controversy if transparent dressings increase the catheter colonisation rate, but the rate of intravascular catheter-related bloodstream infections associated with peripheral lines is so low that both sterile gauze and transparent dressings can be used safely. The more important groups are the central vascular catheters. In this group the controversy builds up. Many studies have been performed, resulting in as many different outcomes. The problems are manifold. First, there are several kinds of different dressings and there are several kind of protocols dealing with those dressings. The variations include the method of skin disinfection and the dressing replacement interval. Considering these variations it is difficult to draw final conclusions. A meta-analysis showed that transparent dressing had a significant higher bacterial colonisation rate of the catheter tip, but the incidence of intravascular device-related infection was not significantly different (39). Newer dressings that permit the escape of moisture should reduce the increased bacterial colonisation rate (7). For central venous lines it is currently considered to be safe and effective to use transparent polyurethane dressings for prolonged periods.

Routinely Changing of Catheters

The risk of intravascular device-related infection increases linearly over time. Therefore, the risk for each successive day is not greater than for any previous day (40–41). Routinely changing of intravascular catheters at certain intervals is therefore not recommended. As an exception to this rule may serve swan-ganz pulmonary artery catheters. The infectious risk of these catheters rises after the fifth day of catheterization and it may therefore not be safe to leave these catheters in place for more than 5 days (42).

Changing Over a Guidewire

Changing a catheter over a guidewire is attractive since it eliminates many non-infectious risks associated with a new puncture site (40). However, if the site of catheterization is infected there is an increased risk of infection associated with changing over the guidewire. In practice the following strategy is an attractive compromise (35,43). When an intravascular catheter is in place for a prolonged period and there is suspicion of infection it is acceptable to change the catheter over a guidewire in the same site. This requires redraping and regloving after removal of the original catheter. It is mandatory to culture the tip of the catheter which is removed and to take blood cultures. When these cultures show that the catheter was significantly colonised, the new catheter should be removed immediately to prevent the development of a bloodstream infection. In this case a new insertion site is mandatory. When there are local signs of infection at the insertion site or when the patient has symptoms of sepsis it is not recommended to use the guidewire technique but to choose another insertion site initially (35).

Routinely Changing of the Infusion Set

The period for which the infusion system can be in place safely is a matter of current investigation. For decades the interval considered to be safe has been 24–48 hours. Recent studies showed that 72 hours gave comparable results (44–46). Also, intervals of 96 and 120 hours have been studied and did not result in higher incidences of intravascular device-related infection (47–48). Nowadays, 72 hour is considered to be safe in general. As an exception to this rule, 24 hour intervals are still recommended when blood or blood products have been administrated and for lipid emulsions. Longer intervals may further reduce the costs associated with intravascular therapy but by increasing the interval, the chance for significant outgrow of contaminating micro-organisms increases. This increases the risk for intravascular device-related infection. The associated risks with additional prolongation of the interval should therefore be studied carefully before being widely implemented.

In Line Filters

In line filters can have a beneficial effect if the infusate is contaminated. As stated above this kind of contamination is nowadays rare. In addition, these filters should be changed regularly and can become blocked, thereby increasing the number of manipulations of the system and thus enhancing the risk of contamination. Moreover, filters increase the cost of infusion therapy. Therefore, in line filters are not recommended for routine use.

The Hub

The importance of the hub as a source of intravascular catheter-related bloodstream infection is often underestimated. Many hospitals still do not have a written policy for care of the hub (49). The longer a catheter remains in place, the greater the importance of the hub as a source of contamination (50). To prevent contamination, it is important to disinfect the hub when manipulating it. New hubs are being designed aimed at reduced contamination. One hub with a iodine tincture reservoir at the connection site resulted in a major reduction in the intravascular catheter-related bloodstream infection rate (50). It must be noted that this study was performed in a setting with a remarkable high intravascular device-related infection rate. The value of this hub in low incidence settings should be further investigated. Another development are needleless connecting systems. Initially these systems were developed to reduce the chance for needlestick accidents. Several anecdotal reports have documented a higher intravascular catheter-related bloodstream infection rate after the introduction of needleless systems (51–55). Danzig et al. performed a case-control as well as a retrospective cohort study to elucidate the cause of an increased intravascular device-related infection rate in home treatment. They found that the combination of total parenteral nutrition with a needleless connection system increased the chance for the development of bacteremia more than 10-fold ($P < 0.001$) (51). Kellerman found similar results in home treatment with children (53). A prospective study was done by Vassalo et al. A significant higher S. aureus infection rate was found after introduction of bionecteur on an intensive care unit (54). Richard and colleagues performed a prospective comparative study and found a three-fold increased risk for intravascular device-related infection associated with the needleless system ($P < 0.0001$) (55). These increased rates may have been caused by inappropriate handling of the needleless connection system. More recently, a randomised, multi-centre study was performed in Belgium and The Netherlands, comparing the infusate contamination rate of a needleless system (Interlink) and the conventional luer-lock system on intensive care units (56). The use of Interlink was associated with a 50% lower contamination rate ($P < 0.05$). The intravascular device-related infection rate was not significantly different between both groups. These results are promising and further investigations are warranted. Because of the uncertainties at this point, the use of needleless systems is not recommended until well-designed trials have proven their safety in clinical practice.

New Catheters and Cuffs

A silver-impregnated tissue-interface barrier has been developed, to prevent migration of micro-organisms from the skin surrounding the insertion site along the catheter surface to the tip. It consists of a detachable, biodegradable collagen cuff with silver ions (VitaCuff, Vitafore Corporation, San Carlos, California, USA). The cuff can be attached to a central vascular catheter and is placed just below the skin. Subcutaneous tissue rapidly grows into the collagen matrix, creating a mechanical barrier against migrating micro-organisms. This mechanical barrier is enforced by a chemical (silver ion) barrier. Several studies found a short-term reduction of the intravascular device-related infection rate using this device (57,58). However, when the duration of catheterization was more than 2 weeks no protective effect of the cuff was found (59,60). This is probably due to the increasing importance of endoluminal contamination when the duration of catheterization increases (50). The extraluminal cuff cannot protect against the endoluminal (i.e. the hub) route.

More recent developments have been aimed at the prevention of adherence to the catheter by using various materials. Both antiseptics and antibiotics have been incorporated in the catheter surface. A catheter impregnated with silver sulfadiazine and chlorhexidine (Arrowgard; Arrow International, Reading, Pensylvania, USA) showed a significant reduction of catheter colonization and intravascular device-related infection in a study by Maki and colleagues (61). The catheter colonization rate was reduced by nearly 50%. The intravascular device-related infection rate was nearly fivefold lower. Another study performed in leukaemic patients found no effect at all (62). A meta-analysis on this subject included 12 randomised, controlled studies (63). Most patients in these studies were considered to be at high risk for intravascular device-related infection. For catheter colonization an odds ratio of 0.44 (95% CI, 0.37–0.84) was found. The odds ratio for catheter-related bloodstream infection was 0.56 (95% CI, 0.37–0.84). Therefore, in patients at high risk, catheters impregnated with silver sulfadiazine and chlorhexidine appear to reduce the intravascular device-related infection rate approximately two-fold. The effect of the impregnation is considered to be most pronounced during the first week of catheterization. With prolonged duration of catheterization the effect largely disappears (35). It is postulated that this is due to the increased importance of the intra-luminal route, the hub, over time. Another approach is coating of catheters with antibiotics. A combination of minocyclin and rifampin was described by Raad and colleagues (64). They performed a multicenter, double-blind, randomised study. A significant reduction of both the catheter colonization rate and of the catheter-related bloodstream infection rate were observed in the group with coated catheters. The same group performed a study comparing two antimicrobial impregnated catheters (65). The earlier mentioned anti-septic catheter impregnated with a combination of chlorhexidine and silver sulfadiazine was compared with the antibiotic catheter coated with minocyclin and rifampin. A threefold reduction of the catheter colonization rate was found in the group of catheters coated with minocyclin and rifampin. The catheter-related bloodstream infection rate was reduced more than tenfold in this group. The reduction was most pronounced in catheters which were in place for more than 7 days. As mentioned above, the effect of the anti-septic catheter decreases over time. The antibiotic catheter is coated on both the inside and the outside and may be more effective with increased duration of catheterization. Two important notes must be made with regard to the use of antimicrobial impregnated catheters. First, the risk for development of resistance with the widespread use of antibiotics. Although the investigators didn't find increased resistance in their study it is a major point of concern. Second, the interpretation of the results of these studies should be done carefully. All studies have used two main outcome measures: catheter colonisation and catheter-related bloodstream infection. By definition, both outcome measures rely on the results of culture of the catheter. The catheters involved are impregnated with antimicrobials which are known to interfere with the outcome of these cultures. It is questionable if this is acceptable. Does the intravascular device-related infection rate really decrease or is it merely a decrease of positive cultures taken from the device, which makes that the bacteremia cannot be attributed to the device anymore? Future studies should at least mention the overall bloodstream infection rates in both groups. On the other hand the development of new strategies to decrease the intravascular device-related infection rate should be strongly encouraged. Most promising developments are to be expected from using new catheter materials which are less prone to adherence by micro-organisms. The use of antibiotics for this preventive strategy is questionable.

CONCLUSIONS

Intravascular device related infection is an important problem with still a high associated morbidity and mortality. Moreover, it causes an hugh increase in the consumption of antibiotics with its associated costs and development of resistance. Certainly, advances have been made over the past decades which have made intravascular therapy and intravascular support more save to the patients. The infusate used to be a serious problem, which has largely been solved. Many preventive measures have been studied to further reduce the intravascular device-related bloodstream infection rate. Some measures have proven their value repeatedly, some have been shown of little or no effect at all. Unfortunately, many measures have shown conflicting results and their value is still uncertain. This causes undesirable differences in local protocols. Measures which are generally accepted include the use of maximal barrier precautions during insertion, the use of skin-antisepsis with a combination of chlorhexidine or povidone-iodine with alcohol 70%, the use of sterile gauze or transparent polyurethane dressings, routinely changing of the infusion set at least every 72 hours, and disinfection of the hub when it is manipulated. Important items for future studies are the effect of topical antimicrobial ointments, new hub design including needleless connection systems, and new catheter materials. Catheters impregnated with anti-septics and with antibiotics have resulted in a reduction of the intravascular device-related infection rates. However, the long-term side-effects of this application of antibiotics are unknown and are an important cause of reluctance to implement this strategy on a large scale. Nevertheless, new catheter materials could offer the most important preventive strategy to further improve the quality of care in the case of intravascular therapy.

REFERENCES

1. Maki DG, Botticelli JT, LeRoy ML, et al. Prospective study of replacing intravenous administration sets for intravenous therapy at 48- vs 72-hour intervals. *JAMA*. 1987;258:1177–1181.
2. Pittet D, Tarara D, Wenzel RP. Nosocomial bloodstream infections in critically ill patients: excess length of stay, extra costs and attributable mortality. *JAMA*. 1994;162:1598–1601.
3. Maki DG. Nosocomial bacteremia. An epidemiologic overview. *Am J Med*. 1981;70:719–732.
4. Nystrom B, larsen SO, Dankert J, et al. Bacteremia in surgical patients with intravenous devices: a European multicenter incidence study. The European Working Party on Control of Hospital Infections. *J Hosp Infect* 1983;4:338–349.
5. Bouza E, Perez-Molina J, Munoz P, et al. Report of ESGNI-001 and ESGNI-002 studies. Bloodstream infections in Europe. *Clin Microbiol Infect* 1999;5:S1–S12.
6. Wischnewski N, Kampf G, Gastmeier P, et al. Prevalence of primary bloodstream infections in representative German hospitals and their association with central and peripheral vascular catheters. *Zent Bl Bakteriol* 1998;287:93–103.
7. Pearson ML. Guideline for the prevention of inttravascular deice related infections. *Am J Infect Control*. 1996;24:262–293.
8. Cooper GL, Schiller Al, Hopkins CC. Possible role of capillary action in the pathogenesis of experimental catheter-associated dermal tunnel infections. *J Clin Microbiol*. 1988;26:8–12.
9. Pittet D, Lew PD, Auckenthaler R, Waldvogel FA. Bacterial spread as a pathogenic factor in catheter-

related infections (abstract). *In: Program and abstracts of the 30th Interscience Conference on Antimicrobial Agents and Chemotherapy. Washington, D.C.: American Society for Microbiology.* 1990:26.
10. Sitges-Serra A, Puig P, Linares J, et al. Hub colonization as the initial step in an outbreak of coagulase-negative staphylococci during parenteral nutrition. *J Parenter Enter Nutr.* 1984;8:668–672.
11. Salzman MB, Isenberg HD, Shapiro JF, et al. A prospective study of the catheter hub as the portal of entry for microorganisms causing catheter-related sepsis in neonates. *J Infect Dis.* 1993;167: 487–490.
12. Moro ML, Vigano EF, Lepri AC and the central venous catheter-related infections study group. Risk factors for central venous catheter-related infections in surgical and intensive care units. *Infect Control Hosp Epidemiol* 1994;15:253–264.
13. Logghe C, Van Ossel C, D'Hoore W, et al. Evaluation of chlorhexidine and silver-sulfadiazine impregnated central venous catheters for the prevention of bloodstream infections in leukaemic patients: a randomized controlled trial. *J Hosp Infect* 1997;37:145–156.
14. Widmer AF. Intravenous related infections. In: Prevention and control of nosocomial infections. Ed: Wenzel RP. 3rd edition 1997. Williams and Wilkins.
15. Crowe MJ, Cooke EM. Review of case definitions for nosocomial infection-Towards a consensus. *J Hosp Infect* 1998;39:3–11.
16. Garner JS, Jarvis WR, Emori TG, Horan TC, Hughes JM. CDC definitions for nosocomial infections, 1988. *Am J Infect Control* 1998;16:128–140.
17. Mermel LA. Defining intravascular catheter-related infections: A plea for uniformity. *Nutrition* 1997;13:2S–4S.
18. Maki DG, Weise CE, Sarafin HW. A semiquantitative culture method for identifying intravenous-catheter-related infection. *N Engl J Med* 1977;296:1305–1309.
19. Cleri DJ, Corrado ML, Seligman SJ. Quantitative culture of intravenous catheters and other intravascular inserts. *J Infect Dis* 1980;141:781–786.
20. Brun-Buissson C, Abrouk F, Legrand P, et al. Diagnosis of central venous catheter-related sepsis. Critical level of quantitative tip cultures. *Arch Intern Med* 1987;147:873–877.
21. Sherertz RJ, Raad II, Belani L, et al. Three year exparience with sonicated vascular catheter cultures in a clinical microbiology laboratory. *J Clin Microbiol* 1990;28:76–82.
22. Douard MC, Clementi E, Arlet G, et al. Negative catheter-tip cultures and diagnosis of catheter-related bacteremia. *Nutrition* 1994;10:397–404.
23. Maki DG, Stolz SS, Wheeler S, Mermel LA. A prospective randomized trial of gauze and two polyurethane dressings for site care of pulmonary catheters: implications for catheter management. *Crit Care Med* 1994;22:1729–1737.
24. Rubie H, Juricic M, Claeyssens S, et al. Morbidity using subcutaneous ports and efficacy of vancomycin flushing in cancer. *Arch Dis Child* 1995;72:325–329.
25. Vassilomanolakis M, Plataniotis G, Koumakis G, et al. Central venous catheter-related infections after bone marrow transplantation in patients with malignancies: a prospective study with short-course vancomycin prophylaxis. *Bone Marrow Transplant* 1995;15:77–80.
26. Ranson MR, Oppenheim BA, Jackson A, et al. Double-blind placebo controlled study of vancomycin prophylaxis for central venous catheter insertion in cancer patients. *J Hosp Infect* 1990;15:95–102.
27. Mermel LA. Prevention of intravascular catheter-related infections. *Infect Dis Clin Pract.* 1994;3: 391–398.
28. Gil RT, Kruse JA, Thill-Baharozian MC, Carlson RW. Triple- versus single-lumen central venous catheters. A prospective study in a critically ill population. *Arch Intern med.* 1989;149:1139–1143.
29. Richet H, Hubert H, Nitemberg G, et al. Prospective multicenter study of vascular-catheter-related complications and risk factors for positive central-catheter cultures in intensive care unit patients. *J Clin Microbiol.* 1990;28:2520–2525.
30. Horowitz HW, Dworkin BM, Savino JA, et al. Central catheter-related infections: comparison of pulmonary artery catheters and triple lumen catheters for the delivery of hyperalimentation in a critical care setting. *J Parenter Enter Nutr.* 1990;14:588–592.
31. Collignon P, Soni N, Pearson I, et al. Sepsis associated with central vein catheters in critically ill patients. *Intensive Care Med.* 1988;14:227–231.
32. Raad I, Hohn DC, Gilbreath BJ, et al. Prevention of central venous catheter-related infections by using maximal sterile barrier precautions. *Infect Control Hosp Epidemiol.* 1994;15:237–238.
33. Maki DG. Yes, Virginia, aseptic technique is very important: maximal barrier precautions during insertion reduce the risk of central venous catheter-related bacteremia. *Infect Control Hosp Epidemiol.* 1994;15:227–230.

34. Bull DA, Neumayer LA, Hunter GC, et al. Improved sterile technique diminishes the incidence of positive line cultures in cardiovascular patients. *J Surg Res*. 1992;52:106–110.
35. Maki DG, Mermel LA. Infections due to infusion therapy. In: Bennett JV, Brachman PS, eds. *Hospital infections 4th ed. Philadelphia, USA*. Lippincott-Raven 1998:689–724.
36. Maki DG, Alvarado CJ, Ringer M. A prospective randomized trial of povidone-iodine, alcohol and chlorhexidine for prevention of infection with central venous and arterial catheters. *Lancet*. 1991;338:339–343.
37. Prager RL, Silva J. Colonization of central venous catheters. *South Med J* 1984;77:458–461.
38. Levin A, Mason AJ, Jindal KK. Prevention of hemodialysis subclavian vein catheter infections by topical povidone-iodine. *Kidney Int* 1991;40:934–938.
39. Hofmann KK, Weber DJ, Samsa GP, Rutala WA. Transparent polyurethane film as an intravenous catheter dressing: a meta-analysis of the infection risks. *JAMA* 1992;267:2072–2076.
40. Cobb DK, High KP, Sawyer RG, et al. A controlled trial of scheduled replacement of central venous and pulmonary artery catheters. *N Engl J Med* 1992;327:1062–1067.
41. Eyer S, Brummitt C, Crossley K, Siegel R, Cerra F. Catheter-related sepsis: a prospective, randomized study of three different methods of long-term catheter maintenance. *Crit Care Med* 1990;18: 1073–1079.
42. Mermel LA, Maki DG. Infectious complications of Swan-Ganz pulmonary artery catheters. *Am J Respir Crit Care Med* 1994;149:1020–1036.
43. Rupp ME. Infections of intravascular catheters and vascular devices. In: Crossley KB, Archer GL, eds. *The staphylocooci in human disease 1 ste ed. New York, USA*. Churchill Livingstone Inc. 1997:379–401.
44. Snydman DR, Reidy MD, Perry LK, et al. Safety of changing intravenous administration sets containing burettes at longer than 48 hours intervals. *Infect Control*. 1987;8:113–116.
45. Maki DG, Botticelli JT, LeRoy ML, et al. Prospective study of replacing intravenous administration sets for intravenous therapy at 48- vs 72-hour intervals. *JAMA*. 1987;258:1177–1181.
46. Josephson A, Gombert ME, Sierra MF, et al. The relationship between intravenous fluid contamination and the frequency of tubing replacement. *Infect Control*. 1985;6:367–370.
47. Pinilla JC, Ross DF, Martin T, et al. Study of the incidence of intravascular catheter infection and associated septicemia in critically ill patients. *Crit Care Med* 1983;11:21–25.
48. Sitges-Serra A, Linares J, Perez JL, et al. A randomized trial on the effect of tubing changes on hub contamination and catheter sepsis during parenteral nutrition. *JPEN J Parenter Enteral Nutr* 1985;9:322–325.
49. Ingliss TJJ, Sproat LJ, Hawkey PM, Knappett P. Infection control in intensive care units: U.K. national survey. *Br J Anaesthesia*. 1992;68:216–220.
50. Sitges-Serra A, Hernandez R, Maestro S, et al. Prevention of catheter sepsis: the hub. *Nutrition*. 1997;13(suppl):30S–35S.
51. Temporado Cookson S, Ihrig M, O'Mara EM, et al. Increased bloodstream infection rates in surgical patients associated with variation from recommended use and care following implementation of a needleless device. *Infect Control Hosp Epidemiol*. 1998;19:23–27.
52. Danzig LE, Short LJ, Collins K, et al. Bloodstream infections associated with a needleless intravenous infusion system in patients receiving home infusion therapy. *JAMA*. 1995;273:1862–1864.
53. Kellerman S, Shay D, Howard J, Feusner J, Goes C, Jarvis W. Bloostream Infections associated with needleless devices used for central venous catheter access in children receiving home health care. 35th Interscience Conference on Antimicrobial Agents and Chemotherapy, Abstract J11, 17–20 september 1995 SanFrancisco USA.
54. Vassallo D, Blanc-Jouvan M, Bret M, Coronel B, Kasparian S, Mosnier S, Mercatello A, Moskovtchenko JF. Staphylococcus aureus septicemia and a needleless system of infusion. 35th Interscience Conference on Antimicrobial Agents and Chemotherapy, Abstract J12, 17–20 september 1995 SanFrancisco USA.
55. Richard P, Plusquellec M, Assicot P. Is intermittent use of peripheral catheters with a needleless injection site a risk factor for catheter-associated-complications. 37th Interscience Conference on Antimicrobial Agents and Chemotherapy, Abstract J56, 28 september—1 October 1997 Toronto, Canada.
56. Boidin R, Kluytmans J and the Interlink study group. Reduction of infusate contamination using the Interlink Needleless IV-access system: A multicenter study. Ninth Annual Meeting of the Society of Healthcare Epidemiology of America. 17–20 april 1999, San Francisco, USA.
57. Maki DG, Cobb L, Garman JK, et al. An attachable silver-impregnated cuff for prevention of

infection with central venous catheters: a prospective randomized multi-center trial. *Am J Med.* 1988;85:307–314.

58. Flowers RH III, Schwenzer KJ, Kopel RJ, et al. Efficacy of an attachable subcutaneous cuff for the prevention of intravascular catheter-related infection. *JAMA*. 1989;261:878–883.
59. Groeger JS, Lucas AB, Coit D, et al. A prospective, randomized evaluation of the effect of silver-impregnated subcutaneous cuffs for preventing tunneled chronic venous access catheter infections in cancer patients. *Ann Surg.* 1993;218:206–210.
60. Dahlberg PJ, Agger WA, Singer JR, et al. Subclavian hemodialysis cahteter infections: a prospective randomized trial of an attachable silver-impregnated cuff for prevention of catheter-related infections. *Infect Control Hosp Epidemiol.* 1995;16:206–210.
61. Maki DG, Stolz SM, Wheeler S, Mermel LA. Prevention of central venous catheter-related bloodstream infection by use of an antiseptic-impregnated catheter: A randomized, controlled trial. *Ann Intern Med* 1997;127:257–266.
62. Logghe C, Van Ossel Ch, D'Hoore W, et al. Evaluation of chlorhexidine ans silver-sulfadiazine impregnated central venous catheters for the prevention of bloodstream infection in leukaemic patients: a randomized controlled trial. *J Hosp Infect* 1997;37:145–156.
63. Veenstra DL, Saint S, Saha S, Lumley T, Sullivan SD. Efficacy of antiseptic-impregnated central venous catheters in preventing catheter-related bloodstream infection: A meta-analysis. *JAMA* 1999;281: 261–267.
64. Raad I, Darouiche R, Dupuis J, et al. Central venous catheters coated with minocycline and rifampin for the prevention of catheter-related colonization and bloodstream infections: A randomized, double blind trial. *Ann Intern Med* 1997;127:267–274.
65. Darouiche R, Raad I, Heard S, et al. A comparison of two antimicrobial-impregnated central venous catheters. *N Engl J Med* 1999;340:1–8.

12. IS PREVENTION OF VENTILATOR-ASSOCIATED PNEUMONIA COST EFFECTIVE

MARIN H. KOLLEF, M.D.

Washington University School of Medicine, St. Louis, MO 63110 USA

INTRODUCTION

Nosocomial infections add significant costs to individual hospitalizations. They are estimated to involve more than 2 million patients annually at a cost of more than 4.5 billion dollars (1). The Centers for Disease Control and Prevention estimated that an episode of nosocomial pneumonia added 5.9 days to the average hospital stay and $5683 dollars in excess costs (1). Other estimates put the excess hospital costs associated with nosocomial pneumonia at $4947 with excess hospital stays ranging from 6.8 to 30 days per episode of nosocomial pneumonia or ventilator-associated pneumonia (VAP) (2). Boyce and colleagues also reported that among 31 of 33 Medicare patients who developed nosocomial pneumonia, hospital costs for the entire admission exceeded reimbursements with a net loss of $5800 per case (3). Therefore, the occurrence of nosocomial infections, including VAP, are associated with excess medical care costs which may, in part, be preventable.

Antibiotic-resistant nosocomial bacterial infections are an increasingly important subgroup of nosocomial infections associated with prolonged hospitalization and increased health care costs relative to antibiotic-sensitive bacterial infections (4–6). Recently, a study from Beth Israel Deaconess Medical Center examined 489 inpatients with positive clinical cultures for *Pseudomonas aeruginosa* (7). The emergence of antibiotic resistance in infections due to *Pseudomonas aeruginosa* was independently associated with greater hospital mortality and longer lengths of hospital stay. These authors estimated that the emergence of antibiotic resistance increased hospital

R.A. Weinstein and M.J.M. Bonten (eds.). INFECTION CONTROL IN THE ICU ENVIRONMENT.

charges by $11,981. Other authors have also reported increased medical care costs associated with antibiotic-resistant infections (8). The overall national costs of antimicrobial resistance have been estimated to be between $100 million and $30 billion annually for the control and treatment of infections caused by antibiotic-resistant bacteria (6,9). The increased costs of infection due to antibiotic-resistant bacteria have been attributed to prolonged hospitalizations and higher antibiotic costs (10). Additionally, the increasing emergence of antibiotic resistance results in the need to develop new antimicrobial agents (11,12). The costs required for the development of new antimicrobial agents, including the necessary clinical research to demonstrate their effectiveness and safety, has also increased in the last decade possibly explaining, in part, the slow development of new antimicrobial agents (13,14).

Nosocomial pneumonia is a leading cause of death from hospital-acquired infections with an associated crude mortality rate of approximately 30% (15). VAP specifically refers to nosocomial pneumonia developing in mechanically ventilated patients. VAP occurring within 48 to 96 hours of tracheal intubation is usually termed early-onset, often resulting from aspiration complicating the intubation process (16). VAP occurring after this time period is considered late-onset. Early-onset VAP is most often due to antibiotic-sensitive bacteria including Oxacillin-sensitive *Staphylococcus aureus*, *Haemophilus influenza*, and *Streptococcus pneumoniae*, while late-onset VAP is frequently caused by antibiotic-resistant pathogens (e.g., Oxacillin-resistant *Staphylococcus aureus*, *Pseudomonas aeruginosa*, *Acinetobacter* species, and *Enterobacter* species) (17–19).

The pathogenesis of VAP usually requires the occurrence of two important processes: bacterial colonization of the aerodigestive tract and the aspiration of contaminated secretions into the lower airway (20). Therefore, the individual strategies aimed at preventing VAP usually attempt to reduce the burden of bacterial colonization within the aerodigestive tract, to decrease the incidence of aspiration, or to accomplish both of these goals. The data describing the excess costs associated with VAP, particularly VAP attributed to antibiotic-resistant bacteria, suggests that infection control activities aimed at the prevention of this nosocomial infection could be cost effective in addition to potentially reducing patient morbidity.

RISK FACTORS AND TREATMENT OF VAP

The need for invasive medical devices during mechanical ventilation are important contributors to the pathogenesis and development of VAP. Many patients have nasogastric tubes in place which predispose to gastric reflux and increase the potential for aspiration to occur. Additionally, endotracheal tubes facilitate bacterial colonization of the tracheobronchial tree, as well as lower airway aspiration of contaminated secretions, due to associated mucosal injury, pooling of contaminated secretions above the endotracheal tube cuff, and elimination of the cough reflex (20). The ventilator circuit and respiratory therapy equipment may also contribute to the pathogenesis of VAP when they become contaminated with bacteria which usually originate from the patient's secretions (20,21).

The risk of VAP appears to be higher in patients with chronic lung disease and the acute respiratory distress syndrome, and as the duration of mechanical ventilation increases (22). Manipulation of the airway and/or ventilator circuit may predispose to aspiration and subsequent VAP, as suggested by the following risk factors: reintubation, tracheostomy, frequent ventilator circuit changes, low intracuff pressure of endotracheal tubes, failed subglottic suctioning, and patient transport out of the intensive care unit (22). Other risk factors also emphasize the role of the gastrointestinal tract in the development of VAP, such as presence of a nasogastric tube, enteral feeding, supine positioning, witnessed aspiration, and stress ulcer prophylaxis with gastric pH-altering agents (22). Antibiotic administration has been associated with both an increased and decreased risk of VAP (23,24). However, a recent study suggests that the prior administration of broad-spectrum antibiotics, particularly in patients requiring prolonged mechanical ventilation, is an important independent risk factor for VAP due to antibiotic-resistant bacteria (25).

Once VAP occurs, treatment is usually supportive along with the administration of antibiotics. Several studies have suggested that the attributable mortality of VAP, particularly late-onset infection due to antibiotic-resistant pathogens, is greater than 10% (18,26,27). However, other investigations have not found an excess mortality while controlling for confounding factors (28). More recently, the importance of adequate initial antibiotic treatment for this infection has become recognized and might influence the estimates of attributable mortality (29–32). These studies suggest that patients with suspected VAP should initially be treated with a broad-spectrum antibiotic regimen aimed at covering all likely bacterial pathogens. This regimen should subsequently be narrowed based on the respiratory culture results and the bacterial antibiotic sensitivity profiles (32). In addition to potentially increasing hospital mortality rates, the occurrence of VAP, especially VAP due to antibiotic-resistant bacteria, is associated with prolonged hospitalizations and increased medical care costs which supports the need for dedicated prevention efforts (20,28).

VAP PREVENTION STRATEGIES

Clinicians caring for mechanically ventilated patients should participate in focused programs aimed at the prevention of VAP as well as other nosocomial infections. A VAP prevention program should incorporate readily available methods whose efficacy and cost-effectiveness are supported by clinical studies, local experience, and the input of experts in this field (21,33). Additionally, such efforts should be tailored to the characteristics and resource availability of individual hospitals in order to increase the likelihood of their acceptance and success. Several resources are available to assist in the development of this type of prevention program (21,33–38).

The benefits derived from implementing a VAP prevention program can be demonstrated both in terms of improved clinical outcomes and reduced medical care costs (35–38). Among the most important elements of this prevention strategy are the presence of a dedicated individual, or group of individuals, who oversee this endeavor (i.e., ownership and accountability for the process) and a mechanism for tracking nosocomial infection rates (21,33). The following clinical recommendations

Table 1. Cost-Effective Strategies for the Prevention of Ventilator-Associated Pneumonia (VAP)*

1. Systematic/formalized VAP prevention program (35–38)
2. Infection control outbreak surveillance (21)
3. Ventilator weaning protocol/ventilator weaning team (41–43)
4. Use of noninvasive mask positive pressure ventilation (44–46)
5. Early removal of endotracheal tubes and naso/orogastric tubes (20)
6. Avoidance of nasal intubation (57,58)
7. Adequate hand washing (49,50)
8. Semirecumbent patient positioning (23,53)
9. Appropriate chemical and physical restraints to avoid self-extubation (54)
10. Adequate nutritional support (56)
11. Avoidance of gastric overdistention (20,55)
12. Routine drainage of ventilator circuit condensate (61)
13. Maintain adequate endotracheal-tube cuff pressure (64)
14. Humidification with heat and moisture exchangers (65)
15. Avoidance of unnecessary antibiotics(19,25)
16. Antibiotic class cycling or rotation (75,76)
17. Vaccination against common respiratory pathogens (84–86)

Numbers in parentheses refer to reference numbers. *Cost-effectiveness determination based on the general lack of additional expenditures associated with the intervention or documented cost savings in the references.

Table 2. Strategies for the Prevention of Ventilator-Associated Demonstrated not to be Cost-Effective

1. Routine ventilator circuit tubing changes (59)
2. Routine changes of in-line suction catheters (60)
3. Dedicated use of disposable suction catheters (21,60)
4. Daily changes of heat and moisture exchangers* (66,67)
5. Routine use of protective gowns and gloves (excludes handling of contaminated equipment or exposure to patients with colonization or infection due to high-risk bacterial pathogens) (21)
6. Routine saline airway lavage with suctioning (21)

Numbers in parentheses refer to reference numbers. *Applies to heat and moisture exchangers demonstrated to maintain their physical properties without degradation beyond 24 hours.

Table 3. Strategies for the Prevention of Ventilator-Associated Pneumonia Requiring Additional Expenditures without Proven Cost-Effectiveness

1. Routine application of continuous subglottic suctioning (62,63)
2. Prophylactic administration of chest physiotherapy (68)
3. Use of heat and moisture exchangers with bacteriologic filter (65)
4. Routine application of kinetic bed therapy (21)
5. Chlorhexidine oral rinse (82)
6. Selective digestive decontamination (78)
7. Prophylactic immune globulin (33)
8. Acidification of enteral feeding solutions (21,33)
9. Routine prophylactic antibiotic administration (aerosolized or systemically administered) following the initiation of mechanical ventilation (21,33)

*These interventions have varying degrees of supportive evidence for the prevention of ventilator-associated pneumonia (see reference number 33).

are presented to serve as a guide for the development of a VAP prevention program employing cost-effective interventions (Table 1). Additionally, interventions which are not considered cost-effective or for which there is limited data are also presented (Table 2 and 3). These recommendations are based on the currently available medical literature, and may need to be changed as additional clinical investigation is performed.

Use of a Quality Improvement Team or Protocol

The application of systematic efforts aimed at improving patient outcomes and the efficiency of the medical care provided to them, by identifying and implementing best available medical practices, is at the heart of the improvement process (39). This usually requires measurement of a clinical outcome (e.g., occurrence of VAP) prior to and during the application of the improvement initiative aimed at that outcome (40). Several clinical trials, and real world examples, have demonstrated the potential for practice guidelines to reduce the rates of VAP in the intensive are unit setting (35–38, 41). In addition to reducing infection rates, substantial cost savings were associated with the use of these guidelines which employed readily available infection control strategies for the prevention of VAP.

The duration of mechanical ventilation has been shown to be an important risk factor for the development of VAP, especially VAP due to antibiotic-resistant bacteria (22,25). Therefore, efforts aimed at reducing the duration of ventilatory assistance could also decrease the incidence of VAP. Unfortunately, specific clinical trials evaluating this preventive strategy have not been performed. Nevertheless, several clinical investigations have demonstrated the ability of weaning teams and protocol guidelines to reduce the length of mechanical ventilation compared to standard medical practices (41–43). Similarly, the application of noninvasive mask positive pressure ventilation has been demonstrated to reduce the occurrence of VAP when systematically substituted for conventional mechanical ventilation with tracheal intubation (44–46). Such efforts should probably be included in prevention guidelines developed for VAP. Additionally, animal data suggests that a strategy of mechanical ventilation which over distends the lung may result in iatrogenic lung injury predisposing to the development of nosocomial pneumonia with resultant blood borne dissemination of the infection (47). These data lend support to the use of protocols aimed at providing mechanical ventilation which does not result in lung unit overdistension (48).

Effective Hand Washing, Protective Gowns, and Gloves

Hand washing is widely recognized as an important but underutilized measure for the prevention of nosocomial infections (49). Unfortunately, increased numbers of patient contacts, as occurs in a busy ICU, can erode the efficiency with which handwashing occurs (50). Therefore, alternative handwashing methods such as the use of alcohol foams or gels may improve handwashing compliance due to shorter durations of time needed for handwashing (51). Failure of strict hand washing techniques, in combination with other infection control measures, to control an outbreak of ventilator-associated pneumonia attributed to a specific high-risk pathogen should suggest the presence of contaminated respiratory therapy equipment or aerosol solutions. The use of protective gowns and gloves has also been shown to reduce the rate of acquired nosocomial infections in pediatric populations (52). However, their use appears to be most effective when directed at specific antibiotic-resistant pathogens, such as Vancomycin-resistant enterococci. Therefore, the routine use of protective gowns and gloves may not be cost-effective for the prevention of VAP. Gloves, and possibly gowns, should be worn when the risk of skin contamination is great such as during the removal of condensate from ventilator circuits.

Semirecumbent Positioning

Aspiration of upper airway secretions is a common event even in normal healthy adults. Positioning of mechanically ventilated patients in the semirecumbent position should be employed in all VAP prevention programs in order to reduce the occurrence of aspiration (53). Additionally, measures aimed at reducing unplanned extubations (e.g., appropriate use of physical and chemical restraints, securing of the endotracheal tube to the patient) and reducing the need for subsequent reintubation performed in the supine position may also be beneficial (54).

Avoidance of Large Gastric Volumes

Although ventilator-associated pneumonia is commonly due to the aspiration of contaminated secretions into the lower airway, the origin of these infected inocula can be variable (20). The stomach, upper airway, teeth, artificial airway, ventilator circuit condensate, and nasal sinuses have all been implicated as potential sources of origin for aspirated secretions. Unfortunately, the relative importance of these sites as a source for the causative agents of pneumonia, particularly the stomach, is not precisely known resulting in considerable controversy (55). This is an important issue since providing adequate nutritional support to ventilated patients is also thought to prevent the occurrence of VAP (56). Therefore, it seems reasonable to administer nutritional support in a manner which minimizes patient risks for bacterial colonization of the aerodigestive tract and subsequent aspiration. Gastric over distention should be avoided by reducing the use of narcotics and anticholinergic agents, monitoring gastric residual volumes following intragastric feedings, using gastrointestinal motility agents (e.g., metoclopramide), and when deemed necessary supplying enteral nutrition with smaller bore feeding tubes directly into the small bowel instead of the stomach. However, the effectiveness of such interventions await validation in clinical trials.

Oral (non-nasal) Intubation

Prolonged nasal intubation (i.e., greater than 48 hours) should be avoided due to the association between the occurrence of nosocomial sinusitis and VAP (57). Nosocomial sinusitis may predispose to the development of pneumonia via the aspiration of infected secretions from the nasal sinuses. Therefore, the preferred route of intubation should be the oropharynx. Additionally, nasal intubation may be associated with a greater need for antibiotics which can further increase medical care costs (58).

Routine Maintenance of Ventilator Circuits

Several clinical studies have demonstrated no benefit from routinely changing ventilator circuit tubing or any of their subcomponents (e.g., in-line suction catheters) (59,60). In large part, this appears to be due to the rapid bacterial colonization of this tubing, usually within 24 hours of its placement. Nevertheless, ventilator circuits will occasionally require replacement due to overt soilage (e.g., emesis, blood) or mechanical malfunction. Additionally, regular monitoring of ventilator circuits for the removal of accumulated tubing condensate should always be performed for the prevention of ventilator-associated pneumonia (61). This is due to the high concentration of pathogenic bacteria found in condensate fluid which if aspirated may result in pneumonia. This condensate can also serve as a reservoir for the spread of nosocomial pathogens to other patients.

Continuous Subglottic Suctioning

Several lines of investigation have suggested that secretions pooling above inflated endotracheal tube cuffs may be a source of aspirated material resulting in ventilator-associated pneumonia. Endotracheal tubes manufactured with a separate dorsal lumen above the endotracheal tube cuff, in order to suction pooled secretions in the subglottic space, are now available for clinical use (62,63). Additionally, endotracheal tube cuff pressures should be adequately maintained to prevent the leakage of colonized subglottic secretions into the lower airway (64).

Humidification with Heat and Moisture Exchangers

Heat and moisture exchangers are attractive alternatives to heated water humidification systems because of their passive operation (i.e., they do not require electricity or active heating elements) and their lower costs. More recent improvements in the performance characteristics of heat and moisture exchangers have resulted in the development of safe and easily applied devices.

In theory, heat and moisture exchangers should reduce the occurrence of ventilator-associated pneumonia by minimizing the development of condensate within ventilator circuits (65). However, they should primarily be considered a cost-effective alternative for providing humidification to ventilated patients when contraindications to their use are not present (e.g., hemoptysis, copious or tenacious secretions, difficulty weaning from mechanical ventilation due to increased airway resistance). Moreover, certain heat and moisture exchangers can be safely left in place for up to one week, further increasing their cost effectiveness relative to heated water humidification (66,67).

Postural Oscillation/Rotation/Chest Physiotherapy

It has long been appreciated that among patients confined to bed there is an increased frequency of pulmonary and nonpulmonary complications. Kinetic therapy (i.e., patient movement achieved with specialized beds or medical devices) is hypothesized to be beneficial for the prevention of VAP by improving the drainage of pulmonary secretions. However, the added expense of such therapy and its lack of demonstrated effectiveness precludes recommending its routine use (21). Similarly, the routine use of chest physiotherapy for the prevention of VAP should be avoided due to its lack of efficacy and associated risks (e.g., arterial oxygen desaturation) (68).

Stress Ulcer Prophylaxis

Mechanically ventilated patients are at high-risk for upper gastrointestinal hemorrhage due to stress ulcer formation and thus require preventive therapy for this potential complication (69). The importance of gastric pH in the pathogenesis of VAP is controversial. Bacterial colonization of the stomach, enhanced by the administration of pH altering drugs (e.g., histamine type-2 receptor antagonists and antacids), is thought to be an important source of pneumonia pathogens (20). Sucralfate administration into the stomach has been demonstrated to prevent stress ulcer bleeding without lowering gastric pH. Several randomized trials have shown sucralfate to be associated with lower rates of VAP compared to the use of antacids or histamine type-2 receptor antagonists (70). The choice of agent for stress ulcer prophylaxis should depend on patient factors (e.g., presence or absence of a nasogastric tube), the potential for unwanted drug interactions, and the local costs associated with providing the various forms of therapy (71).

Antibiotic Administration

Colonization of the lower respiratory tract by antibiotic-resistant organisms such as Pseudomonas aeruginosa and Oxacillin-resistant Staphylococcus aureus has been shown to be closely correlated with the subsequent development of overt pneumonia (72,73). In an attempt to reverse the trend of increasing antimicrobial resistance among hospital-acquired infections, more effective antibiotic utilization strategies have been advocated which restrict antibiotic use or offer practice guidelines for their administration (34,74). Changing or rotating the use of antibiotic classes for the treatment of suspected bacterial infections (i.e., avoiding the use of a single class of antimicrobial agents in an intensive care unit) may also be effective at reducing the rates of nosocomial pneumonia due to antibiotic-resistant pathogens (75,76). However, the elimination or reduction of the unnecessary use of antibiotics should be seen as the primary goal in preventing antibiotic-resistant nosocomial infections (34).

Prophylactic Antibiotic Therapy

The use of aerosolized antibiotics for the prevention of VAP has been abandoned due to its lack of efficacy and the subsequent emergence of antibiotic-resistant infections (21). Similarly, the routine use of selective digestive decontamination, with nonabsorbable antibiotics applied to the orodigestive tract, has not gained acceptance in the United States due to its lack of demonstrated impact on mortality, the emergence of antibiotic-resistant infections, and additional toxicity (77). A recent metaanalysis of selective digestive decontamination did not demonstrate a survival advantage for selective digestive decontamination as compared with parenteral antibiotic prophylaxis which is commonly administered in the perioperative period (78). Therefore, a definitive recommendation cannot be made on the cost effectiveness of routine selective digestive decontamination for the prevention of VAP.

The routine use of broad-spectrum parenteral antibiotics for the prevention of VAP also cannot be recommended at the present time due to concerns over increasing antibiotic resistance among subsequent hospital-acquired infections (25,80). Nevertheless, one recent investigation suggests that the administration of such therapy to patients with coma may reduce the incidence of VAP (79). Further investigations are required to determine the general applicability of this observation. At present, antibiotics directed against specific infections for patients requiring mechanical ventilation may protect against the development of VAP (24).

Chlorhexidine Oral Rinse

Chlorhexidine is an antiseptic solution used by dentists since 1959 for the control of dental plaques. Bacteria accumulating in dental plaques have been implicated as a source of pathogens for VAP. Chlorhexidine has been shown to be effective in the control of ventilator circuit colonization and pneumonia due to antibiotic-resistant bacteria (81). The use of oropharyngeal decontamination with chlorhexidine solution has also been shown to reduce the occurrence of VAP in patients undergoing cardiac surgery (82). Preventative oral washes with chlorhexidine seems reasonable in selected high-risk patients given its ease of administration. However, overuse could result in patient colonization and superinfection with chlorhexidine-resistant pathogens (83).

Vaccines

Various vaccination programs in adults and children have been demonstrated to be successful in reducing the incidence of pneumonia due to specific pathogens including Haemophilus influenza type b strains, Streptococcus pneumoniae, and the influenza virus (84–86). It would be expected that vaccination against infection with these pathogens may also prevent some hospital-acquired infections as well. Indeed, the difference between nosocomial and community-acquired infections is becoming "grayer", particularly in the era of managed care where patients with acute and chronic illnesses are often medically managed outside of the hospital setting. Therefore, pneumococcal vaccination and if indicated, influenza vaccination should be considered prior to hospital discharge or included in the discharge planning of all patients at risk for subsequent respiratory infections, including VAP.

SUMMARY

The prevention of VAP appears to be a cost effective endeavor based on the healthcare costs and morbidity associated with this nosocomial infection. Infection control measures should be integrated into a systematic program for general application to all patients requiring mechanical ventilation at a particular hospital (36,37). Additionally, attention needs to be focused on the emergence of antibiotic-resistant bacterial infections in the intensive care unit setting (87,88). The prevention of antibiotic-resistant bacterial infections should result in fewer overall nosocomial infections including VAP (75). At present, VAP prevention programs should employ practices which are readily accepted by local practitioners, safe for patients, and associated with acceptable costs to the institution.

SUPPORT INFORMATION

This work was supported in part by a grant from the American Lung Association of Eastern Missouri and CDC Grant #UR8/CCU715087.

REFERENCES

1. Public health focus: Surveillance, prevention, and control of nosocomial infections. *MMWR* 1992;41:783–787.
2. Jarvis WR. Selected aspects of the socioeconomic impact of nosocomial infections: morbidity, mortality, cost, and prevention. *Infect Control Hosp Epidemiol* 1996;17:552–557.
3. Boyce JM, Potter-Bynoe G, Dziobek L, Solomon SL. Nosocomial pneumonia in Medicare patients. Hospital costs and reimbursement patterns under the prospective payment system. *Arch Intern Med* 1991;151:1109–1114.
4. Ascar JF. Consequences of bacterial resistance to antibiotics in medical practice. *Clin Infect Dis* 1997; 24;S17–S18.
5. Cohen ML. Epidemiology of drug resistance: implications for a post-antimicrobial era. *Science* 1992;257:1050–1055.
6. Impacts of antibiotic-resistant bacteria: Thanks to Penicillin—He will come home! Washington, DC; Office of Technology Assessment, Congress; 1995. Publication OTC-H-629.
7. Carmeli Y, Troillet N, Karchmer AW, Somore MH. Health and economic outcomes of antibiotic resistance in Pseudomonas aeruginosa. *Arch Intern Med* 1999;159:1127–1132.
8. Holemberg SD, Solomon SL, Blake PA. Health and economic impact of antimicrobial resistance. *Rev Infect Dis* 1987;9:1065–1078.
9. Phelps CE. Bug-drug resistance: Sometimes less is more. *Med Care* 1989;27:194–203.
10. Einarsson S, Kristjansson M, Kristinsson KG, Kjartansson G, Jonsson S. Pneumonia caused by penicillin-non-susceptible and penicillin-susceptible pneumococci in adults: a case-control study. *Scand J Infect Dis* 1998;30:253–256.
11. Moellering RC. A novel antimicrobial agent joins the battle against resistant bacteria. *Ann Intern Med* 1999;130:155–157.
12. Hancock RE. The role of fundamental research and biotechnology in finding solutions to the global problem of antibiotic resistance. *Clin Infect Dis* 1997;24:S148–S150.
13. Bax RP. Antibiotic resistance: A view from the pharmaceutical industry. *Clin Infect Dis* 1997;24: S151–S153.
14. Jones RN. The emergent needs for basic research, education, and surveillance of antimicrobial resistance. Problems facing the report from the American Society for Microbiology Task Force on Antibiotic Resistance. *Diag Microbiol Infect Dis* 1996;25:153–161.
15. Leu HS, Kaiser DL, Mori M, Woolson RF, Wenzel RP. Hospital-acquired pneumonia. Attributable mortality and morbidity. *Am J Epidemiol* 1989;129:1258–1267.
16. Pingleton SK, Fagon JY, Leeper KV Jr. Patient selection for clinical investigation of ventilator-associated pneumonia. Criteria for evaluating diagnostic techniques. *Chest* 1992;102:553S–556S.
17. Niederman MS, Craven DE, Fein AM, Schultz DE. Pneumonia in the critically ill hospitalized patient. *Chest* 1990;97:170–181.
18. Kollef MH, Silver P, Murphy DM, Trovillion E. The effect of late-onset ventilator-associated pneumonia in determining patient mortality. *Chest* 1995;108:1655–1662.
19. Rello J, Ausina V, Ricart M, Castella J, Prats G. Impact of previous antimicrobial therapy on the etiology and outcome of ventilator-associated pneumonia. *Chest* 1993;104:1230–1235.
20. Craven DE, Steger KA. Epidemiology of nosocomial pneumonia. New perspectives on an old disease. *Chest* 1995;108:1S–16S.
21. Tablan OC, Anderson LJ, Arden NH, Breiman RF, Butler JC, McNeil MM. Guideline for preven-

tion of nosocomial pneumonia. The Hospital Infection Control Practices Advisory Committee, Centers for Disease Control and Prevention. *Infect Control Hosp Epidemiol* 1994;15:587–627.
22. Cook DJ, Kollef MH. Risk factors for ICU-acquired pneumonia. *JAMA* 1998;279:1605–1606.
23. Kollef MH. Ventilator-associated pneumonia: a multivariate analysis. *JAMA* 1993;270:1965–1970.
24. Cook DJ, Walter SD, Cook RJ, Griffith LE, Guyatt GH, Leasa D, Jaeschke RZ, Brun-Buison C. Incidence and risk factors for ventilator-associated pneumonia in critically ill patients. *Ann Intern Med* 1998;129:433–440.
25. Trouillet JL, Chastre J, Vuagnat A, Joly-Guillou ML, Combaux D, Dombret MC, Gibert C. Ventilator-associated pneumonia caused by potentially drug-resistant bacteria. *Am J Respir Crit Care Med* 1998;157:531–539.
26. Fagon JY, Chastre J, Hance AJ, Montravers P, Novara A, Gibert C. Nosocomial pneumonia in ventilated patients: a cohort study evaluating attributable mortality and hospital stay. *Am J Med* 1993;94: 281–288.
27. Crouch Brewer S, Wunderink RG, Jones CB, Leeper KV Jr. Ventilator-associated pneumonia due to Pseudomonas aeruginosa. *Chest* 1996;109:1019–1029.
28. Papazian L, Bregeon F, Thirion X, Gregoire R, Saux P, Denis JP, Perin G, Charrel J, Dumon JF, Affray JP, Gouin F. Effect of ventilator-associated pneumonia on mortality and morbidity. *Am J Respir Crit Care Med* 1996;154:91–97.
29. Rello J, Gallego M, Mariscal D, Sonora R, Valles J. The value of routine microbial investigation in ventilator-associated pneumonia. *Am J Respir Crit Care Med* 1997;156:196–200.
30. Luna CM, Vujacich P, Niederman MS, Vay C, Gherardi C, Matera J, Jolly EC. Impact of BAL data on the therapy and outcome of ventilator-associated pneumonia. *Chest* 1997;111:676–685.
31. Kollef MH, Ward S. The influence of mini-BAL cultures on patient outcomes: implications for the antibiotic management of ventilator-associated pneumonia. *Chest* 1998;113:412–420.
32. Kollef MH, Sherman G, Ward S, Fraser VJ. Inadequate antimicrobial treatment of infections: A risk factor for hospital mortality among critically ill patients. *Chest* 1999;115:462–474.
33. Kollef MH. The prevention of ventilator-associated pneumonia. *N Engl J Med* 1999;340:627–634.
34. Goldmann DA, Weinstein RA, Wenzel RP, Tablan OC, Duma RJ, Gaynes RP, Schlosser J, Martone WJ. Strategies to prevent and control the emergence and spread of antimicrobial-resistant microorganisms in hospitals. A challenge to hospital leadership. *JAMA* 1996;275:234–240.
35. Boyce JM, White RL, Spruill EY, Wall M. Cost-effective application of the Centers for Disease Control Guideline for Prevention of Nosocomial Pneumonia. *Am J Infect Control* 1985;13:228–232.
36. Joiner GA, Salisbury D, Bollin GE. Utilizing quality assurance as a tool for reducing the risk of nosocomial ventilator-associated pneumonia. *Am J Medical Quality* 1996;11:100–103.
37. Kelleghan SI, Salemi C, Padilla S, McCord M, Mermilliod G, Canola T, Becker L. An effective continuous quality improvement approach to the prevention of ventilator-associated pneumonia. *Am J Infect Control* 1993;21:322–330.
38. Gaynes RP, Solomon S. Improving hospital-acquired infection rates: the CDC experience. *Joint Commission Journal on Quality Improvement*. 1996;22:457–467.
39. Berwick DM. Continuous improvement as an idea in healthcare. *N Engl J Med* 1989;320:53–56.
40. Booth FV. ABCs of quality assurance. *Crit Care Clin* 1993;9:477–498.
41. Kollef MH, Horst HM, Prang L, Brock WA. Reducing the duration of mechanical ventilation: Three examples of change in the intensive care unit. *New Horizons* 1998;6:52–60.
42. Ely EW, Baker AM, Dunagan DP, Burke HL, Smith AC, Kelley PT, Johnson MM, Browder RW, Bowton DL, Haponik EF. Effect on the duration of mechanical ventilation of identifying patients capable of breathing spontaneously. *N Engl J Med* 1996;335:1864–1869.
43. Kollef MH, Shapiro SD, Silver P, St. John RE, Prentice D, Sauer S, Ahrens TS, Shannon W, Baker-Clinkscale D. A randomized, controlled trial of protocol-directed versus physician-directed weaning from mechanical ventilation. *Crit Care Med* 1997;25:567–574.
44. Nava S, Ambrosino N, Clini E, Prato M, Orlando G, Vitacca M, Brigada P, Fracchia C, Rubini F. Noninvasive mechanical ventilation in the weaning of patients with respiratory failure due to chronic obstructive pulmonary disease. A randomized, controlled trial. *Ann Intern Med* 1998;128:721–728.
45. Antonelli M, Conti G, Rocco M, Bufi M, Deblasi RA, Vivino G, Gasparetto A, Meduri GV. A comparison of noninvasive positive-pressure ventilation and conventional mechanical ventilation in patients with acute respiratory failure. *N Engl J Med* 1998;339:429–435.
46. Nourdine K, Combes P, Carton MJ, Beuret P, Cannamela A, Ducreux JC. Does noninvasive ventilation reduce the ICU nosocomial infection risk? A prospective clinical survey. *Intensive Care Med* 1999;25:567–573.

47. Nahum A, Hoyt J, Schmitz L, Schmitz L, Moody J, Shapiro R, Marini JJ. Effect of mechanical ventilation strategy on dissemination of intratracheally instilled Escherichia coli in dogs. *Crit Care Med* 1997;25:1733–1743.
48. Amato MB, Barbas CS, Medeiros DM, Magaldi RB, Schettino GP, Lorenzi-Filho G, Kairalla RA, Deheinzelin D, Munoz C, Oliveira R, Takagaki TY, Carvalho CR. Effect of a protective-ventilation strategy on mortality in the acute respiratory distress syndrome. *N Engl J Med* 1998;338:347–354.
49. Doebbeling BN, Stanley GL, Sheetz CT, Pfaller MA, Houston AK, Annis L, Li N, Wenzel RP. Comparative efficacy of alternative hand-washing agents in reducing nosocomial infections in intensive care units. *N Engl J Med* 1992;327:88–93.
50. Pittet D, Mourouga P, Perneger TV, and the Members of the Infection Control Program. Compliance with handwashing in a teaching hospital. *Ann Intern Med* 1999;130:126–130.
51. Pereira LJ, Lee GM, Wade KJ. An evaluation of five protocols for surgical handwashing in relation to skin condition and microbial counts. *J Hosp Infect* 1997;36:49–65.
52. Klein BS, Perloff WH, Maki DG. Reduction of nosocomial infection during pediatric intensive care by protective isolation. *N Engl J Med* 1989;320:1714–1721.
53. Torres A, Serra-Batlles J, Ros E, Piera C, Puig de la Bellacasa J, Cobos A, Lomena F, Rodriguez-Roisin R. Pulmonary aspiration of gastric contents in patients receiving mechanical ventilation: the effect of body position. *Ann Intern Med* 1992;116:540–543.
54. Torres A, Gatell JM, Aznar E, el-Ebiary M, Puig de la Bellacasa J, Gonzalez J, Ferrer M, Rodriguez-Roisin R. Re-intubation increases the risk of nosocomial pneumonia in patients needing mechanical ventilation. *Am J Respir Crit Care Med* 1995;152:137–41.
55. Niederman MS, Craven DE. Devising strategies for preventing nosocomial pneumonia—should we ignore the stomach? *Clin Infect Dis* 1997;24:320–323.
56. Niederman MS, Mantovani R, Schoch P, Papas J, Fein AM. Patterns and routes of trancheobronchial colonization in mechanically ventilated patients. The role of nutritional status in colonization of the lower airway by Pseudomonas species. *Chest* 1989;95:155–161.
57. Rouby JJ, Laurent P, Gosnach M, Cambau E, Lamas G, Zouaoui A, Leguillou JL, Bodin L, Khac TD, Marsault C. Risk factors and clinical relevance of nosocomial maxillary sinusitis in the critically ill. *Am J Respir Crit Care Med* 1994;150:776–783.
58. Holzapfel L, Chastang C, Demingeon G, Bohe J, Piralla B, Coupry A. A randomized study assessing the systematic search for maxillary sinusitis in nasotracheally mechanically ventilated patients. Influence of nosocomial maxillary sinusitis on the occurrence of ventilator-associated pneumonia. *Am J Respir Crit Care Med* 1999;159:695–701.
59. Kollef MH. Prolonged use of ventilator circuits and ventilator-associated pneumonia. A model for identifying the optimal clinical practice. *Chest* 1998;113:267–269.
60. Kollef MH, Prentice D, Shapiro SD, Fraser VJ, Silver P, Trovillion E, Weilitz P, von Harz B, St. John R. Mechanical ventilation with or without daily changes of in-line suction catheters. *Am J Respir Crit Care Med* 1997;156:466–472.
61. Craven DE, Goularte TA, Make BJ. Contaminated condensate in mechanical ventilator circuits. A risk factor for nosocomial pneumonia. *Am Rev Respir Dis* 1984;129:625–628.
62. Valles J, Artigas A, Rello J, Bonsoms N, Fontanals D, Blanch L, Fernandez R, Baigorri F, Mestre J. Continuous aspiration of subglottic secretions in preventing ventilator-associated pneumonia. *Ann Intern Med* 1995;122:179–186.
63. Kollef MH, Skubas NJ, Sundt TM. A randomized clinical trial of continuous aspiration of subglottic secretions (CASS) in cardiac surgery patients. *Chest* (In Press).
64. Rello J, Sonora R, Jubert P, Artigas A, Rue M, Valles J. Pneumonia in intubated patients: role of respiratory airway care. *Am J Respir Crit Care Med* 1996;154:111–115.
65. Kirton OC, DeHaven B, Morgan J, Morejon O, Civetta J. A prospective randomized comparison of an in-line heat moisture exchange filter and heated wire humidifiers: rates of ventilator-associated early-onset (community-acquired) or late-onset (hospital acquired) pneumonia and incidence of endotracheal tube occlusion. *Chest* 1997;112:1055–1059.
66. Kollef MH, Shapiro SD, Boyd V, Silver P, Von Harz B, Trovillion E, Prentice D. A randomized clinical trial comparing an extended-use hygroscopic condenser humidifier to heated water humidification in mechanically ventilated patients. *Chest* 1998;113:759–767.
67. Djedaini K, Billiard M, Mier L, Le Bourdelles G, Brun P, Markowicz P, Estagnasie P, Coste F, Boussougant Y, Dreyfuss D. Changing heat and moisture exchangers every 48 hours rather than 24 hours does not affect their efficacy and the incidence of nosocomial pneumonia. *Am J Respir Crit Care Med* 1995;152:1562–1569.

68. Hall JC, Tarala RA, Tapper J, Hall JL. Prevention of respiratory complications after abdominal surgery: a randomized clinical trial. *BMJ* 1996;312:148–152.
69. Cook DJ, Fuller HD, Guyatt GH, Marshall JC, Leasa D, Hall R. Risk factors for gastrointestinal bleeding in critically ill patients. Canadian Critical Care Trials Group. *N Engl J Med* 1994;330: 377–381.
70. Cook DJ, Reeve BK, Guyatt GH, Heyland DK, Griffith LE, Buckingham L, Tryba M. Stress ulcer prophylaxis in critically ill patients. Resolving discordant meta-analysis. *JAMA* 1996;275:308–314.
71. Cook D, Guyatt G, Marshall J, Leasa D, Fuller H, Hall R, Peters S, Rutledge F, Griffith L, McLellan A, Wood G, Kirby A. A comparison of sucralfate and ranitidine for the prevention of upper gastrointestinal bleeding in patients requiring mechanical ventilation. Canadian Critical Care Trials Group. *N Engl J Med* 1998;338:791–797.
72. Johanson WG Jr, Pierce AK, Sandford JP, Thomas GD. Nosocomial respiratory infections with gram-negative bacilli. The significance of colonization of the respiratory tract. *Ann Intern Med* 1972;77: 701–706.
73. Garrouste-Orgeas M, Chevret S, Arlet G, Marie O, Rouveau M, Popoff N, Schlemmer B. Oropharyngeal or gastric colonization and nosocomial pneumonia in adult intensive care unit patients. A prospective study based on genomic DNA analysis. *Am J Respir Crit Care Med* 1997;156:1647–1655.
74. Evans RS, Pestotnik SL, Classen DC, Clemmer TP, Weaver LK, Orme JF, Lloyd JF, Burke JP. A computer-assisted management program for antibiotics and other antiinfective agents. *N Engl J Med* 1998;338:232–238.
75. Kollef MH, Vlasnik J, Sharpless L, Pasque C, Murphy D, Fraser V. Scheduled change of antibiotic classes: a strategy to decrease the incidence of ventilator-associated pneumonia. *Am J Respir Crit Care Med* 1997;156:1040–1048.
76. Rahal JJ, Urban C, Horn D, Freeman K, Segal-Maurer S, Maurer J, Mariano N, Marks S, Burns JM, Dominick D, Lim M. Class restriction of cephalosporin use to control total cephalosporin resistance in nosocomial Klebsiella. JAMA 1998;280:1233–1237.
77. Gastinne H, Wolff M, Delatour F, Faurisson F, Chevret S. A controlled trial in intensive care units of selective decontamination of the digestive tract with nonabsorbable antibiotics. The French Study Group of Selective Decontamination of the Digestive Tract. *N Engl J Med* 1992;326:594–599.
78. D'Amico R, Pifferi S, Leonetti C, Torri V, Tinazzi A, Liberati A. Effectiveness of antibiotic prophylaxis in critically ill adult patients: systematic review of randomized controlled trials. BMJ 1998;316: 1275–1285.
79. Sirvent JM, Torres A, El-Ebiary M, Castro P, de Batlle J, Bonet A. Protective effect of intravenously administered cefuroxime against nosocomial pneumonia in patients with structural coma. *Am J Respir Crit Care Med* 1997;155:1729–1734.
80. Tenover FC, McGowan JE Jr. Reasons for the emergence of antibiotic resistance. Am J Med Sci 1996;311:9–16.
81. Rumbak MJ, Cancio MR. Significant reduction in methicillin-resistant Staphylococcus aureus ventilator-associated pneumonia associated with the institution of a prevention protocol. *Crit Care Med* 1995;23:1200–1203.
82. DeRiso AJ 2nd, Ladowski JS, Dillon TA, Justice JW, Peterson AC. Chlorhexidine gluconate 0.12% oral rinse reduces the incidence of total nosocomial respiratory infection and nonprophylactic systemic antibiotic use in patients undergoing heart surgery. *Chest* 1996;109:1556–1561.
83. Russell AD. Plasmids and bacterial resistance to biocides. *J Applied Microbiology* 1997;83:155–165.
84. Herceg A. The decline of Haemophilus influenza type b disease in Australia. *Communicable Diseases Intelligence* 1997;21:173–176.
85. Gross PA, Hermogenes AW, Sacks HS, Lau J, Levandowoski RA. The efficacy of influenza vaccine in elderly persons. A meta-analysis and review of the literature. *Ann Intern Med* 1995;123:518–527.
86. Nuorti JP, Butler JC, Crutcher JM, Guevara R, Welch D, Holder P, et al. An outbreak of multidrug-resistant pneumococcal pneumonia and bacteremia among unvaccinated nursing home residents. *N Engl J Med* 1998;338:1861–1868.
87. Richards MJ, Edwards JR, Culver DH, Gaynes RP. Nosocomial infections in medical intensive care units in the United States. Crit Care Med 1999;27:887–892,
88. Hanberger H, Garcia-Rodriguez JA, Gobernado M, Goossens H, Nilsson LE, Struelens MJ. Antibiotic susceptibility among aerobic gram-negative bacilli in intensive care units in 5European Countries. JAMA 1999;281:67–71.

13. VENTILATOR-ASSOCIATED PNEUMONIA: IS PREVENTION COST-EFFECTIVE?

RICARD FERRER, TORSTEN BAUER, ANTONI TORRES

Institut Clinic de Pneumologia i Cirugia Toràcica, Hospital Clínic.
Institut d'Investigacions Biomèdiques August Pi i Sunyer (IDIBAPS)
Universitat de Barcelona, Barcelona, Spain

INTRODUCTION

Nosocomial pneumonia (NP) is regarded as the infection of lung parenchyma that was neither present not incubated at hospital admission. Ventilator-associated pneumonia (VAP) is a NP that occurs after the first 48 hours of initiating mechanical ventilation and can be further differentiated in early (<5 days after tracheal intubation) and late-onset (>5 days) VAP (1). NP still remains the leading cause of death from hospital-acquired infections. Crude mortality rates range from 24% to 76% depending on the population and clinical setting studied (2–9).

The average additional cost for NP was estimated as high as U.S. $1,255 per patient in 1982 (10). A similar study in 1985, reported an average extra cost of U.S. $2,863 per patient and case of NP (11). In trauma patients this figure may reach eventually U.S. $40,000 (12). However, it is almost impossible to directly evaluate extra costs associated with NP but the excess morbidity as a direct consequence of pneumonia may be a good measurement, as well. Initial reports found that pneumonia extended the Intensive Care Unit (ICU) stay threefold (13), whereas Jimenez and co-workers estimated the excess morbidity attributable to NP between 10 to 32 days (14). This figure was later corroborated by others: Leu et al. reported 9.2 days of additional hospital stay (15) and Fagon and co-workers calculated the median length of stay in the ICU for the patients that developed VAP with 21 days, versus a median of 15 days for control patients (16). Comparable figures were also reported for trauma patients with VAP (12).

From this data we may conclude that prevention of NP is the most important step towards reducing hospitalisation costs. A variety of measures has been suggested for prevention of NP depending on the setting and the individual risk profile. In order to estimate the cost-effectiveness we would like to discuss of these preventive strategies with respect to the cost of the measurement itself and the potential to reduce the incidence of pneumonia and the length of hospital stay. For this purpose we used an arbitrary classification of low cost, intermediate cost and high cost measures. We assumed a low cost, when the measure is not associated with direct costs. Intermediate costs were hypothesised when the average daily expense does probably not exceed 50 Euros, and other measures were classified as high cost items. In addition, we will present the preventive measures again in tabular form according to the efficacy as it has been proposed by the Center for Diseases Control (CDC) (17). This report comprises three classes of evidence, recommended strategies are based on strong rationale and suggestive evidence, suggested strategies may be supported by suggestive clinical or epidemiologic studies, and no recommendations are given for practices for which insufficient evidence or consensus regarding efficacy exists. However, this report has been published in 1994 and recent evidence has not been reviewed. We therefore indicated also measures that have not been included previously.

LOW-COST MEASURES

Hand Washing

Cross-contamination via the inoculation of bacteria into upper and lower airways is an exogenous mechanism in the aetiopathogenesis of NP especially in the ICU. Bacterial contamination of respiratory equipment, condensed water in ventilator-circuit tubing, excessive manipulation of ventilator circuits are potential sources of inoculation of highly contaminated material. Hand washing is an important yet underused measure to prevent nosocomial infections.

Some data indicate that an antimicrobial hand washing agent may be more effective than a non-medicated soap in reducing the rates of nosocomial infection in the ICU (18). Clearly, hand washing is simple and should be routinely adopted based on its efficacy and low cost.

Adjustment of Sedatives, Immunosupresive Drugs and Antibiotics

Aspiration is an important aetiopathological factor in patients with coma and an altered level of consciousness and can significantly contribute to the development of lung infections (19–21). Accordingly, sedative agents should be adjusted to the individual patient using e.g. a sedation score. The use of excessive sedation could be reduced in this way.

Immunosuppressive agents such as corticosteroids and cytotoxic agents impair host defence mechanisms, and immunosupression have been identified as a risk factor for NP (22). Immunosuppressive agents should be avoided wherever possible and, when necessary, the minimal effective dose should be used and treatment should be regularly reviewed and stopped at the earliest opportunity.

Previous antibiotic treatment is a risk factor for the presence of potentially drug-resistant bacteria, requiring a much more potent antimicrobial regimen (23). It is therefore important to be rational in our choice and use of antibiotics, restricting excessive and inappropriate use. When antibiotics are needed, an adequate and no expensive measure could be to change the antibiotic class according to an annual schedule to avoid the development of local resistance. Data from a study investigating this issue for suspected Gram-negative bacterial infections in patients undergoing cardiac surgery suggested that scheduled changes can reduce the incidence of VAP attributed to antibiotic-resistant Gram-negative bacteria (24).

Semirecumbent Body Position of Patients

In supine position aspiration of upper-airway secretions is common even in healthy adults. Two studies with radioactive-labelled gastric content showed that reflux can be reduced and subsequent aspiration avoided by positioning mechanically ventilated patients in a semirecumbent position (25,26). An elevated head position (>30° angle) was also a protective factor of nosocomial infection in an epidemiological study (27) and Kollef and co-workers demonstrated that a supine body position during the first 24 hours of mechanical ventilation was an independent risk factor of mortality in patients with NP (9). It has also been documented in a recently published randomised clinical trial that a persistent semirecumbent body position reduced the incidence of NP in intubated and mechanically ventilated patients, but without a significant decrease in morbidity or mortality (28). If there is no contraindication to the manoeuvre, patients receiving mechanical ventilation and have a enteral tube in place, the head of the bed should be elevated at an angle of 30–45 degrees.

Gastric Overdistension

Gastric overdistension may facilitate the reflux of bacteria from the gut and should be avoided by reduction by the use of narcotics and anticholinergic agents, monitoring gastric residual volumes after intragastric feeding, use of gastric prokinetic agents (e.g., metoclopramide), and when necessary supplying enteral feeding via nasojejunal intubation (17,29,30). Gastric overdistension has especially to be avoided when non-invasive mechanical ventilation is applied. However, the effectiveness of this interventions awaits validation in clinical trials.

Correct Respiratory Airway Care

Not only gross but also micro-aspiration to lower airway can facilitate the development of NP despite the presence of an artificial airway. It is therefore important to maintain an adequate tube cuff pressure to reduce micro-aspiration. Rello and associates found a higher risk for VAP in patients with cuff pressures less than 20 cm H_2O (31). Clearly, maintaining cuff pressure is simple and should be routinely adapted based on its efficacy and low cost.

Two types of suction-catheter systems are available: the open, single-use system and the closed, multiple use system; the risk of VAP appears to be similar with both systems (17). The main advantages of the closed, multiple use catheters are lower costs and decreased environmental cross-contamination.

Prolonged nasal intubation (≥48 hours) should be avoided because nosocomial sinusitis may predispose the patient to pneumonia through the aspiration of infected secretions from de nasal sinuses (32), and using endotracheal tube has no extra cost. In cases where nasal intubation can not be avoided (e.g., maxillar surgery), early tracheostomy may still be a cost-effective measure to prevent NP.

Re-intubation is a risk factor for VAP as was shown in a case-control study (33). The careful evaluation during the weaning trial of the patient's ability to sustain spontaneous breathing might therefore reduce the number of extubation failures, and thus may prove to be a cost-effective measure, as well.

INTERMEDIATE-COST MEASURES

Use of Protective Gowns and Gloves

As with hand washing, the use of protective gowns and gloves during patient contact has also been found to reduce the rate of acquired nosocomial infections (34), but their use appears to be most effective when directed at specific antibiotic-resistant pathogens. Therefore, the use of protective gowns and gloves during patient contact can not be recommended for the routine prevention of VAP, but must be considered when handling respiratory secretions or during patient contact when the patient carries an antibiotic-resistant pathogen (for instance MRSA).

Chlorhexidine Oral Rinse

Bacteria accumulated in dental plaque have been implicated as pathogens of VAP when aspirated to lower airways. Chlorhexidine is an antiseptic solution for the control of dental plaque. Oro-pharyngeal decontamination with chlorhexidine solution has also been shown to reduce the incidence of VAP in patients undergoing cardiac surgery (35) and has also been shown to be effective in the control of colonisation and VAP caused by antibiotic-resistant bacteria (36). The use of preventive oral washes with chlorhexidine seems therefore reasonable in selected high-risk patients, given the easy administration and the reasonable costs.

Preventive Systemic Antibiotic Therapy

Unlike topical antibiotic therapy (e.g., SDD) a preventive systemic antibiotic strategy can not be recommended, because it has been shown that the prior administration of antibiotics contributes to the development of nosocomial pneumonia and increases mortality (9). However, the administration of cefuroxime (two 1,500-mg doses 12 hours apart after intubation) to patients with structural coma after head injury or stroke represents an effective prophylactic strategy (37). The incidence of microbiologically confirmed pneumonia could be reduced from 50% in the control group to 24% in the group of patients, who had received cefuroxime. No difference was found with regard to morbidity in the two study arms, but the authors reported a decrease in total hospital stay when patients with pneumonia were compared to those without. Our personal view is that the administration of short term and high doses of antibiotics is a useful preventive measure for early-onset aspiration pneumonia. We can not extrapolate these results to late-onset pneumonia.

Stress-Ulcer Prophylaxis

The stomach is a reservoir of nosocomial pathogens with the potential to colonise the upper respiratory tract. When gastric pH increases from the normal levels to ≥4, microorganisms are able to multiply to high concentrations in the stomach. The gastro-pulmonary route of infection has therefore been proposed as an important aetiopathogenic factor, but this issue is controversial (25,38–42). Mechanical ventilated patients are at risk for stress ulcers with gastrointestinal haemorrhage and preventive treatment with H_2-blockers, antacids or sucralfate is employed routinely. However, H_2-blockers raise the intragastric pH, which in turn enhances gastric colonisation with pathogens that can cause pneumonia. The evidence on the effects of H_2-blockers on the development of VAP is conflicting with some studies saying a definite increased incidence (43), and other reporting no increased risk (44,45) of nosocomial pneumonia. A recently published large randomised study, however, failed to identify an increased risk for pneumonia in either the sucralfate or ranitidine group (46). However, use of sucralfate instead of H_2-blockers provides less efficient anti-ulcer prophylaxis so that the risks have to be well balanced in order to provide cost-effective treatment.

Nasogastric Tubes

Providing adequate enteral nutritional support to intensive care patients is a important point in the prevention of NP. However, it has been suggested that placement of a nasogastric tube in the stomach may facilitate the reflux of bacteria from the gut, and hence be a risk factor for the development of VAP (21). The nasogastric tube does impair the closure of the upper oesophagus sphincter (47) and some investigators have suggested to use smaller nasogastric tubes (48). Ferrer and co-workers compared reflux pattern in intubated and mechanically ventilated patients with a large-bore and a small-bore nasogastric tube (49). They used a radioactive colloid instilled into the stomach to trace gastro-pharyngeal reflux and subsequent microaspiration and found no significant differences between the two types of nasogastric tubes. The results of this study guide prevention measures directly towards better cost-effectiveness, since the standard tube is less expensive than the small-bore device.

Nutritional Support

By impairing host defence, malnutrition has been shown to be a major contributing factor to the development of pneumonia (48,50). Providing adequate nutritional support to intensive care patients is therefore important for the prevention of NP. However, as pointed out above by rising the pH in the stomach, enteral fees may encourage bacterial colonisation and increase the risk of NP. The acidification of the enteral nutrient may results in decrease bacterial colonization of the stomach in critically ill patients. Enteral nutrition is generally preferred to parenteral feeding and is associated with fewer septic complications (51). In addition, enteral feeding could increase the risk of NP when the patient remains in supine body position (28). Some authors suggested the use of oro-jejunal feeding by-passing the stomach as a better way of nutrition in ICU patients (52). Moreover, this measure is associated with increased costs due to the catheter and the control measures required. As general recommendation, early enteral nutrition should be provided to patients in intensive care, initially supplemented by parenteral nutrition when enteral nutrition can only be tolerated in low volumes (51).

Recently the use of immune enhancing feeds enriched with a variety of nutrients including amino acids, arginine, glutamine, and nucleotides has been associated with fewer acquired infections (53). However, whether this measure is cost-effective remains to be proven.

Non-invasive Ventilation

Several recent investigations have attempted to examine directly the influence of eliminating tracheal intubation on the incidence of NP. Nourdine and co-workers report an observational cohort study to determine the influence of different types of ventilatory support on occurrence of NP, and based on their study results, the use of non-invasive positive pressure ventilation, adjusted for severity of the illness, was associated with a lower risk of NP (54). Previous studies of Nava and et al. in patients with chronic obstructive pulmonary disease (55) and Antonelli and colleagues in patients with acute hypoxic respiratory failure (56) also demonstrated a lower incidence of NP. These studies suggest that prevention strategies should include efforts aimed at eliminating or at least reducing the frequency of tracheal intubation. However, it is very important to avoid gastric overdistention during non-invasive mechanical ventilation to reduce the risk of gross aspiration, and thus pneumonia.

Continuous Subglotic Suctioning

Stagnant oropharyngeal secretions pooled above the cuff can easily gain access to lower airways when the pressure of the cuff decreases spontaneously or there is a temporally deflation of the cuff providing in that way a direct route for tracheal colonisation and bolus aspiration from the oropharynx. Endotracheal tubes with an extra lumen designed to suction secretions pooled above endotracheal tube cuffs are available. This have been found able to decrease the incidence of nosocomial pneumonia in mechanically-ventilated patients (57,58).

Maintenance of Ventilator Equipment. Heat and Moisture Exchangers

Although transmission of bacteria via the respirator equipment was identified as a cause of pulmonary infections more than 15 years ago, current systems are rarely a major source of bacteria. Several studies have found no advantage to changing ventilator circuits more frequently than every 48 hours (59). Heat and moisture exchangers reduce the incidence of VAP by minimising the development of condensate within ventilator circuits (60), are well tolerated by most patients and are easy to use. Therefore heat and moisture exchangers should be preferred to heated-water humidificators.

Sterile water should be used for rinsing nebulization devices and other semicritical respiratory-care equipment after they have been cleaned and/or disinfected because of the risk of nosocomial transmission of *Legionella* spp. (61,62).

HIGH-COST MEASURES

Selective Digestive Decontamination (SDD)

Bacterial oropharingeal and gastric colonization is an important aetiopathogenic mechanism to develop VAP. The systematic use of topical antibiotics (usually polymyxin, tobramycin and amphotericin B) in oropharynx and stomach, together with intravenous administration of cefotaxime, has been shown to reduce the incidence of nosocomial pneumonia (63–65), although not all studies have confirmed this finding (66–68). A recent meta-analysis (69) concluded that SDD can reduce respiratory tract infections and overall mortality in critically ill patients. The daily charge for the antibiotics used for SDD has been estimated with U.S. $66.50 in 1992, but additional costs for imperative bacterial surveillance cultures have to be taken into account (70). In the study by Sanchez and coworkers SDD reduced the incidence of VAP, the incidence of nonrespiratory infections, the length of ICU stay and the hospital costs ($11,926 for treated patients versus $16,296 for control-group patients) (71). However, SDD approach has not gained widespread acceptance. Nevertheless, the use of SDD may be appropriate in particular clinical conditions including immunosuppressed patients and those undergoing liver or lung transplantation.

Postural Changes by Rotating Beds

Kinetic therapy that changes the patient's position may also prevent VAP by enhancing pulmonary drainage. Automated position changes during the first five days in the ICU reduced the incidence of early NP in traumatic patients and non-traumatic patients, alike (72,73). However, this form of automated position changes does not reduce significantly the number of days of mechanical ventilation, length of ICU stay or hospital stay, or in-hospital mortality. Nevertheless, rotating beds are much more expensive than standard ICU beds which limit the use of these systems.

Administration of Standard Immune Globulin

Immune-enhancement may reduce the incidence of NP, by reducing translocation and improving host defence. The administration of standard immune globulin (400 mg per kilogram of body weight weekly) in surgical patients reduced the incidence of NP in a placebo controlled study (74). This was especially the case for NP due to Gram-negative bacteria. In addition this measure significantly reduced the number of ICU days and the total days spent in the hospital. However, the use of standard immune globulin should be limited to clinical trials or selected groups of high-risk patients, because of its costs and potential side effects.

Administration of Granulocyte Colony-Stimulating Factor

The presence of neutropenia is associated with an increased risk of both community-acquired and nosocomial infections. Granulocyte colony-stimulating factor (G-CSF) has been found to amplify the immune response by regulating the number and function of neutrophils and may also have a role in prevention nosocomial infections.

In neutropenic patients G-CSF should be administered to patients receiving ventilation who have neutropenic fever in an attempt to decrease the incidence of acquired infections, including VAP (75). However, in non-neutropenic patients, a recent randomised, placebo controlled, clinical study using prophylactic G-CSF in patients with acute traumatic brain injury or cerebral haemorrhage reported no difference in the incidence of NP compared with placebo treated patients (76).

Administration of Cytokines

An immunosuppression is a major factor in the development of NP, the restoration of the adequate immune response may represent an important strategy to prevent nosocomial lung infections. The administration of interferon-γ may restore monocyte function (77), although clinical studies of the effects of prophylactic systemic interferon-γ on infections rates are inconclusive (78).

Interleukin-12, a pro-inflammatory cytokine, can stimulate the Th-1 type immune responses and the administration of interleukin-12 has been shown to protect animals against lung infections (79).

Prophylactic immunomodulating agents represent an exiting area of ongoing research but many more studies are required before any recommendations can be made regarding their routine use in intensive care patients.

SUMMARY

A variety of measures for the prevention of NP have been reviewed according to their costs and mode of action. However, an additional issue has to be taken into account, when the goal is to rank the measures according to cost effectiveness. Not all measures have the same estimated efficacy therefore a "high cost" measure that is proven effective may be more cost effective than an "intermediate cost" measure of uncertain efficacy. We will therefore present the reviewed measures again in tabular form according to the efficacy as it has been proposed by the Center for Diseases Control (CDC) (17). This report comprises three classes of evidence, recommended strategies are based on strong rationale and suggestive evidence, suggested strategies may be supported by suggestive clinical or epidemiologic studies, and no recommendations are given for practices for which insufficient evidence or consensus regarding efficacy exists. However, this report has been published in 1994 and recent evidence has not been reviewed. We therefore indicated also measures that have not been included previously. This table will further help to identify mea-

Table 1. Strategies for Prevention of ventilator-associated Pneumonia. Strategies are classified by cost and on the basis of existing scientific evidence following the CDC recommendations (17).

CDC category	Low Cost No cost associated	Intermediate Cost <50 Euros	High Cost >50 Euros
Recommended strategies	Semirecumbent body position of patients	No use of preventive systemic antibiotic therapy	
	Avoid gastric overdistension	Adequate maintenance of ventilator equipment	
	Hand washing	Use of protective gowns and gloves	
Suggested strategies		Stress-ulcer prophylaxis	Postural changes in rotating beds G-CSF in neutropenics
Unresolved issues	Adjustment of medication	Continuous subglottic suctioning	Selective digestive decontamination
	Type of suction catheter	Type of nasogastric tubes	
	Avoid prolonged nasal intubation		
not mentioned	Adequate cuff pressure	Nutritional support	
	Avoid re-intubation	Non-invasive ventilation	Cytokines
		Chlorhexidine Oral Rinse	Standard immune globulins

G-CSF, granulocyte colony-stimulating factor.

sures that are probably cost effective (e.g., low cost item that is rated recommended strategy, Table 1).

CONCLUSION

The appropriate use of the discussed techniques can reduce the incidence of NP in ICU patients. While simple methods without extra cost as hand washing or placing the patients in semirecumbent position should be part of routine practice, the use of more invasive and expensive preventive measures should be used only in patients who are at high risk of NP. The results of ongoing research, particularly targeting at techniques to modulate immune defence, may strengthen our preventative capabilities and help to limit further the number of patients who currently develop NP with a reduction in medical care costs.

REFERENCES

1. American Thoracic Society. Hospital-acquired pneumonia in adults: Diagnosis, assessment, initial therapy, and prevention: A consensus statement. Am J Respir Crit Care Med 1996;153:1711–1725.
2. Stevens RM, Teres D, Skillman JJ, Feingold DS. Pneumonia in an intensive care unit. Arch Intern Med 1974;134:106–111.
3. Fagon JY, Chastre J, Domart Y, Trouillet JL, Pierre J, Darne C, Gilbert C. Nosocomial pneumonia in patients receiving continuous mechanical ventilation. Prospective analysis of 52 episodes with use of a protected specimen brush and quantitative culture techniques. Am Rev Respir Dis 1989;139: 877–884.
4. Torres A, Aznar R, Gatell JM, Jiménez P, González J, Ferrer M, Celis R, Rodriguez-Roisin R. Incidence, risk, and prognosis factors of nosocomial pneumonia in mechanically ventilated patients. Am Rev Respir Dis 1990;142:523–528.
5. Craven DE, Kuncher LM, Lichtenberg DA, Kollisch NR, Barry MA, Heeren TC, McCabe WR. Nosocomial infection and fatality in medical and surgical intensive care unit patients. Arch Intern Med 1988;148:1161–1168.
6. Kerber AJH, Rommes JH, Mevissen-Verhage EAE, Hulstaert PF, Vos A, Verhoef J. Colonization and infection in surgical intensive care patients. Intensive Care Med 1987;13:347–351.
7. Constantini M, Donisi PM, Turrin MG, Diana L. Hospital acquired infections surveillance and control in intensive care services. Results of an incidence study. Eur J Epidemiol 1987;3:347–355.
8. Craven DE, Kunches LM, Kilinsky V, Lichtenberg DA, Make BJ, McCabe WR. Risk factors for pneumonia and fatality in patients receiving mechanical ventilation. Am Rev Respir Dis 1986;133: 792–796.
9. Kollef MH. Ventilator-associated pneumonia: A multivariate analysis. JAMA 1993;270:1965–1970.
10. Pinner RW, Haley RW, Blumenstein BA, Schaberg DR, Von Allmen SD, McGowan JE Jr. Hight cost nosocomial infection. Infect Control 1982;3:143–149.
11. Beyt BE, Troxler S, Caveness J. Prospective payment and infection control. Infect Control 1985;6: 161–164.
12. Baker AM, Meredith JW, Haponik EF. Pneumonia in intubated trauma patients. Microbiology and outcomes. Am J Respir Crit Care Med 1996;153:343–349.
13. Craig CP, Connelly S. Effect of intensive care unit nosocomial pneumonia on duration of stay and mortality. Am J Infect Control 1984;12:233–238.
14. Jimenez P, Torres A, Rodriguez RR, de-la-Bellacasa JP, Aznar R, Gatell JM, Agusti VA. Incidence and etiology of pneumonia acquired during mechanical ventilation. Crit Care Med 1989;17(9): 882–885.
15. Leu HS, Kaiser DL, Mori M, Woolson RF, Wenzel RP. Hospital-acquired pneumonia. Attributable mortality and morbidity. Am J Epidemiol 1989;129:1258–1267.
16. Fagon JY, Chastre J, Hance AJ, Montravers P, Novara A, Gibert C. Nosocomial pneumonia in ventilated patients: A cohort study evaluating attributable mortality and hospital stay. Am J Med 1993;94: 281–288.
17. Tablan OC, Andreson LJ, Arden NH, Breiman RF, Butler JC, McNeil MM. Guideline for prevention of nosocomial pneumonia. The Hospital Infection Control Practices Advisory Committee, Centers for Disease Control and Prevention. Infect Control Hosp Epidemiol 1994;15:588–625.
18. Doebbeling GN, Stanley GL, Sheetz CT, Pfaller MA, Houston AK, Annis L, Li N, Wenzel RP. Comparative efficacy of alternative hand-washing agents in reducing nosocomial infections in intensice care units. N Engl J Med 1992;327:88–93.
19. Celis R, Torres A, Gatell JM, Almela M, Rodriguez-Roisin R. Nosocomial pneumonia: A multivariate analysis of risk and prognosis. Chest 1988;93:318–324.
20. Rello J, Ausina V, Castella J, Net A, Prats G. Nosocomial respiratory tract infections in multiple trauma patients. Influence of level of consciousness with implications for therapy. Chest 1992;102:525–529.
21. Joshi N, Localio AR, Hamory BH. A predictive index for nosocomial pneumonia in the intensive care unit. Am J Med 1992;93:135–142.
22. Fayon MJ, Tucci M, Lacroix J, et al. Nosocomial pneumonia and thacheitis in a pediatric intensive care unit: a prospective study. Am J Respir Crit Care Med 1997;155:162–169.
23. Trouillet JL, Chastre J, Vuagnat A, Joly-Guillou ML, Combaux D, Dombret MC, Gibert C. Ventilator-associated pneumonia caused by potentially drug-resistant bacteria. Am Rev Respir Dis 1998; 157(2):531–539.
24. Kollef MH, Vlasnik J, Sharpless L, Pasque C, Murphy D, Fraser V. Scheduled change of antibiotic

classes: a strategy to decrease the incidence of ventilator-associated pneumonia. Am J Respir Crit Care Med 1997;156:1040–1048.

25. Torres A, Serra-Batlles J, Ros E, Piera C, Puig de la Bellacasa J, Cobos A, Lomena F, Rodriguez-Roisin R. Pulmonary aspiration of gastric contents in patients receiving mechanical ventilation: the effect of body position. Ann Intern Med 1992;116:540–543.
26. Orozco-Levi M, Torres A, Ferrer M, Piera C, El-Ebiary M, Puig de la Bellacasa J, Rodriguez-Roisin R. Semirecumbent position protects from pulmonary aspiration but not completely from gastroesophageal reflux in mechanically ventilated patients. Am J Respir Crit Care Med 1995;152: 1387–1390.
27. Fernández-Crehuet R, Diáz-Molina C, De Irala J, Martínez-Concha D, Salcedo-Leal I, Masa-Calles J. Nosocomial infection in an intensive-care unit: Identification of risk factors. Infect Control Hosp Epidemiol 1997;18:825–830.
28. Drakulovic M, Torres A, Bauer TT, Nicolas JM, Nogué S, Ferrer M. Supine body position is a risk factor of nosocomial pneumonia in mechanically ventilated patients: a randomised clinical trial. Lancet. In press.
29. Inglis TJ, Sherratt MJ, Sproat LJ, Gibson JS, Hawkey PM. Gastroduodenal dysfunction and bacterial colonisation of the ventilated lung. Lancet 1993;341:911–913.
30. Craven DE, Steger KA. Epidemiology of nosocomial pneumonia: New concepts on an old disease. Chest 1995;108:1S–16S.
31. Rello J, Sonora R, Jubert P, Artigas A, Rue M, Valles J. Pneumonia in intubated patients: Role of respiratory airway care. Am J Respir Crit Care Med 1996;154:111–115.
32. Rouby JJ, Laurent P, Gosnach M, Cambau E, Lamas G, Zouaoui A, Leguillou JL, Dodin L, Khac TD, Marsault C. Risk factors and clinical relevance of nosocomial maxillary sinisitis in the critically ill. Am J Respir Crit Care Med 1994;150:776–783.
33. Torres A, Gatell JM, Aznar R, El-Ebiary M, Puig de la Bellacasa J, González J, Ferrer M, Rodriguez-Roisin R. Re-intubation increases the risk of nosocomial pneumonia in patients needing mechanical ventilation. Am J Respir Crit Care Med 1995;152:137–141.
34. Klein BS, Perloff WH, Maki DG. Reduction of nosocomial infection during pediatric intensive care by protective isolation. N Engl J Med 1989;320:1714–1721.
35. DeRiso AJ II, Ladowski JS, Dillion TA, Justice JW, Peterson AC. Clorhexidine gluconate 0.12% oral rinse reduces the incidence of total nosocomial respiratory infection and nonprophylactic systemic antibiotic use in patients undergoing heart surgery. Chest 1996;109:1556–1561.
36. Rumbak MJ, Cancio MR. Significant reduction in methicillin-resistant Staphylococcus aureus ventilator-associated pneumonia associated with the isntitution of a prevention control. Crit Care Med 1995;23:1200–1203.
37. Sirvent JM, Torres A, El-Ebiary M, Castro P, de Batlle J, Bonet A. Protective effect of intravenously administered cefuroxime against nosocomial pneumonia in patients with structural coma. Am J Respir Crit Care Med 1997;155(5):1729–1734.
38. Bonten MJ, Gaillard CA, van Thiel FH, Smeets HG, van der Geest S, Stobberingh EE. The stomach is not a source for colonization of the upper respiratory tract and pneumonia in ICU patients. Chest 1994;(105):878–884.
39. de Latorre FJ, Pont T, Ferrer A, Rosselló J, Palomar M, Planas M. Pattern of tracheal colonization during mechanical ventilation. Am J Respir Crit Care Med 1995;152:1028–1033.
40. Reusser P, Zimmerli W, Scheideggeder D, Marbet GA, Buser M, Klaus G. Role of gastric colonization in nosocomial infections and endotoxemia: A prospective study in neurosurgical patients on mechanical ventilation. J Infect Dis 1989;160:414–421.
41. Prod hom G, Leuenberger P, Koerfer J, Blum A, Chiolero R, Schaller MD, Perret C, Spinnler O, Blondel J, Siegrist H, Saghaffi L, Blanc D, Francioli P. Nosocomial pneumonia in mechanically ventilated patients receiving antacid, ranitidine, or sucralfate as prophylaxis for stress ulcer. Ann Intern Med 1994;120:653–662.
42. Ewig S, Torres A, El-Ebiary M, Fàbregas N, Hernández C, González J, Nicolas JM, Soto L. Bacterial colonization patterns in mechanically ventilated patients with traumatic and medical head injury. Am J Respir Crit Care Med 1999;159(1):188–198.
43. Apte NM, Karnad DR, Medhekar TP, Tilve GH, Morye S, Bhave GG. Gastric colonization and pneumonia in intubated critically ill patients receiving stress ulcer prophylaxis: a randomized, controlled trial. Crit Care Med 1992;80:590–593.
44. Martin LF, Booth FV, Karlstadt RG. Continuous intravenous cimetidine decreases stress-related gastrointestinal hemorrhage without promoting pneumonia. Crit Care Med 1993;21:19–30.

45. Metz CA, Livingston DH, Smith JS, Larson GM, Wilson TH. Impact of multiple risk factors and ranitidine prophylaxis on the development of stress-related gastrointestinal bleeding: a prospective, multicenter, double-blind randomized trial. Crit Care Med 1993;21:1844–1849.
46. Cook DJ, Guyatt GH, Marshall J, Leasa D, Fuller H, Hall R, Peters S, Rutledge F, Griffith L, McLellan A, Wood G, Kirby A. A comparison of sucralfate and ranitidine for the prevention of upper gastrointestinal bleeding in patients requiring mechanical ventilation. N Engl J Med 1998;338: 791–797.
47. Hardy JF. Large volume gastroesophageal reflux: A rational for risk reduction in the perioperative period. Can J Anaesth 1988;35:162–173.
48. Valles J. Severe pneumonia: sources of infection and implications for treatment. Sepsis 1998;1: 199–209.
49. Ferrer M, Bauer TT, Torres A, Hernández C, Piera C. Gastro-esophgeal reflux and microaspiration to lower airways in intubated patients: Impact of nasogastric tube size. Ann Intern Med 1999;130(12): 991–994.
50. Hanson LC, Weber DJ, Rutala WA. Risk factors for nosocomial pneumonia in the elderly. Am J Med 1992;92:161–166.
51. Heyland DK, Cook DJ, Guyatt GH. Enteral nutrition in the critically ill patient: A critical review of the evidence. Intensive Care Med 1993;19:435–442.
52. Montecalvo MA, Steger KA, Farber HW, Smith BF, Dennis RC, Fitzpatrick GF Pollack S, Korsberg TZ, Birkett DH, Hirsch EF. Nutritional outcome and pneumonia in critical care patients radomized to gastric versus jejunal tube feedings. Crit Care Med 1992;20:1377–1387.
53. Bower RH, Cerra FB, Bershadsky B, Licari JJ, Hoyt DB, Jensen GL, Van Buren CT, Rothkopf MM, Daly JM, Adelsberg BR. early enteral administration of a formula (Impact) supplemented with arginine, nucleotides, and fish oil in intensive care unit patients: results of a multicenter, prospective, randomized trial. Crit Care Med 1995;23:436–449.
54. Nourdine K, Combes P, Carton MJ, Beuret P, Cannamela A, Ducreux JC. Does noninvasive ventilation reduce the ICU nosocomial infection risk? A prospective clinical survey. Intensive Care Med 1999;25:567–573.
55. Nava S, Ambrosini N, Clini E, Prato M, Orlando G, Vitacca M, Brigada P, Fracchia C, Rubini F. Noninvasive mechanical ventilation in the weaning of patients with respiration failure due to chronic obstructive pulmonary disease. A randomized, controlled trial. Ann Intern Med 1998;128:721–728.
56. Antonelli M, Conto G, Rocco M, Bufi M, Deblasi RA, Vivino G, Gasparetto A, Meduri GV. A comparison of noninvasive positive-pressure ventilation and conventional mechanical ventilation in patients with acute respiratory failure. N Engl J Med 1998;339:429–435.
57. Mahul PH, Auboyer C, Jospe R, Ros A, Guerin C, el Khouri Z, Galliez M, Dumont A, Gaudin O. Prevention of nosocomial pneumonia in intubated patients: Respective role of mechanical subglottic secretions drainage and stress ulcer prophylaxis. Intensive Care Med 1992;18:20–25.
58. Vallés J, Artigas A, Rello J. Continuous aspiration of subglottic secretions in preventing ventilator-associated pneumonia. Ann Intern Med 1995;122:179–186.
59. Kollef MH. Prolonged use of ventilator circuits and ventilator-associated pneumonia: a model for identifying clinical practice. Chest 1998;113:267–269.
60. Kirton OC, DeHaven B, Morgan J, Morejon O, Civetta J. A prospective randomized comparison of an in-line heat moisture exchang filter and heated wire humidifiers: rates of ventilator-associated early-onset (community- acquired) or late-onset (hospital-acquired) pneumonia and incidence of endotracheal tube occlusion. Chest 1997;112:1055–1059.
61. Mastro TD, Fields BS, Breiman RF, Campbell J, Plikaytis BD, Spika JS. Nosocomial Legionnaires' disease and use of medication nebulizers. J Infect Dis 1991;163:667–670.
62. Alary MA, Joly JR. Factors contributing to the contamination of hospital water distribution systems by Legionellae. J Infect Dis 1992;165:565–569.
63. Abele-Horn M, Dauber A, Bauernfeind A, Russwurm W Seyfarh-Metzger I, Gleich P, Ruckdeschel G. Decrease in nosocomial pneumonia in ventilated patients by selective oropharyngeal decontamination. Intensive Care Med 1997;23:187–195.
64. Vandenbroucke-Grauls CM, Vandenbroucke JP. Effect of selective decontamination of the digestive tract on respiratory tract infections and mortality in the intensive care unit. Lancet 1991;338: 859–862.
65. Cockerill FRI, Muller SR, Ahnalt JP, Marsh HM, Farnell MB, Mucha P, Gillespie DJ, Ilstrup DM, Larson-Keller JJ, Thompson RL. Prevention of infection in critically ill patients by selective decontamination of the digestive tract. Ann Intern Med 1992;117:545–553.

66. Ferrer M, Torres A, González J, Puig de la Bellacasa J, El-Ebiary M, Roca M, Gatell JM, Rodriguez-Roisin R. Utility of selective digestive decontamination in mechanically ventilated patients. Ann Intern Med 1994;120(5):389–395.
67. Wiener J, Itozaku G, Nathan C, Kabins SA, Weinstein RA. A randomized, double-blind, placebo-controled trial of selective digestive decontamination in a medical-surgical intensive care unit. Clin Infect Dis 1995;20:861–867.
68. Hammond JM, Potgieter PD, Saunders GL, Forder AA. Double-blind study of selective decontamination of the digestive tract in intensive care. Lancet 1992;340:5–9.
69. D'Amico R, Pifferi S, Leonetti C, Torri V, Tinazzi A, Liberati A. Effectiveness of antibiotic prophylaxis in critically ill adult patients. BMJ 1998;316:1275–1285.
70. Gastinne H, Wolff M, Delatour F, Faurisson F, Chevret S. A controled trial in intensive care units of selective decontamination af the digestive tract with nonabsorbable antibiotics. N Engl J Med 1992;326:594–599.
71. Sanchez Garcia M, Cambronero Galache JA, Lopez Diaz J, Cerda Cerda E, Rubio Blasco J, Gomez Aguinaga MA, Nunez Reiz A, Rogero Marin S, Sacristan del Castillo JA. Effectiveness and cost of selective decontamination of the digestive tract in critically ill intubated patients. A randomized, double-blind, placebo-controlled, multicenter trial. Am J Respir Crit Care Med 1998;158(3): 908–916.
72. de Boisblanc BP, Castro M, Everret B, Grender J, Walker CD, Summer WR. Effect of air-supported, continuous, postural oscillation on the risk of early ICU pneumonia in nontraumatic critical illness. Chest 1993;103(5):1543–1547.
73. Nelson LD, Choi SC. Kinetic therapy in critically ill trauma patients. Clin Intensive Care 1992;37: 248–252.
74. The Intravenous Immunoglobulin Collaborative Study Group. Prophylactic intravenous administration of standard immune globulin as compared with core-lipopolysaccharide immune globulin in patients at high risk of postsurgical infection. N Engl J Med 1992;327(4):234–240.
75. Maher DW, Lieschke GJ, Green M, Bishop J, Stuart-Harris R, Wolf M, Sheridan WP, Kefford RF, Cebon J, Olver I. Filgastrim in patients with chemotherapy-induced febrile neutropenia: a double-blind, placebo-controlled trial. Ann Intern Med 1994;121:492–501.
76. Heard SO, Fink MP, Gamelli RL, Solimkin JS, Joshi M, Trask AL, Fabian TC, Hudson LD, Gerold KB, Logan ED. Effect of prophylactic administration of recombinant human granulocyte colony-stimulating factor (filgastrim) on the frequency of nosocomial infections in patients with acute traumatic brain injury or cerebral haemorrhage. Crit Care Med 1998;26:748–754.
77. Docke WD, Randow F, Syrbe HP, Krausch D, Asadullah K, Reinke P, Volk HD, Kox W. Monocyte deactivation in septic patients: restoration by INF-gamma treatment. Nature Med 1997;3:678–681.
78. Dries DJ, Jurkovich GJ, Maier RV, Clemmer TP, Struve SN, Weigelt JA, Stanford GG, Herr DL, Champion HR, Lewis FR. Effect of interferon gamma on infection-related death in patients with severe injuries. A randomized, double-blind, placebo-controlled trial. Arch Surg 1994;129:1031–1041.
79. Greenberger MJ, Kunkel SL, Strieter RM, Lukacs NW, Brmson J, Gauldie J, Graham FL, Hitt M, Danforth JM, Standiford TJ. IL-12 gene therapy protects mice in lethal *Klebsiella* pneumonia. J Immunol 1996;157:3006–3012.

14. CROSS-COLONIZATION IN INTENSIVE CARE UNITS: FACT OR FICTION?

MATTHEW SAMORE, M.D.

University of Utah, Salt Lake City, UT 84132 USA

INTRODUCTION

The central issue addressed in this chapter is the origin of microorganisms colonizing patients in the intensive care unit (ICU) (1). To what extent are organisms acquired in the ICU via patient-to-patient transmission and to what extent are they brought into the ICU because of pre-existing colonization? These questions could equally well be directed toward other types of settings such as non-ICU acute-care wards or extended care facilities. The underlying characteristics that establish the dynamics of microbial transmission within an ICU population—a) entry into and discharge from a geographically-confined area of persons who are ill, receive antibiotics and other gastrointestinal flora-altering medications, and undergo invasive procedures; and b) a work-force of caregivers who inadvertently serve as vectors for transmission of microorganisms via transient hand carriage—are also operational in other epidemiologic settings. The distinction of the ICU is that it is the environment where the factors which promote spread and acquisition of microorganisms are most highly concentrated.

SOURCES OF COLONIZATION

Most infections acquired in ICUs are caused by organisms that attach to and occupy ecologic niches on mucosal body surfaces or the skin before causing invasive disease (2). As such, colonization can be viewed as a critical intermediate step prior to inva-

R.A. Weinstein and M.J.M. Bonten (eds.). INFECTION CONTROL IN THE ICU ENVIRONMENT.

sive disease. Only a minority of individuals colonized with these organisms ever manifest overt disease, a phenomenon which is often referred to as the iceberg effect (3). As a corollary, asymptomatically colonized individuals are presumed to be the source of most transmission-events in the ICU.

Every patient admitted to the ICU at the outset carries enormous numbers of endogenous microbial flora, which live in diverse anatomic sites such as the alimentary, upper respiratory, and genitourinary tracts as well as the skin (4,5). When an organism is found to be associated with a clinical infection, the difficulty is in determining whether the organism was originally part of the endogenous flora or acquired subsequent to admission (1). To the degree that patient-to-patient transmission contributes to colonization with pathogens associated with symptomatic infection and with increased antibiotic resistance, programs that focus on limiting cross-colonization should rise in priority. On the other hand, if cross-colonization is not a frequent event in ICUs, interventions directed toward reducing host susceptibility or altering other modifiable individual risk factors may be more deserving of resources and investigation.

It is worth noting that organisms may be endogenous with respect to the ICU, that is, present on admission to the ICU, but exogenous with respect to another part of the hospital where acquisition may have taken place prior to ICU transfer. It should also be kept in mind that not every potential transmission event is associated with clinical harm. For instance, if an endogenous strain of *Escherichia coli* in an individual's alimentary tract is replaced by an exogenous, but equally susceptible, *E. coli* strain, the effect is presumably neutral. One could even envision a situation where cross-transmission would be advantageous, if the circulating organism lowered the risk of acquisition of a more pathogenic organism. For instance, there are some data to suggest that non-toxigenic *C. difficile* may be protective against infection due to virulent, toxigenic *C. difficile* strains (6). If this strategy ever proved to be effective and safe in humans, the spread of non-toxigenic strains within the hospital via cross-colonization could be beneficial.

EVIDENCE FOR AND AGAINST CROSS-COLONIZATION

The most abundant, albeit indirect evidence, for cross-colonization in ICUs comes from descriptive analyses of data from clinical microbiology laboratories (table 1). The distribution of organisms recovered from ICU patients differs substantially, with respect to both species categories and antibiotic susceptibility patterns, from the distribution of organisms recovered from patients housed in non-ICU wards and even more so from healthy individuals in the community (7,8). The longer the interval of time from admission to recovery of the organism the more divergent the type of organism, relative to the community setting.

In general, pathogens associated with infection in ICUs are more likely to be antibiotic resistant than organisms that cause infection in other populations (9–11). There also is a shift toward greater frequency of aerobic gram negative rods and *Candida sp* as causes of bloodstream infection, pneumonia, and other categories of infection (12,13). However, the limitation of these comparisons is that they do not

Table 1. Evidence for and against role of cross-colonization in intensive care units (ICUs)

Type of evidence	Interpretation of results	Limitations
Comparison of organisms associated with infections in ICUs versus other settings	Support concept that a distinctive ICU flora exists	Source of organisms not discerned
Molecular typing of organisms associated with outbreaks	Illustrate potential of many kinds of organisms to spread either from environmental reservoirs or presumptively via health care worker hands	Average or usual frequency of cross-colonization not addressed
Molecular typing of clinical isolates during non-outbreak periods	Demonstrate diversity of strains, particularly gram negative rods	Sources of transmission may be missed if comprehensive surveillance cultures not done
Serial surveillance cultures	Verify that some resistant flora are found on admission while others are acquired in the ICU	Does acquisition always indicate cross-colonization?
Cultures of health care worker hands	Indicate the transferability of microorganisms to health care worker hands during routine patient care activities	Potential for cross-colonization demonstrated but not necessarily its frequency
Trials of improved handwashing or stricter barrier precautions	Have not yet provided strong causal evidence of magnitude of benefit	Studies have had limited power; successful implementation of intervention difficult

address the source of organisms. Increased resistance could be due to emergence of resistance during antibiotic therapy rather than cross-colonization. The increased rate of gram negative infection could be attributed to enhanced host susceptibility to infection because of invasive devices and altered patterns of colonization, for instance, transfer of endogenous gastrointestinal flora to the oropharygneal tract (14).

Knowledge about organism biology and genetics can be useful for evaluating the plausibility of these various explanations. For instance, emergence of resistance during antibiotic therapy is feasible for *Enterobacter cloacae*, *E. aerogenes*, *Serratia marcescens*, and *Citrobacter freundii*, organisms which have the capacity to become resistant to non-carbepenem beta-lactam antibiotics as a result of a single mutation that de-represses production of ampC beta-lactamase, and for *Pseudomonas aeruginosa*, which also has the capacity to become resistant on the basis of a single mutation and often exists as multiple subpopulations (15,16). In contrast, de novo emergence from endogenous strains is much less likely, and exogenous acquisition more likely, for vancomycin-resistant enterococci (VRE) and methicillin-resistant *S. aureus* (MRSA), because a new set of genes acting in concert is necessary for the resistant phenotype to become manifest (17). In the case of VRE, even though these genes may be delivered into endogenous strains on plasmids, an exogenous source of the resistance plasmid is still needed, and hence transmission from another individual is likely if the patient was not already colonized with VRE on admission.

The application of molecular typing techniques has been critically important in the evaluating the potential for microorganisms to spread between individuals within ICUs. Many ICU-based outbreaks have been described where an analysis of DNA restriction profiles strongly suggested patient-to-patient dissemination of a microorganism. These studies suggest that a myriad of species are capable of cross-colonization, ranging from bacteria such as coagulase negative staphylococci which are normal skin colonizers to species such as *Acinetobacter baumanii* which are rarely associated with disease or colonization outside of the hospital setting (18–30). These investigations have also been useful for identifying mechanisms of cross-colonization, particularly when personnel and environmental cultures are employed. However, these studies do not address the occurrence of cross-colonization apart from the special circumstance of a reported outbreak. Robust data on the average number of well-defined outbreaks that are attributable to cross-colonization per ICU per year are lacking (31,32).

Molecular analyses of organisms recovered from clinically-directed cultures or from point prevalence surveys have yielded useful but less-than-definitive information about cross-colonization during non-outbreak periods. An extreme diversity of types or, alternatively, a lack of epidemiologic links between the few patients who harbor the same type, argue against patient-to-patient transmission, although to the extent that the population of individuals colonized with the flora of interest are incompletely captured, this conclusion is weakened (33–35). For instance, if only isolates recovered from clinical cultures are analyzed it is possible that molecular types which appear to be unique and therefore of endogenous origin are in fact acquired from asymptomatically colonized contacts.

STUDIES UTILIZING SERIAL SURVEILLANCE CULTURES

To address sources of colonization more thoroughly, the laborious and resource-intensive approach of performing serial surveillance cultures in a patient cohort is necessary, to determine which organisms are present on admission and which are newly acquired. The proportion of organisms of a particular category that are acquired, coupled with the risk of disease after acquisition, provides an estimate of the fraction of symptomatic infections due to the organism which might be directly prevented by elimination of cross-colonization. This formulation assumes that each acquisition event represents an instance of direct or indirect patient-to-patient transmission. In some studies, the inference of cross-colonization is only made when the patient with the acquired strain is temporo-spatially linked to another patient with the same strain (36,37). It should be kept in mind, however, that operational criteria to define transmission always involve an element of probabilistic inference. Regardless of the molecular epidemiology or whether a likely source of the acquired strain is identified, pinpointing the moment of contact or transmission is virtually never possible. Even the question of whether the transmission event took place in the ICU is difficult to prove. The critical contact with a contaminated individual may have occurred when the patient was transported elsewhere in the hospital for a test or procedure. Another caveat is that exposure to a common environmental reservoir, the contamination of which may have been external to the ICU, can closely mimic patient-to-patient transmission with respect to geographic clustering and similarity of molecular types.

Defining acquisition on the basis of serial cultures has additional limitations due to sampling error. For instance, even selective culture techniques to detect small numbers of resistant enterococci in stool cultures do not have 100% sensitivity (38,39). The consequence of a less-than-perfect assay is misclassification in both directions. Patients who were falsely negative on their baseline culture may be misidentified as representing acquisition if follow-up cultures are positive. Alternatively, patients who acquire the organism during their hospital stay may have falsely negative follow-up cultures.

Despite these imperfections, the serial surveillance culture study design remains better than the alternatives. Studies relying on serial surveillance cultures have generally focused on patients within a single institution and monitored a restricted subset of organisms. Organisms most often studied in ICU and non-ICU acute care settings include VRE, *Clostridium difficile*, MRSA, *Candida sp.*, and aerobic gram negative rods, particularly those that are resistant to broad spectrum beta-lactam antibiotics (29,40–51). In studies that applied this methodology to VRE in cohorts of ICU patients, the prevalence of VRE colonization at the time of ICU admission varied from 12 to 15% and the cumulative incidence of acquisition among patients not already colonized on admission varied from 13% to 41% (42,43,52). Molecular typing analyses supported the hypothesis that acquisition predominantly occurred as a result of cross-colonization. Patients who were colonized with VRE at the time of ICU admission presumably either acquired the organism in non-ICU wards (53,54), or less likely, had been VRE colonized prior to hospitalization.

For gram negative rods, results have pointed toward a greater role of endogenous colonization. A substantial fraction of resistant organisms either colonized patients at the time of ICU admission or emerged from endogenous strains as a consequence of antibiotic selection pressure. Studies of *P. aeruginosa* and *E. cloacae* conducted in the 1980s suggested that even when these organisms were acquired following ICU admission, cross-colonization was often not the mechanism of acquisition (36,37). In a more recent study, 18% of patients were colonized with ceftazidime-resistant gram negative rods at the time of admission and 26% of patients with negative baseline cultures who underwent follow-up cultures acquired ceftazidime-resistant gram negative rods (44). However, in 21% of instances of acquisition, it was possible to document that the same strain, albeit susceptible, had been present on admission (55). Studies of broad spectrum beta-lactam resistant gram negative rods in other ICU settings, such as a pediatric hospital, have also suggested a primary role of endogenous colonization (41,56,57). A major exception appears to be extended-spectrum beta-lactamase producing *Klebsiella pneumoniae*. In an extended study at a French hospital, patient-to-patient spread was the dominant mechanism of colonization (58).

Except in the situation of a common, external environmental source, transmission of an organism depends on the presence of other individuals with the organism. If no patients with VRE exist within an institution or population, transmission of VRE will not occur. The mass action principle of transmission-dynamic theory predicts that rate of occurrence of new infections among susceptible members of the population will be a function of the proportion of infected individuals in the population. Empirical data on VRE from a study performed at Cook County Hospital support this hypothesis (59). Colonization pressure was defined as the average point prevalence of VRE colonization in the ICU from admission until acquisition of VRE or discharge. In a Cox proportional hazards regression model, colonization pressure was a significant predictor of acquisition of VRE (59).

MECHANISMS OF CROSS-COLONIZATION

Health care worker hand carriage is the most plausible and well-supported mechanism of cross-colonization (60,61). It has been demonstrated on many occasions that health care worker hands are readily contaminated with pathogenic microorganisms following patient care activities or, alternatively, from touching environmental surfaces in patient rooms (62–65). It is more difficult to directly link health care worker hand contamination to acquisition of the same organism by exposed patients. The most definitive studies were conducted in the 1960s in which it was demonstrated that antiseptic handwashing largely prevented the high rate of transmission of *S. aureus* to infants by colonized health care workers (66,67). Another study published in the 1970s found high rates of *Klebsiella* hand carriage among health care workers and that increased handwashing rates were associated with a sustained reduction in frequency of *Klebsiella* colonization in patients (68).

The mediation of organism transmission by health care workers bears some similarity to vector-borne infections such as malaria with respect to population dynamics and spread (69). A health care worker is contaminated by contact with an infected patient and in turn transmits the organism to an uninfected patient during the period of transient hand colonization. The prediction from transmission models is that the average number of secondary cases per primary case will be proportional to the square of the average contact rate between health care workers and patients (69). This carries the implication that interventions which alter worker-patient contact patterns such as nurse cohorting will be particularly effective control measures, a forecast that has not yet been adequately confirmed by empirical data.

Contamination of environmental surfaces promotes cross-colonization either by acting as a source for personnel hand carriage (65) or, for some types of objects such as electronic rectal thermometers, by coming in direct contact with multiple patients (70). It is likely environmental contamination plays a more important role for certain types of organisms than others. Contamination of room surfaces with enterococci and *C. difficile* has generally been more commonly found than contamination with enteric gram negative rods and *S. aureus* (65,71–74). Patients with diarrhea appear to contaminate the room environment more heavily than patients who do not have diarrhea (65,75). Gram negative rods, particularly non-fermenting organisms such as *Stenotrophomoas maltophilia*, *Acinetobacter sp.*, and *Pseudomonas sp.*, are prone to colonize liquid reservoirs associated with equipment, such as ventilator tubing, resuscitation bags, and nebulizers (76–79). The contribution of these environmental reservoirs to patient acquisition has been most clearly demonstrated in the context of outbreaks.

Apart from the special outbreak settings described above, direct links between contaminated environmental surfaces and subsequent patient acquisition are infrequently found. Environmental contamination in the room is rarely documented prior to acquisition of the environmental strain by the patient housed in the room (43,65). Thus, the evidence that environmental contamination contributes to patient-to-patient transmission is still often indirect and circumstantial.

EFFECT OF MEASURES TO REDUCE CROSS-COLONIZATION

It is clear that with rates of handwashing compliance typically less than 50%, opportunities exist to reduce personnel hand carriage and therefore transmission mediated by health care workers. Most studies that attempted to demonstrate benefits of improved handwashing in ICUs yielded relatively weak causal evidence because of limitations in study design (60). A major problem is that it has been remarkably difficult to achieve sustained improvement in handwashing compliance (80). For instance, in a cross-over trial comparing chlorhexidine and alcohol-based hand antisepsis, even though healthcare workers attended educational programs and knew their practices were being monitored, overall compliance with handwashing was still less than 50% (81,82). More recent studies targeting health care worker compliance with infection control guidelines have reported greater success at inducing change in behavior, so there is reason for cautious optimism (83,84).

In studies of other types of interventions in ICUs such as imposition of barrier precautions, benefits have also not been conclusively demonstrated. One trial conducted in a pediatric ICU found that children randomized to protective isolation had lower nosocomial infection rates than children receiving standard care (85). Another study conducted in a different setting failed to find a significant difference between universal glove and gown use together and glove use alone with respect to nosocomial acquisition of VRE in the ICU (42).

CONCLUSION

Cross-colonization occurs in ICUs but there are many unresolved questions. The most important and clinically relevant unanswered question pertains to the effect of better control of cross-colonization in ICUs, on either antibiotic resistance or on nosocomial infection rates. It is probably only in the context of carefully done experimental studies of effectively implemented interventions across multiple medical centers that the question of the frequency and importance of cross-colonization can be unambiguously resolved. It is possible that infection control measures will need to be coupled with changes in other practices such as antibiotic prescribing for benefits on antibiotic resistance to be fully realized (86). These trials will be costly and difficult to implement but the dividends are likely to be substantial.

REFERENCE LIST

1. Bonten MJ, Weinstein RA. The role of colonization in the pathogenesis of nosocomial infections. Infect Control Hosp Epidemiol 1996;17:193–200.
2. Boyce JM. Treatment and control of colonization in the prevention of nosocomial infections. Infect Control Hosp Epidemiol 1996;17:256–261.
3. Weinstein RA. Epidemiology and control of nosocomial infections in adult intensive care units. Am J Med 1991;91:179S–184S.
4. Niederman MS. Gram-negative colonization of the respiratory tract: pathogenesis and clinical consequences. Semin Respir Infect 1990;5:173–184.
5. Nord CE. Studies on the ecological impact of antibiotics. Eur J Clin Microbiol Infect Dis 1990;9:517–518.
6. Shim JK, Johnson S, Samore MH, Bliss DZ, Gerding DN. Primary symptomless colonisation by Clostridium difficile and decreased risk of subsequent diarrhoea. Lancet 1998;351:633–636.
7. Flaherty JP, Weinstein RA. Nosocomial infection caused by antibiotic-resistant organisms in the intensive-care unit. Infect Control Hosp Epidemiol 1996;17:236–248.
8. Fridkin SK, Steward CD, Edwards JR, Pryor ER, McGowan JEJ, Archibald LK, et al. Surveillance of antimicrobial use and antimicrobial resistance in United States hospitals: project ICARE phase 2. Project Intensive Care Antimicrobial Resistance Epidemiology (ICARE) hospitals. Clin Infect Dis 1999;29:245–252.
9. Weber DJ, Raasch R, Rutala WA. Nosocomial infections in the ICU: the growing importance of antibiotic-resistant pathogens. Chest 1999;115:34S–41S.
10. Archibald L, Phillips L, Monnet D, McGowan JEJ, Tenover F, Gaynes R. Antimicrobial resistance in isolates from inpatients and outpatients in the United States: increasing importance of the intensive care unit. Clin Infect Dis 1997;24:211–215.
11. Jarlier V, Fosse T, Philippon A. Antibiotic susceptibility in aerobic gram-negative bacilli isolated in intensive care units in 39 French teaching hospitals (ICU study). Intensive Care Med 1996;22:1057–1065.
12. Jarvis WR. Epidemiology of nosocomial fungal infections, with emphasis on Candida species. Clin Infect Dis 1995;20:1526–1530.
13. Richards MJ, Edwards JR, Culver DH, Gaynes RP. Nosocomial infections in medical intensive care units in the United States. National Nosocomial Infections Surveillance System. Crit Care Med 1999;27:887–892.
14. Bonten MJ, Gaillard CA, de Leeuw PW, Stobberingh EE. Role of colonization of the upper intestinal tract in the pathogenesis of ventilator-associated pneumonia. Clin Infect Dis 1997;24:309–319.
15. Livermore DM. beta-Lactamases in laboratory and clinical resistance. Clin Microbiol Rev 1995;8:557–584.
16. Bush K, Jacoby GA, Medeiros AA. A functional classification scheme for beta-lactamases and its correlation with molecular structure. Antimicrob Agents Chemother 1995;39:1211–1233.
17. Gold HS, Moellering RCJ. Antimicrobial-drug resistance. N Engl J Med 1996;335:1445–1453.
18. John JFJ, Grieshop TJ, Atkins LM, Platt CG. Widespread colonization of personnel at a Veterans Affairs medical center by methicillin-resistant, coagulase-negative Staphylococcus. Clin Infect Dis 1993;17:380–388.
19. Nystrom B, Ransjo U, Ringertz S, Faxelius G, Tunell R, Ohman G, et al. Colonization with coagulase-negative staphylococci in two neonatal units. J Hosp Infect 1992;22:287–298.
20. Cook LN, Davis RS, Stover BH. Outbreak of amikacin-resistant Enterobacteriaceae in an intensive care nursery. Pediatrics 1980;65:264–268.

21. Mutton KJ, Brady LM, Harkness JL. Serratia cross-infection in an intensive therapy unit. J Hosp Infect 1981;2:85–91.
22. Rutala WA, Kennedy VA, Loflin HB, Sarubbi FAJ. Serratia marcescens nosocomial infections of the urinary tract associated with urine measuring containers and urinometers. Am J Med 1981;70:659–663.
23. Husni RN, Goldstein LS, Arroliga AC, Hall GS, Fatica C, Stoller JK, et al. Risk factors for an outbreak of multi-drug-resistant Acinetobacter nosocomial pneumonia among intubated patients. Chest 1999;115:1378–1382.
24. Lortholary O, Fagon JY, Buu HA, Mahieu G, Gutmann L. Colonization by Acinetobacter baumanii in intensive-care-unit patients. Infect Control Hosp Epidemiol 1998;19:188–190.
25. Harbarth S, Sudre P, Dharan S, Cadenas M, Pittet D. Outbreak of Enterobacter cloacae related to understaffing, overcrowding, and poor hygiene practices. Infect Control Hosp Epidemiol 1999;20:598–603.
26. Herra CM, Knowles SJ, Kaufmann ME, Mulvihill E, McGrath B, Keane CT. An outbreak of an unusual strain of Serratia marcescens in two Dublin hospitals. J Hosp Infect 1998;39:135–141.
27. Meier PA, Carter CD, Wallace SE, Hollis RJ, Pfaller MA, Herwaldt LA. A prolonged outbreak of methicillin-resistant Staphylococcus aureus in the burn unit of a tertiary medical center. Infect Control Hosp Epidemiol 1996;17:798–802.
28. Tilley PA, Roberts FJ. Bacteremia with Acinetobacter species: risk factors and prognosis in different clinical settings. Clin Infect Dis 1994;18:896–900.
29. Vazquez JA, Dembry LM, Sanchez V, Vazquez MA, Sobel JD, Dmuchowski C, et al. Nosocomial Candida glabrata colonization: an epidemiologic study. J Clin Microbiol 1998;36:421–426.
30. Widmer AF, Wenzel RP, Trilla A, Bale MJ, Jones RN, Doebbeling BN. Outbreak of Pseudomonas aeruginosa infections in a surgical intensive care unit: probable transmission via hands of a health care worker. Clin Infect Dis 1993;16:372–376.
31. Wenzel RP, Reagan DR, Bertino JSJ, Baron EJ, Arias K. Methicillin-resistant Staphylococcus aureus outbreak: a consensus panel's definition and management guidelines. Am J Infect Control 1998;26:102–110.
32. Wenzel RP, Thompson RL, Landry SM, Russell BS, Miller PJ, Ponce dL, et al. Hospital-acquired infections in intensive care unit patients: an overview with emphasis on epidemics. Infect Control 1983;4:371–375.
33. Samore MH, Bettin KM, DeGirolami PC, Clabots CR, Gerding DN, Karchmer AW. Wide diversity of Clostridium difficile types at a tertiary referral hospital. J Infect Dis 1994;170:615–621.
34. Chetchotisakd P, Phelps CL, Hartstein AI. Assessment of bacterial cross-transmission as a cause of infections in patients in intensive care units. Clin Infect Dis 1994;18:929–937.
35. Sabria-Leal M, Pfaller MA, Morthland VH, Young SA, Hollis RJ, Werkmeister L, et al. Molecular epidemiology of gastric colonization by Enterococcus faecalis in a surgical intensive care unit. Diagn Microbiol Infect Dis 1994;19:197–202.
36. Flynn DM, Weinstein RA, Nathan C, Gaston MA, Kabins SA. Patients' endogenous flora as the source of "nosocomial" Enterobacter in cardiac surgery. J Infect Dis 1987;156:363–368.
37. Olson B, Weinstein RA, Nathan C, Chamberlin W, Kabins SA. Epidemiology of endemic Pseudomonas aeruginosa: why infection control efforts have failed. J Infect Dis 1984;150:808–816.
38. Roger M, Faucher MC, Forest P, St-Antoine P, Coutlee F. Evaluation of a vanA-specific PCR assay for detection of vancomycin-resistant Enterococcus faecium during a hospital outbreak. J Clin Microbiol 1999;37:3348–3349.
39. Satake S, Clark N, Rimland D, Nolte FS, Tenover FC. Detection of vancomycin-resistant enterococci in fecal samples by PCR. J Clin Microbiol 1997;35:2325–2330.
40. Schimpff SC, Young VM, Greene WH, Vermeulen GD, Moody MR, Wiernik PH. Origin of infection in acute nonlymphocytic leukemia. Significance of hospital acquisition of potential pathogens. Ann Intern Med 1972;77:707–714.
41. Toltzis P, Yamashita T, Vilt L, Green M, Morrissey A, Spinner-Block S, et al. Antibiotic restriction does not alter endemic colonization with resistant gram-negative rods in a pediatric intensive care unit. Crit Care Med 1998;26:1893–1899.
42. Slaughter S, Hayden MK, Nathan C, Hu TC, Rice T, van Voorhis J, et al. A comparison of the effect of universal use of gloves and gowns with that of glove use alone on acquisition of vancomycin-resistant enterococci in a medical intensive care unit. Ann Intern Med 1996;125:448–456.

43. Bonten MJ, Hayden MK, Nathan C, van Voorhis J, Matushek M, Slaughter S, et al. Epidemiology of colonisation of patients and environment with vancomycin-resistant enterococci. Lancet 1996;348:1615–1619.
44. D'Agata E, Venkataraman L, DeGirolami P, Burke P, Eliopoulos G, Karchmer AW, et al. Colonization with broad spectrum cephalosporin-resistant gram negative bacilli during a non-outbreak period: Prevalence, risk factors, and rate of infection. Crit Care Med 1999;
45. McFarland LV, Mulligan ME, Kwok RY, Stamm WE. Nosocomial acquisition of Clostridium difficile infection. N Engl J Med 1989;320:204–210.
46. Samore MH, DeGirolami PC, Tlucko A, Lichtenberg DA, Melvin ZA, Karchmer AW. Clostridium difficile colonization and diarrhea at a tertiary care hospital. Clin Infect Dis 1994;18:181–187.
47. Clabots CR, Johnson S, Olson MM, Peterson LR, Gerding DN. Acquisition of Clostridium difficile by hospitalized patients: evidence for colonized new admissions as a source of infection. J Infect Dis 1992;166:561–567.
48. Girou E, Pujade G, Legrand P, Cizeau F, Brun-Buisson C. Selective screening of carriers for control of methicillin-resistant Staphylococcus aureus (MRSA) in high-risk hospital areas with a high level of endemic MRSA. Clin Infect Dis 1998;27:543–550.
49. Bergmans DC, Bonten MJ, van Tiel FH, Gaillard CA, van der Geest S, Wilting RM, et al. Cross-colonisation with Pseudomonas aeruginosa of patients in an intensive care unit. Thorax 1998;53:1053–1058.
50. Pena C, Pujol M, Ricart A, Ardanuy C, Ayats J, Linares J, et al. Risk factors for faecal carriage of Klebsiella pneumoniae producing extended spectrum beta-lactamase (ESBL-KP) in the intensive care unit. J Hosp Infect 1997;35:9–16.
51. Arbo MD, Hariharan R, Nathan C, Barefoot L, Weinstein RA, Snydman DR. Utility of serial rectal swab cultures for detection of ceftazidime- and imipenem-resistant gram-negative bacilli from patients in the intensive care unit. Eur J Clin Microbiol Infect Dis 1998;17:727–730.
52. Ostrowsky BE, Venkataraman L, D'Agata EM, Gold HS, DeGirolami PC, Samore MH. Vancomycin-resistant enterococci in intensive care units: high frequency of stool carriage during a non-outbreak period. Arch Intern Med 1999;159:1467–1472.
53. Bonten MJ, Slaughter S, Hayden MK, Nathan C, van Voorhis J, Weinstein RA. External sources of vancomycin-resistant enterococci for intensive care units. Crit Care Med 1998;26:2001–2004.
54. Farr BM. Hospital wards spreading vancomycin-resistant enterococci to intensive care units: returning coals to Newcastle. Crit Care Med 1998;26:1942–1943.
55. D'Agata E, Venkataraman L, DeGirolami P, Samore M. Molecular epidemiology of acquisition of ceftazidime-resistant gram-negative bacilli in a nonoutbreak setting. J Clin Microbiol 1997;35:2602–2605.
56. Bonten MJ, Bergmans DC, Speijer H, Stobberingh EE. Characteristics of polyclonal endemicity of Pseudomonas aeruginosa colonization in intensive care units. Implications for infection control. Am J Respir Crit Care Med 1999;160:1212–1219.
57. Toltzis P, Yamashita T, Vilt L, Blumer JL. Colonization with antibiotic-resistant gram-negative organisms in a pediatric intensive care unit. Crit Care Med 1997;25:538–544.
58. Decre D, Gachot B, Lucet JC, Arlet G, Bergogne-Berezin E, Regnier B. Clinical and bacteriologic epidemiology of extended-spectrum beta-lactamase-producing strains of Klebsiella pneumoniae in a medical intensive care unit. Clin Infect Dis 1998;27:834–844.
59. Bonten MJ, Slaughter S, Ambergen AW, Hayden MK, van Voorhis J, Nathan C, et al. The role of "colonization pressure" in the spread of vancomycin-resistant enterococci: an important infection control variable. Arch Intern Med 1998;158:1127–1132.
60. Larson E. Skin hygiene and infection prevention: more of the same or different approaches? Clin Infect Dis 1999;29:1287–1294.
61. Bauer TM, Ofner E, Just HM, Just H, Daschner FD. An epidemiological study assessing the relative importance of airborne and direct contact transmission of microorganisms in a medical intensive care unit. J Hosp Infect 1990;15:301–309.
62. Ehrenkranz NJ, Alfonso BC. Failure of bland soap handwash to prevent hand transfer of patient bacteria to urethral catheters. Infect Control Hosp Epidemiol 1991;12:654–662.
63. Ehrenkranz NJ. Bland soap handwash or hand antisepsis? The pressing need for clarity. Infect Control Hosp Epidemiol 1992;13:299–301.
64. Eckert DG, Ehrenkranz NJ, Alfonso BC. Indications for alcohol or bland soap in removal of aerobic

gram-negative skin bacteria: assessment by a novel method. Infect Control Hosp Epidemiol 1989;10:306–311.
65. Samore MH, Venkataraman L, DeGirolami PC, Arbeit RD, Karchmer AW. Clinical and molecular epidemiology of sporadic and clustered cases of nosocomial Clostridium difficile diarrhea. Am J Med 1996;100:32–40.
66. Mortimer EAJ, Wolinsky E, Hines D. The effect of rooming-in on the acquisition of hospital staphylococci by newborn infants. Pediatrics 1966;37:605–609.
67. Mortimer EAJ, Wolinsky E, Gonzaga AJ, Rammelkamp CHJ. Role of airborne transmission in staphylococcal infections. Br Med J 1966;5483:319–322.
68. Casewell M, Phillips I. Hands as route of transmission for Klebsiella species. Br Med J 1977;2:1315–1317.
69. Austin DJ, Bonten MJ, Weinstein RA, Slaughter S, Anderson RM. Vancomycin-resistant enterococci in intensive-care hospital settings: transmission dynamics, persistence, and the impact of infection control programs. Proc Natl Acad Sci U S A 1999;96:6908–6913.
70. Jernigan JA, Siegman-Igra Y, Guerrant RC, Farr BM. A randomized crossover study of disposable thermometers for prevention of Clostridium difficile and other nosocomial infections. Infect Control Hosp Epidemiol 1998;19:494–499.
71. Boyce JM, Potter-Bynoe G, Chenevert C, King T. Environmental contamination due to methicillin-resistant Staphylococcus aureus: possible infection control implications. Infect Control Hosp Epidemiol 1997;18:622–627.
72. Byers KE, Durbin LJ, Simonton BM, Anglim AM, Adal KA, Farr BM. Disinfection of hospital rooms contaminated with vancomycin-resistant Enterococcus faecium. Infect Control Hosp Epidemiol 1998;19:261–264.
73. Mayhall CG. The epidemiology and control of VRE: still struggling to come of age. Infect Control Hosp Epidemiol 1999;20:650–652.
74. D'Agata EM, Venkataraman L, DeGirolami P, Samore M. Molecular epidemiology of ceftazidime-resistant gram-negative bacilli on inanimate surfaces and their role in cross-transmission during nonoutbreak periods. J Clin Microbiol 1999;37:3065–3067.
75. Boyce JM, Opal SM, Chow JW, Zervos MJ, Potter-Bynoe G, Sherman CB, et al. Outbreak of multidrug-resistant Enterococcus faecium with transferable vanB class vancomycin resistance. J Clin Microbiol 1994;32:1148–1153.
76. Alfieri N, Ramotar K, Armstrong P, Spornitz ME, Ross G, Winnick J, et al. Two consecutive outbreaks of Stenotrophomonas maltophilia (Xanthomonas maltophilia) in an intensive-care unit defined by restriction fragment-length polymorphism typing. Infect Control Hosp Epidemiol 1999;20:553–556.
77. Weber DJ, Rutala WA, Blanchet CN, Jordan M, Gergen MF. Faucet aerators: A source of patient colonization with Stenotrophomonas maltophilia. Am J Infect Control 1999;27:59–63.
78. Hartstein AI, Rashad AL, Liebler JM, Actis LA, Freeman J, Rourke JWJ, et al. Multiple intensive care unit outbreak of Acinetobacter calcoaceticus subspecies anitratus respiratory infection and colonization associated with contaminated, reusable ventilator circuits and resuscitation bags. Am J Med 1988;85:624–631.
79. Hamill RJ, Houston ED, Georghiou PR, Wright CE, Koza MA, Cadle RM, et al. An outbreak of Burkholderia (formerly Pseudomonas) cepacia respiratory tract colonization and infection associated with nebulized albuterol therapy. Ann Intern Med 1995;122:762–766.
80. Simmons B, Bryant J, Neiman K, Spencer L, Arheart K. The role of handwashing in prevention of endemic intensive care unit infections. Infect Control Hosp Epidemiol 1990;11:589–594.
81. Goldmann D, Larson E. Hand-washing and nosocomial infections. N Engl J Med 1992;327:120–122.
82. Doebbeling BN, Stanley GL, Sheetz CT, Pfaller MA, Houston AK, Annis L, et al. Comparative efficacy of alternative hand-washing agents in reducing nosocomial infections in intensive care units. N Engl J Med 1992;327:88–93.
83. Sherertz RJ, Ely EW, Westbrook DM, Gledhill KS, Streed SA, Kiger B, et al. Education of physicians-in-training can decrease the risk for vascular catheter infection. Ann Intern Med 2000;132:641–648.
84. Eggimann P Harbarth S, Constantin MN, Touveneau S, Chevrolet JC, Pittet. Reduction of intensive care unit-acquired infections following an over-all prevention strategy targeted at vascular access care. Lancet 2000; In press.

85. Klein BS, Perloff WH, Maki DG. Reduction of nosocomial infection during pediatric intensive care by protective isolation [see comments]. N Engl J Med 1989;320:1714–1721.
86. Lipsitch M, Bergstrom CT, Levin BR. From the cover: the epidemiology of antibiotic resistance in hospitals: paradoxes and prescriptions. Proc Natl Acad Sci U S A 2000;97:1938–1943.

15. CROSS-COLONIZATION: FACT OR FICTION?

MIGUEL SÁNCHEZ GARCÍA, M.D., PH.D.

Hospital Universitario Príncipe de Asturias. 28805 Alcalá de Henares (Madrid) Spain

INTRODUCTION

Cross-colonization refers to the transmission of potentially-pathogenic microorganisms (PPM) from colonized to other concurrent patients in an intensive care unit (ICU). Genotyping has provided the necessary reliable tool for the epidemiological studies that confirm the existence of cross-colonization of a certain strain type. It has been shown to occur during epidemic outbreaks (1), as well as in non-outbreak situations (2,3). The spread of multidrug-resistant PPM is particularly relevant and has therefore been studied more extensively for strains of *Pseudomonas aeruginosa* and *Acinetobacter baumanii* (4), extended-spectrum beta-lactamases producing *enterobacteriaceae* (5), methicillin-resistant *Staphylococcus aureus* (MRSA) (6,7), and vancomycin-resistant enterococci (VRE) (8). Cross-colonization has not only been shown to occur within ICUs, but spread of multidrug-resistant microorganisms has also been observed to other wards of the hospital (5) and to the community (9).

The importance of the study of the reservoirs and the dissemination of PPM is underlined by the fact that colonization is the most relevant risk factor for nosocomial infection (10–15). Studies of cross-colonization, however, are usually based on culture results of diagnostic samples obtained upon clinical indications (16), rather than on scheduled microbiological surveillance of colonization of the aerodigestive tract. This approach only detects the "tip of the iceberg" and ignores the majority of colonized patients (17,18), who constitute 60 to 75% of the carriers. Unfortunately, only a minority of epidemiological studies performed in the ICU setting

R.A. Weinstein and M.J.M. Bonten (eds.). INFECTION CONTROL IN THE ICU ENVIRONMENT.

(2,8,18–20) have addressed ICU-acquired colonization or infection appropriately, i.e. performing scheduled surveillance cultures. These studies are extremely important, because the information about the exact role of each reservoir and route of transmission of PPM in ICUs is a prerequisite for instituting effective preventive measures of nosocomial infections. If secondary exogenous infections predominate (direct inoculation to the site of infection, not preceded by colonization), barrier precautions and/or adequate disinfection of medical devices have to be implemented. A high incidence of secondary endogenous infections (infection is preceded by colonization of the digestive tract by PPM originating from the patient's own flora or by cross-colonization) requires attempts to eradicate the carrier state (21), as well as barrier precautions which prevent acquisition. Most ICU-acquired nosocomial infections are secondary endogenous (14,15,22,23).

The present review will focus on the factors involved in acquisition of PPM from exogenous sources in the ICU setting, either to colonize or, in a minority of cases, to directly cause infection. The two components of the epidemiological event of cross-colonization are the reservoir of the PPM and the vector providing the route of transmission.

RESERVOIRS

Colonized Patients

A patient may become colonized by a strain originating from his own flora, which has been subjected to the selective pressure of antibiotics. Although definite confirmation of endogenous colonization is never possible, it is accepted to occur whenever the same strain type, as evidenced by genotyping, has not been previously isolated from another patient (2). Colonization may also begin after cross-colonization from another patient, an event called exogenous colonization.

The early detection and the identification of all colonized patients requires surveillance cultures to avoid underestimation of colonization based on isolates of clinical samples. Several studies using molecular typing techniques confirm the existence of occult carriers. For example, D'Agata et al. (18) report that only three of sixty (5%) patients who were colonized at admission had also positive clinical diagnostic cultures for ceftazidime-resistant Gram-negative bacilli within 2 days before admission. In that study, clinical cultures would also have missed most of the patients later acquiring and carrying ceftazidime-resistant Gram-negative bacilli. Data from our ICU show that three quarters of critically ill intubated patients with MRSA in surveillance cultures go undetected (17), because they never develop clinical infections. Moreover, those MRSA carriers who finally develop infection, are identified late, as clinical samples are drawn 10 to 12 days after the index culture. A certain time period of colonization seems to be required for most PPM to invade and infect (15). Girou et al. (24) report that within 72 hours before or after admission to a medical ICU only 49.3% of 150 imported MRSA carriers were identified by clinical samples. The other 50.7% of patients colonized at admission grew MRSA in surveillance cultures.

The population of occult carriers constitutes the main determinant of cross-colonization and of the persistence of an endemic situation or an epidemic outbreak. The magnitude of the influence of the human reservoir is illustrated by studies with the highest compliance scores for infection control measures that have ever been reported (19,25). Scheduled surveillance cultures and genotyping performed during these studies show that colonization pressure, i.e. the point prevalence of colonized patients present in the ICU, is the most significant risk factor for ICU-acquired colonization. Of note is that Bonten et al. (19) studied the case of the vancomycin-resistant enterococcus, which almost exclusively colonizes the rectum. Colonization pressure may be even higher for other multidrug-resistant PPM like *Pseudomonas aeruginosa*, *Acinetobacter baumanii*, *enterobacteriaceae*, and MRSA, which reportedly are not only carried in the rectum, but also in the upper and lower respiratory tract (18,26), providing additional chances for contamination of the hands of health care workers. In neonates MRSA may colonize extensive areas of the skin surface (27). Pittet et al. (28) recently showed that respiratory care constitutes an independent risk factor for contamination of the hands of health care workers (HCW).

The importance of the human reservoir in cross-colonization was brilliantly documented by Bonten in 1994 (29). He observed that if colonization pressure is reduced by applying selective decontamination of the digestive tract to the oropharynx and stomach of half of the patients of an ICU, colonization and infection are reduced and delayed in the other half of the patients who are simultaneously present in the unit. In this study the control group was composed of patients of another unit, in which no topical antibiotic prophylaxis was given. Brun-Buisson et al. (30) published a randomized trial in 1989 which showed that reducing intestinal carriage, i.e. reducing colonization pressure, with multidrug-resistant *Enterobacteriaceae* with selective decontamination of the digestive tract (SDD) administered to half of the patients of an intensive care unit, was associated with a significant reduction of colonization and infection not only in the group of patients receiving SDD, but also in a concurrent control group. The patients of the control group received no topical antibiotics and had a 10 percent incidence of colonization and a 3 percent incidence of infection, compared to 19.6 and 9 percent incidence, respectively, in an immediately previous historical control group, representing the baseline situation which prompted the interventional trial. No infection with multidrug-resistant Gram-negative bacilli was observed during 4 months of follow-up. Taylor et al. (31) reported that after traditional infection control measures failed to control an outbreak of infections with a multidrug-resistant *Enterobacter aerogenes,* the administration of SDD rapidly ended the outbreak. No new isolates were identified during an 8 weeks follow-up period.

The decisive role for cross-colonization played by the colonization pressure is also supported by results presented by De Gheldre et al. (32), who report an epidemic outbreak with *Enterobacter aerogenes* that persists in spite of early institution of isolation measures, until colonized patients are discharged from the intensive care unit. The spread of two *Acinetobacter baumanii* clones could not be prevented in a burns unit, in spite of strict control measures (33), and Wells et al. (22) report a stable incidence of stool carriage with VRE in spite of prompt institution of contact precautions. Zafar et al. detected (27) MRSA only in samples obtained from patients and HCW, but never from environmental sites of a neonatal nursery. Pelke et al. (34) and Slaughter et al. (35) found that the addition of gowns to the universal use of gloves does not reduce infection rates and acquisition of VRE, respectively.

ICUs are generally considered the epicenter of the hospital for bacterial resistance. However, careful study of the aerodigestive flora at admission (18–20) revealed the presence of VRE in 14% (20), MRSA in 4% (24), and ceftazidime-resistant Gram-negative bacilli in 18% (18) of the patients admitted to different ICUs, respectively. Therefore, it seems that the pool of colonized patients exerting colonization pressure is maintained both by cross-colonization within the ICU and by external sources (16,20).

Colonization Patterns

The different colonization patterns of PPM microorganisms may influence the frequency and routes of cross-colonization (11,36). Whereas VRE preferentially colonizes the gut (rectum), and is identified in rectal cultures (8,15,19,22,25,37), other organisms, like *Pseudomonas aeruginosa* (36) are also carried in the upper and lower airway. The distribution of MRSA is wide and hands of HCW may be contaminated during respiratory care, contact with oropharyngeal secretions, feces (26), as well as the skin surface (27,38). This may explain the difficulty of the control of endemicity and outbreaks of MRSA (39). *Acinetobacter baumanii* has also been reported to colonize the aerodigestive tract, as well as large areas of the skin surface (23,40). For those microorganisms with preferential colonization of the upper airway, the oropharynx may also be an important port of entry of cross-colonization. In addition, survival on hands of HCW or inanimate surfaces may influence the rate of cross-colonization of a PPM. Long periods of survival have been reported for *Acinetobacter* (41), *Serratia* (42), and VRE (15). However, whether the incidence of cross-colonization is influenced by the colonization pattern remains to be proven. The hands of hospital personnel are generally considered to be only transient carriers, not a reservoir, of PPM. At most, they may be a source of what is considered resident "normal skin flora". However, non-transient carriage of Gram-negative rods (43) and yeast (44) has been observed on the hands of nurses, suggesting the existence of a chronic skin reservoir for hospital colonization and infection. During non-outbreak situations endogenous colonization with Gram-negative bacilli may play a more important role than cross-colonization in the pathogenesis of nosocomial infections (3,16).

Inanimate Reservoirs

Microorganisms may spread from colonized patients to the environment (42,45,46) and to medical instruments, which, if not adequately disinfected, act as inanimate reservoirs for cross-colonization. Many different devices have repeatedly been reported to serve as sources of PPM during epidemic outbreaks (15,42,46–48). PPM may also be acquired from contaminated enteral feedings. Even contaminated hand-washing machines have been made responsible for an epidemic outbreak (49).

ROUTES

Information about the routes of dissemination is available mainly for multidrug-resistant PPM.

Health Care Personnel

Cross-colonization via the hands of health care personnel is considered to be the main route of spread of PPM. Microorganisms contaminate the hands and are transiently carried on the skin, only rarely causing cutaneous diseases, but probably being responsible for most of the episodes leading to cross-colonization and infection. Contrary to "resident" flora, "transient" flora is not able to multiply on the skin and usually does not survive for long periods of time. However, chronic contamination with Gram-negative bacilli (43) and yeasts (44) has also been identified on the hands of nurses.

The determinants of bacterial contamination of the hands of HCW during routine patient care has recently been studied by Pittet et al. (28). They observed 417 episodes of care, half of which were performed after patient care on intensive care wards. Although normal skin flora was identified after most observations, *Staphylococcus aureus* was cultured in 10.5% and Gram-negative bacilli in 14.5%, a finding which confirms other previous observations (43,44). Wearing gloves largely prevented bacterial contamination, whereas bacterial counts increased significantly over time on ungloved hands as a direct function of the duration of patient contact, rupture in the sequence of care, performing respiratory care, and handling of body fluid secretions. In addition, significant reductions of bacterial counts were observed in those cases in which hand washing included the use of an antiseptic agent.

The circumstances associated with low compliance with hand washing were also recently investigated by Pittet et al. (50), who report discouraging results. According to these investigators, ICU-HCW of a tertiary care center wash their hands only on 36% of situations in which it is indicated, according to the written guidelines of the hospital. The authors hypothesize that the real percentage may even be lower when HCW don't realize that they are being observed. Multivariate analysis showed that compliance was significantly worse when high-risk procedures (before patient contact or care, or between a dirty and a clean site on the patient) were performed. Compliance with hand washing was only 11% between care of a dirty and clean body site. Busyness was also significantly associated with poor compliance with hand washing in this and other reports (51,52). Compliance with hand washing and barrier precautions has been extensively reviewed by Larson and Kretzer (51), who report data from 47 published studies. Hand washing in intensive care units ranged from 17 to 75% in different studies and, typically, non-compliance was significantly higher for physicians and other HCW than for nurses. Similarly, only 40% of procedures were followed by hand washing in a study performed in 4 scandinavian ICUs (53).

Cross-colonization has been documented in most cases by molecular typing methodology, mainly during outbreaks, and almost always for multidrug-resistant microorganisms like *Acinetobacter* (1,4,41), *Serratia* and *Klebsiella* (54), *Enterobacter* (32), methicillin-resistant *Staphylococcus aureus* (7,27), vancomycin-resistant enterococi (15,22).

Inanimate Vectors

Inanimate objects may not only be a reservoir in a particular, anecdotal, situation, but also be the vector for PPM to the mucosa and skin of another patient. Many reports can be found describing instances of exogenous colonization or infection via contaminated medical devices like electric thermometers, tap water (54), faucet, bed-pan macerator (47), indoor air (48), environmental contamination (42,46), enteral feeding, and saline flush solution (55).

Survival of PPM on the hands of HCW and inanimate surfaces may determine the incidence of cross-colonization of each species. Vancomycin-resistant enterococci, for example, have been shown to survive on the fingertips of volunteers and different inanimate surfaces (56).

Risk Factors

In addition to the existence of reservoirs and routes of spread of PPM, specific conditions that may contribute to and increase the incidence of cross-colonization have been identified.

Understaffing, as cited above, is a contributory factor because it reduces compliance with infection control measures (50,57–59). Overcrowding an acute medical ward, i.e. increasing the number of beds in a fixed area, increased the incidence of colonization with MRSA in a study by Kibbler et al. (60).

Harvey (61) critically reviewed the available data from the literature about the impact of critical-care-unit bedside design and furnishing on nosocomial infections. No definite data seem to exist on this topic. However, she suggests that, compared to open units, private rooms may contribute to reduce infection rates. Mulin et al. (62) report of a remarkable drop of colonization rates for *Acinetobacter baumanii* from 28.1% to 5.0% of intubated patients in chronological association with conversion from an open design to individual rooms of a 15-bed surgical ICU. The finding that 4 strains, as identified by pulsed-field gel electrophoresis, colonized 44 of the 47 colonized patients of the study, strongly suggests that the remodeling of the ICU caused a reduction in cross-colonization. No correlations with nosocomial infections have been demonstrated for different types of coverings (ceiling, walls, floor, windows) (61), or for the design and placement of bedside hand washing facilities. Inadequate placement of hand washing facilities, however, has been mentioned as a cause of poor compliance (63).

Table 1. Proposal of intensive care unit guidelines for the prevention of cross-colonization

1. No multidrug-resistant PPM in clinical cultures.
   - ➢ Routine hand washing with plain soap between patient contact.
   - ➢ Hand washing with antiseptic agent before invasive procedure.
   - ➢ Surveillance cultures at admission in certain high-risk groups.
2. Low colonization pressure (For example, less than 20% of patients colonized with multidrug-resistant PPM)
   - ➢ Hand washing with antiseptic agent between patient contact and before invasive procedure.
   - ➢ Surveillance cultures at admission and once per week (for example oropharyngeal and rectal swab inoculated in selective media with gentamicin and/or methicillin).
3. High colonization pressure (For example, more than 20% of patients colonized with multidrug-resistant PPM)
   - ➢ Hand washing with antiseptic agent between patient contact and before invasive procedure.
   - ➢ Consider other barrier precautions, like masks, gloves and gowns (for example, a surgical patient with positive cultures of several different sites, like abdominal drains, oropharynx and rectum).
   - ➢ Attempt to eradicate carriage with topical antimicrobial agents applied to the oropharynx and gut (nasogastric tube or per os) of colonized patients.
4. Outbreak
   - ➢ Hand washing with antiseptic agent between patient contact and before invasive procedure.
   - ➢ Consider other barrier precautions, like masks, gloves and gowns (for example, a surgical patient with positive cultures in many different sites, like abdominal drains, oropharynx and rectum).
   - ➢ Eradicate carriage with topical antimicrobial agents applied to the oropharynx and gut (nasogastric tube or per os) of all patients.

PREVENTION

The primary objective of preventing cross-colonization is obviously reducing the incidence of nosocomial infections, with its associated morbidity and mortality. In addition it is worthwhile considering the important financial and psychological costs of attempting to control outbreaks (27). These include antibiotics, increased workload due to barrier precautions, cohorting of nurses and patients, and even removing HCW from duty (27).

Only a few comparative trials of the control and prevention of outbreaks with multidrug-resistant PPM are available, probably because it is difficult to design and perform controlled studies during outbreaks. These studies were performed after all conventional infection control measures had failed (30,31). Uncontrolled interventions in which termination of an epidemic outbreak is attributed to implementation of strict, or stricter than usual (27), infection control measures are difficult to interpret, because outbreaks tend to wean spontaneously, probably due to discharge and death of most of the carriers (4), or because the inanimate source is decontaminated. Controlled trials of eradication of endemicity are also not available.

Prevention of cross-colonization should be based on the information provided by microbiological surveillance and specifically concentrate on 1) adequate barrier precautions, mainly hand washing, and 2) eradication of the carrier state (Table 1). Once an ICU reaches a certain level of colonization pressure, cross-colonization cannot be prevented if the source of the microorganisms is not controlled by reducing colonization pressure (27). In practice this usually stands for: "If more than x percent of patients are colonized, spread cannot be prevented if the microorganism is not eradicated from the aerodigestive tract of carriers". The percentage "x" is probably different for each species of microorganism, as a function of colonization pattern and adherence and survival on skin and inanimate surfaces.

Prompt institution of adequate infection control strategies requires early detection of colonization (15,17,24) as well as identification of occult carriers of PPM. As patients may be colonized on admission, surveillance cultures should be performed in high-risk patients who are admitted from other wards of the hospital and have received broad-spectrum antibiotics (20,24). Further scheduled surveillance cultures during ICU stay may be simplified by employing selective culture media (64), but its frequency depends on local incidence and type of infectious problems (18).

Barrier Precautions (Routes)

Already 150 years ago, Semmelweis in Hungary recognized the importance of the hands for the transmission of infectious disease in the hospital setting. Microbiological confirmation, as well as universal recognition and acceptance of his epidemiological observations occurred several decades later. That contamination of the hands of HCW is the main route of cross-colonization in the hospital is actually a well known fact for nurses and physicians (51), who also are aware that, amongst all barrier precautions, hand washing is the single most important measure for the prevention of spread. To narrow the gap between theory and practice, a universally poor compliance, educational and behavioral approaches have been investigated and proposed (65–69). However, even the most intensive efforts to enhance hand washing practice have had poor results (67,70).

It seems appropriate that written general recommendations for non-outbreak situation, adapted to local conditions, should be issued (50,63). Guidelines for the control of specific multidrug-resistant microorganisms may be required (6,71). Compliance with specific guidelines to be implemented during outbreaks will be higher if they are kept simple (72). For example, boxed, clean, non-sterile gloves may be equivalent to antiseptic hand washing if gloves are removed after each patient contact (28,72). Important aspects of effective hand washing should be mentioned in those guidelines, like the use of an antiseptic agent (28,73), the duration of hand washing (74,75), and removal of wrist watches (76) and rings (77). New formulations (78) may improve compliance, but it still has to be proven if its use reduces nosocomial infections (79).

Simple measures like placement of warning labels (80) have been proposed to improve adherence to barrier precautions. The use of mathematical models that predict the spread of multidrug-resistant bacteria and the impact of hand washing (81,82), or the impact of infection control measures necessary to eradicate VRE (83) and MRSA (84) has recently been suggested.

Reservoirs

The decisive role of the human reservoir for cross-colonization has already been mentioned (19,29,82). Therefore, strategies to prevent cross-colonization should include measures that reduce colonization-pressure (19,24,29,38,85) if a certain percentage is reached. Eradication of PPM should certainly be attempted whenever all conventional infection control measures have failed (27,86). Selective decontamination of the digestive tract has been shown to be extremely effective in controlling outbreaks with multidrug-resistant Gram-negative bacilli (30,31). In addition, topical antibiotics applied to the digestive tract may prevent acquisition of multidrug-resistant PPM during high-risk periods of ICU stay, like intubation and mechanical ventilation (85,87). We recently concluded a double-blind randomized placebo controlled trial in our general ICU (85). Topical vancomycin was added to the usual SDD regimen (gentamicin, polymyxin E, and amphotericin B) that is applied to the oropharynx and through the nasogastric tube in critically ill long-term intubated patients. In the test group vancomycin completely prevented acquisition and infection with methicillin-resistant *Staphylococcus aureus*, and significantly reduced other Gram-positive infections.

SUMMARY AND CONCLUSIONS

The existence of cross-colonization has been established beyond doubt. Cross-colonization occurs during epidemic outbreaks, as well as in non-outbreak situations. Its magnitude is a direct function of colonization pressure. However, for a given level of colonization pressure, poor compliance with infection control practice may further increase the incidence of cross-colonization and nosocomial infection. Cross-colonization has been proven to take place via the contaminated hands of health care personnel. Contamination of the hands is a direct consequence of non-compliance with barrier precautions. Non-compliance, in turn, is favored under circumstances like understaffing, overcrowding, and design of intensive care units. Scheduled surveillance cultures of the aerodigestive tract are the fundamental tool to design preventive strategies. With the information they provide, efforts to prevent cross-colonization should be addressed both at eradication of the carrier state, as well as at improving barrier precautions, mainly hand washing.

REFERENCES

1. Husni RN, Goldstein LS, Arroliga AC, et al. Risk factors for an outbreak of multi-drug-resistant Acinetobacter nosocomial pneumonia among intubated patients. Chest. 1999;115: 1378–1382.
2. Bergmans DC, Bonten MJ, van Tiel FH, et al. Cross-colonisation with Pseudomonas aeruginosa of patients in an intensive care unit. Thorax. 1998;53:1053–1058.
3. D'Agata EM, Venkataraman L, DeGirolami P, Samore M. Molecular epidemiology of ceftazidime-resistant gram-negative bacilli on inanimate surfaces and their role in cross-transmission during nonoutbreak periods. J Clin Microbiol. 1999;37:3065–3067.
4. Marques MB, Waites KB, Mangino JE, Hines BB, Moser SA. Genotypic investigation of multidrug-resistant Acinetobacter baumannii infections in a medical intensive care unit. J Hosp Infect. 1997;37:125–135.
5. Arpin C, Coze C, Rogues AM, Gachie JP, Bebear C, Quentin C. Epidemiological study of an outbreak due to multidrug-resistant Enterobacter aerogenes in a medical intensive care unit. J Clin Microbiol. 1996;34:2163–2169.
6. Herwaldt LA. Control of methicillin-resistant Staphylococcus aureus in the hospital setting. Am J Med. 1999;106:11S–18S.

7. Andersen BM, Bergh K, Steinbakk M, et al. A Norwegian nosocomial outbreak of methicillin-resistant Staphylococcus aureus resistant to fusidic acid and susceptible to other antistaphylococcal agents. J Hosp Infect. 1999;41:123–132.
8. Bonten MJ, Hayden MK, Nathan C, et al. Epidemiology of colonisation of patients and environment with vancomycin-resistant enterococci. Lancet. 1996;348:1615–1619.
9. Anonymous Guidelines on the control of methicillin-resistant Staphylococcus aureus in the community. Report of a combined Working Party of the British Society for Antimicrobial Chemotherapy and the Hospital Infection Society. J Hosp Infect. 1995;31:1–12.
10. Johanson WGJ, Pierce AK, Sanford JP, Thomas GD. Nosocomial respiratory infections with gram-negative bacilli. The significance of colonization of the respiratory tract. Ann Intern Med. 1972;77:701–706.
11. Bonten MJ, Gaillard CA, van Tiel FH, Smeets HG, van der Geest S, Stobberingh EE. The stomach is not a source for colonization of the upper respiratory tract and pneumonia in ICU patients. Chest. 1994;105:878–884.
12. Bonten MJ, Gaillard CA, van der Geest S, et al. The role of intragastric acidity and stress ulcus prophylaxis on colonization and infection in mechanically ventilated ICU patients. A stratified, randomized, double-blind study of sucralfate versus antacids. Am J Respir Crit Care Med. 1995;152:1825–1834.
13. Pittet D, Monod M, Filthuth I, Frenk E, Suter PM, Auckenthaler R. Contour-clamped homogeneous electric field gel electrophoresis as a powerful epidemiologic tool in yeast infections. Am J Med. 1991;91:256S–263S.
14. Bonten MJ, Bergmans DC, Ambergen AW, et al. Risk factors for pneumonia, and colonization of respiratory tract and stomach in mechanically ventilated ICU patients. Am J Respir Crit Care Med. 1996;154:1339–1346.
15. Edmond MB, Ober JF, Weinbaum DL, et al. Vancomycin-resistant Enterococcus faecium bacteremia: risk factors for infection [see comments]. Clin Infect Dis. 1995;20:1126–1133.
16. Chetchotisakd P, Phelps CL, Hartstein AI. Assessment of bacterial cross-transmission as a cause of infections in patients in intensive care units. Clin Infect Dis. 1994;18:929–937.
17. Sánchez M, Mir N, Cantón R, López B, Baquero F. The importance of surveillance cultures (SVC) for the detection of carriage of methicillin-resistant *Staphylococcus aureus* (MRSA) in critically ill patients. 38th Interscience Conference on Antimicrobial Agents and Chemotherapy (ICAAC). 1998;September 24–27; San Diego, California.:[Abstract].
18. D'Agata EMC, Venkatraman L, DeGirolami P, et al. Colonization with broad-spectrum cephalosporin-resistant Gram-negative bacilli in intensive care units during a nonoutbreak period: Prevalence, risk factors, and rate of infection. Crit Care Med. 1999;27:1090–1095.
19. Bonten MJ, Slaughter S, Ambergen AW, et al. The role of "colonization pressure" in the spread of vancomycin-resistant enterococci: an important infection control variable. Arch Intern Med. 1998;158:1127–1132.
20. Bonten MJ, Slaughter S, Hayden MK, Nathan C, van Voorhis J, Weinstein RA. External sources of vancomycin-resistant enterococci for intensive care units. Crit Care Med. 1998;26:2001–2004.
21. van Saene HK, Damjanovic V, Murray AE, de la Cal MA. How to classify infections in intensive care units—the carrier state, a criterion whose time has come? J Hosp Infect. 1996;33:1–12.
22. Wells CL, Juni BA, Cameron SB, et al. Stool carriage, clinical isolation, and mortality during an outbreak of vancomycin-resistant enterococci in hospitalized medical and/or surgical patients. Clin Infect Dis. 1995;21:45–50.
23. Corbella X, Pujol M, Ayats J, et al. Relevance of digestive tract colonization in the epidemiology of nosocomial infections due to multiresistant Acinetobacter baumannii. Clin Infect Dis. 1996;23:329–334.
24. Girou E, Pujade G, Legrand P, Cizeau F, Brun-Buisson C. Selective screening of carriers for control of methicillin-resistant Staphylococcus aureus (MRSA) in high-risk hospital areas with a high level of endemic MRSA. Clin Infect Dis. 1998;27:543–550.
25. Lai KK, Kelley AL, Melvin ZS, Belliveau PP, Fontecchio SA. Failure to eradicate vancomycin-resistant enterococci in a university hospital and the cost of barrier precautions. Infect Control Hosp Epidemiol. 1998;19:647–652.
26. Sánchez García M, Cambronero Galache JA, Rogero Marín S, Daguerre Talou M, De la Fuente O'Connor E, Nuñez Reiz A. Methicillin-resistant *Staphylococcus aureus* (MRSA) colonizes the airway as well as the gut in critically ill intubated patients. 33rd Interscience Conference on Antimicrobial Agents and Chemotherapy (ICAAC). 1993;October 17–20; New Orleans, Louisiana.:[Abstract].

27. Zafar AB, Butler RC, Reese DJ, Gaydos LA, Mennonna PA. Use of 0.3% triclosan (Bacti-Stat) to eradicate an outbreak of methicillin-resistant Staphylococcus aureus in a neonatal nursery. Am J Infect Control. 1995;23:200–208.
28. Pittet D, Dharan S, Touveneau S, Sauvan V, Perneger TV. Bacterial contamination of the hands of hospital staff during routine patient care. Arch Intern Med. 1999;159:821–826.
29. Bonten MJ, Gaillard CA, Johanson WGJ, et al. Colonization in patients receiving and not receiving topical antimicrobial prophylaxis. Am J Respir Crit Care Med. 1994;150:1332–1340.
30. Brun-Buisson C, Legrand P, Rauss A, et al. Intestinal decontamination for control of nosocomial multiresistant gram-negative bacilli. Study of an outbreak in an intensive care unit. Ann Intern Med. 1989;110:873–881.
31. Taylor ME, Oppenheim BA. Selective decontamination of the gastrointestinal tract as an infection control measure. J Hosp Infect. 1991;17:271–278.
32. De Gheldre Y, Maes N, Rost F, et al. Molecular epidemiology of an outbreak of multidrug-resistant Enterobacter aerogenes infections and in vivo emergence of imipenem resistance. J Clin Microbiol. 1997;35:152–160.
33. Lyytikainen O, Koljalg S, Harma M, Vuopio VJ. Outbreak caused by two multi-resistant Acinetobacter baumannii clones in a burns unit: emergence of resistance to imipenem. J Hosp Infect. 1995;31:41–54.
34. Pelke S, Ching D, Easa D, Melish ME. Gowning does not affect colonization or infection rates in a neonatal intensive care unit. Arch Pediatr Adolesc.Med. 1994;148:1016–1020.
35. Slaughter S, Hayden MK, Nathan C, et al. A comparison of the effect of universal use of gloves and gowns with that of glove use alone on acquisition of vancomycin-resistant enterococci in a medical intensive care unit [see comments]. Ann Intern Med. 1996;125:448–456.
36. Bergmans DC, Bonten MJ, Stobberingh EE, et al. Colonization with Pseudomonas aeruginosa in patients developing ventilator-associated pneumonia. Infect Control Hosp Epidemiol. 1998; 19:853–855.
37. Sánchez M, Mir N, Cantón R, Luque R, López B, Baquero F. Incidence of carriage and colonization pattern of vancomycin-resistant *enterococcus* (VRE) in intubated patients (Pts) receiving topical vancomicin (V). 37th Interscience Conference on Antimicrobial Agents and Chemotherapy (ICAAC). 1997;September 28–October 1, 1997; Toronto, Ontario, Canada. [Abstract]
38. Talon D, Rouget C, Cailleaux V, et al. Nasal carriage of Staphylococcus aureus and cross-contamination in a surgical intensive care unit: efficacy of mupirocin ointment. J Hosp Infect. 1995;30:39–49.
39. Boyce JM, Causey WA. Increasing occurrence of methicillin-resistant Staphylococcus aureus in the United States. Infect Control. 1982;3:377–383.
40. Ayats J, Corbella X, Ardanuy C, et al. Epidemiological significance of cutaneous, pharyngeal, and digestive tract colonization by multiresistant Acinetobacter baumannii in ICU patients. J Hosp Infect. 1997;37:287–295.
41. Jawad A, Seifert H, Snelling AM, Heritage J, Hawkey PM. Survival of Acinetobacter baumannii on dry surfaces: comparison of outbreak and sporadic isolates. J Clin Microbiol. 1998;36:1938–1941.
42. Peltroche-Llacsahuanga H, Lutticken R, Haase G. Temporally overlapping nosocomial outbreaks of Serratia marcescens infections: an unexpected result revealed by pulsed-field gel electrophoresis [letter]. Infect Control Hosp Epidemiol. 1999;20:387–388.
43. Guenthner SH, Hendley JO, Wenzel RP. Gram-negative bacilli as nontransient flora on the hands of hospital personnel. J Clin Microbiol. 1987;25:488–490.
44. Strausbaugh LJ, Sewell DL, Ward TT, Pfaller MA, Heitzman T, Tjoelker R. High frequency of yeast carriage on hands of hospital personnel. J Clin Microbiol. 1994;32:2299–2300.
45. van Saene HK, Van Putte JC, Van Saene JJ, Van de Gronde TW, Van Warmerdam EG. Sink flora in a long-stay hospital is determined by the patients' oral and rectal flora. Epidemiol Infect. 1989;102:231–238.
46. Udo EE, al-Obaid IA, Jacob LE, Chugh TD. Molecular characterization of epidemic ciprofloxacin- and methicillin-resistant Staphylococcus aureus strains colonizing patients in an intensive care unit. J Clin Microbiol. 1996;34:3242–3244.
47. Herra CM, Knowles SJ, Kaufmann ME, Mulvihill E, McGrath B, Keane CT. An outbreak of an unusual strain of Serratia marcescens in two Dublin hospitals. J Hosp Infect. 1998;39:135–141.
48. Chandrashekar MR, Rathish KC, Nagesha CN. Reservoirs of nosocomial pathogens in neonatal intensive care unit. J Indian Med Assoc. 1997;95:72–74, 77.

49. Wurtz R, Moye G, Jovanovic B. Handwashing machines, handwashing compliance, and potential for cross-contamination. Am J Infect Control. 1994;22:228–230.
50. Pittet D, Mourouga P, Perneger TV. Compliance with handwashing in a teaching hospital. Ann Intern Med. 1999;130:126–130.
51. Larson E, Kretzer EK. Compliance with handwashing and barrier precautions. J Hosp Infect. 1995;30 Suppl:88–106.
52. Sproat LJ, Inglis TJ. A multicentre survey of hand hygiene practice in intensive care units. J Hosp Infect. 1994;26:137–148.
53. Zimakoff J, Stormark M, Larsen SO. Use of gloves and handwashing behaviour among health care workers in intensive care units. A multicentre investigation in four hospitals in Denmark and Norway. J Hosp Infect. 1993;24:63–67.
54. Pegues DA, Arathoon EG, Samayoa B, et al. Epidemic gram-negative bacteremia in a neonatal intensive care unit in Guatemala. Am J Infect Control. 1994;22:163–171.
55. Chodoff A, Pettis AM, Schoonmaker D, Shelly MA. Polymicrobial gram-negative bacteremia associated with saline solution flush used with a needleless intravenous system. Am J Infect Control. 1995;23:357–363.
56. Noskin GA, Stosor V, Cooper I, Peterson LR. Recovery of vancomycin-resistant enterococci on fingertips and environmental surfaces. Infect Control Hosp Epidemiol. 1995;16:577–581.
57. Archibald LK, Manning ML, Bell LM, Banerjee S, Jarvis WR. Patient density, nurse-to-patient ratio and nosocomial infection risk in a pediatric cardiac intensive care unit. Pediatr Infect Dis J. 1997;16:1045–1048.
58. Fridkin SK, Pear SM, Williamson TH, Galgiani JN, Jarvis WR. The role of understaffing in central venous catheter-associated bloodstream infections. Infect Control Hosp Epidemiol. 1996;17:150–158.
59. Farrington M, Redpath C, Trundle C, Coomber S, Brown NM. Winning the battle but losing the war: methicillin-resistant Staphylococcus aureus (MRSA) infection at a teaching hospital. QJM. 1998;91:539–548.
60. Kibbler CC, Quick A, O'Neill AM. The effect of increased bed numbers on MRSA transmission in acute medical wards. J Hosp Infect. 1998;39:213–219.
61. Harvey MA. Critical-care-unit bedside design and furnishing: impact on nosocomial infections. Infect Control Hosp Epidemiol. 1998;19:597–601.
62. Mulin B, Rouget C, Clement C, et al. Association of private isolation rooms with ventilator-associated Acinetobacter baumanii pneumonia in a surgical intensive-care unit. Infect Control Hosp Epidemiol. 1997;18:499–503.
63. Kesavan S, Barodawala S, Mulley GP. Now wash your hands? A survey of hospital handwashing facilities. J Hosp Infect. 1998;40:291–293.
64. Mir N, Sanchez M, Baquero F, Lopez B, Calderon C, Canton R. Soft salt-mannitol agar-cloxacillin test: a highly specific bedside screening test for detection of colonization with methicillin-resistant Staphylococcus aureus. J Clin Microbiol. 1998;36:986–989.
65. Kretzer EK, Larson EL. Behavioral interventions to improve infection control practices. Am J Infect Control. 1998;26:245–253.
66. Connolly J. Finding ways to encourage health care workers to wash hands often. Product placement and health care worker education on compliance were not enough to change behaviors. Todays.Surg.Nurse. 1998;20:36–38.
67. Larson EL, Bryan JL, Adler LM, Blane C. A multifaceted approach to changing handwashing behavior. Am J Infect Control. 1997;25:3–10.
68. Handwashing Liaison Group. Hand washing. BMJ. 1999;318:686
69. Boyce JM. It is time for action: improving hand hygiene in hospitals. Ann Intern Med. 1999;130:153–155.
70. Simmons B, Bryant J, Neiman K, Spencer L, Arheart K. The role of handwashing in prevention of endemic intensive care unit infections. Infect Control Hosp Epidemiol. 1990;11:589–594.
71. Perl TM. The threat of vancomycin resistance. Am J Med. 1999;106:26S–37S.
72. Rossoff LJ, Borenstein M, Isenberg HD. Is hand washing really needed in an intensive care unit? Crit Care Med. 1995;23:1211–1216.
73. Huang Y, Oie S, Kamiya A. Comparative effectiveness of hand-cleansing agents for removing methicillin-resistant Staphylococcus aureus from experimentally contaminated fingertips. Am J Infect Control. 1994;22:224–227.
74. Rotter ML. Hand washing and hand disinfection. In: Mayhall CG, ed. Hospital Epidemiology and Infection Control. Baltimore: Williams & Wilkins; 1996:1052–1068.

75. Larson EL. APIC guideline for handwashing and hand antisepsis in health care settings. Am J Infect Control. 1995;23:251–269.
76. Hartley JC, Mackay AD, Scott GM. Wrist watches must be removed before washing hands. BMJ. 1999;318:328.
77. Salisbury DM, Hutfilz P, Treen LM, Bollin GE, Gautam S. The effect of rings on microbial load of health care workers' hands. Am J Infect Control. 1997;25:24–27.
78. Hobson DW, Woller W, Anderson L, Guthery E. Development and evaluation of a new alcohol-based surgical hand scrub formulation with persistent antimicrobial characteristics and brushless application. Am J Infect Control. 1998;26:507–512.
79. Zaragoza M, Salles M, Gomez J, Bayas JM, Trilla A. Handwashing with soap or alcoholic solutions? A randomized clinical trial of its effectiveness. Am J Infect Control. 1999;27:258–261.[Abstract]
80. Khatib M, Jamaleddine G, Abdallah A, Ibrahim Y. Hand washing and use of gloves while managing patients receiving mechanical ventilation in the ICU. Chest. 1999;116:172–175.
81. Sebille V, Valleron AJ. A computer simulation model for the spread of nosocomial infections caused by multidrug-resistant pathogens. Comput Biomed Res. 1997;30:307–322.
82. Sebille V, Chevret S, Valleron AJ. Modeling the spread of resistant nosocomial pathogens in an intensive-care unit. Infect Control Hosp Epidemiol. 1997;18:84–92.
83. Austin DJ, Bonten MJ, Weinstein RA, Slaughter S, Anderson RM. Vancomycin-resistant enterococci in intensive-care hospital settings: transmission dynamics, persistence, and the impact of infection control programs. Proc Natl Acad Sci U S A. 1999;96:6908–6913.
84. Austin DJ, Anderson RM. Transmission dynamics of epidemic methicillin-resistant Staphylococcus aureus and vancomycin-resistant enterococci in England and Wales. J Infect Dis. 1999;179:883–891.
85. Sánchez M, Mir N, Cantón R, uque R, López B, Baquero F. The effect of topical vancomycin on acquisition, carriage and infection with methicillin-resistant *staphylococcus aureus* in critically ill patients (Pts). A double-blind, randomized, placebo-controlled study. 37th Interscience Conference on Antimicrobial Agents and Chemotherapy (ICAAC). 1997;September 28–October 1, 1997; Toronto, Ontario, Canada:[Abstract]
86. Mylotte JM. Control of methicillin-resistant Staphylococcus aureus: the ambivalence persists. Infect Control Hosp Epidemiol. 1994;15:73–77.
87. Sanchez GM, Cambronero GJ, Lopez DJ, et al. Effectiveness and cost of selective decontamination of the digestive tract in critically ill intubated patients. A randomized, double-blind, placebo-controlled, multicenter trial. Am J Respir Crit Care Med. 1998;158:908–916.

16. CONVENTIONAL INFECTION CONTROL MEASURES: VALUE OR RITUAL?

JOHN P. FLAHERTY, JANIS WIENER, ROBERT A. WEINSTEIN

University of Chicago, Chicago, IL; MacNeal Hospital, Berwyn, IL; Cook County Hospital and Rush Medical College, Chicago, IL

INTRODUCTION

Nosocomial infections complicate the hospital course of 20% or more of intensive care unit (ICU) patients resulting in substantial mortality, prolonged length of stay, and increased utilization of resources (1,2). Is the development of nosocomial infection an inevitable consequence of modern intensive medical care or can traditional infection control practices reduce the risk of hospital-acquired infection? Reports of surprisingly poor compliance with traditional infection control procedures by healthcare workers in ICUs raise questions about the perceived value, and the practicality of these measures. Do handwashing, barrier precautions, and traditional isolation procedures provide enough value in reducing infection risk to warrant more strenuous efforts to improve compliance or do we need to develop new methods of infection control? In this chapter we review the value of these and other common control measures.

SURVEILLANCE

Infection surveillance is the systematic collection, tabulation, and analysis of data on nosocomial infection occurrences. The usual goals of surveillance are to ascertain the incidence of nosocomial infections and to provide sufficient detail about those infections so that problems can be recognized. Surveillance activities include monitoring culture results (microbiology laboratory-based surveillance), monitoring

R.A. Weinstein and M.J.M. Bonten (eds.). INFECTION CONTROL IN THE ICU ENVIRONMENT.

antimicrobial use (pharmacy-based surveillance), monitoring patients for clinical evidence of infection (ward-based surveillance), and screening for evidence of colonization with particular problem pathogens. Nosocomial infection rates may be reported per patient admissions (e.g., per 100 patient admits), per patient-days (e.g., per 1000 patient-days), or per device days. To reasonably compare units or hospitals, infection rates should be stratified for underlying disease, device use, length of stay, the type of ICU, and the hospital size.

The routine use of screening cultures to identify colonization of patients with particular problem pathogens is controversial. Although ICUs generally are considered epicenters of antibiotic resistance, sources outside the ICU also contribute. A study of the epidemiology of *Pseudomonas aeruginosa* in ICU patients identified colonization of 25% of patients on admission to the unit (3). Screening of patients in a medical ICU by Bonten and coworkers found that 14% were colonized with vancomycin-resistant enterococci (VRE) on admission to the unit (4). By the time antibiotic resistance among clinical isolates becomes apparent, colonization with resistant microorganisms may well be endemic. Studies of VRE have demonstrated that clinical cultures identify only 10%–20% of patients colonized or infected with VRE (5,6). During an outbreak of drug-resistant gram-negative infection in an ICU, 60 (18%) of 333 patients were colonized with ceftazidime-resistant gram-negative bacilli on admission to the unit (7). Routine clinical cultures detected only 5% (3/60) of colonization or infection.

Limiting surveillance to clinical cultures results provides an incomplete perspective of the scope of antibiotic-resistant pathogen prevalence in a unit. But does detection of "occult" resistance facilitate infection control? Routine screening for methicillin-resistant *Staphylococcus aureus* (MRSA) colonization on admission and weekly thereafter in a pediatric ICU resulted in a decrease in MRSA carriage from 34% to 2% and MRSA infection from 5.9 to 0.8 per 1000 patient-days (8). The heightened awareness of MRSA colonization led to improved handwashing although no particular effort was taken to improve handwashing compliance. Girou and coworkers employed selective screening for MRSA for patients admitted to their ICU and reported a decrease from 5.6% to 1.4% in acquired colonization and infection with MRSA (9). Screening cultures have been recommended for patients admitted to the ICU during outbreak situations. A complementary approach is routine screening of patients transferred from epicenters of antimicrobial-resistant pathogens (e.g., other hospitals and nursing homes). The latter procedure has not yet been adopted widely by hospital infection control programs because it requires significant resources and has not yet been proven to be cost-effective (10) or lead to a measurable reduction in infection incidence. Surveillance can require the expenditure of significant resources and only when improvements in patient care are documented through measurable outcomes can the costs of surveillance be justified.

HAND DISINFECTION

Hand carriage of pathogens by healthcare personnel is a perennial problem in hospitals. A study assessing the relative importance of airborne and direct contact in the transmission of nosocomial microorganisms in an ICU identified pathogenic bacteria in hand samples from 31% of physicians and 17% of nurses and strains recovered from patients and their caretakers were often indistinguishable. In contrast, isolates obtained from air samples could not be correlated with patient infections (11). An investigation of the hand flora of 103 hospital personnel showed that one or more of 22 different species of gram negative bacteria were carried persistently on the hands of 21% of personnel (12). Persons who washed their hands less than eight times daily were significantly more likely to carry the same species of gram-negative bacteria throughout the day. Over a seven-month period, 21% of 541 nosocomial infections were caused by species found on the hands of personnel. In laboratory studies, *Klebsiella* artificially inoculated onto hands survived for up to 150 minutes (13). A multiply-resistant strain of *Enterobacter cloacae* and an outbreak strain of VRE survived for up to 30 minutes on the fingertips of volunteers after inoculation (14). The transmission of bacteria via the hands of healthcare workers has been implicated in numerous outbreaks of infection caused by gram-negative bacteria (15,16), MRSA (17), and VRE (18).

Hand disinfection has been recognized to reduce the risk of transmission of microbial pathogens since the time of Semmelweis, more than 150 years ago. Improved handwashing has been linked to decreased nosocomial infection rates (19,20) and a number of ICU infection outbreaks have been controlled with simple reinforcement of handwashing (15). Nevertheless, audits of handwashing in hospitals and ICUs repeatedly show poor compliance (28%–56%) by healthcare workers (20,21,22). Even the quality of handwashing may be important. Noskin and coworkers showed that a 5 second handwash with soap and water failed to decrease counts of VRE inoculated on the hands of volunteers; a 30 second wash with soap and water was necessary to eradicate VRE from hands completely (23). Actual handwashing time averages 9–20 seconds which may be too short to be fully effective (21). Surveys of healthcare workers identify two important factors associated with decreased handwashing: being too busy and the damaging effects of frequent handwashing on the skin (24). Frequent and infrequent handwashers did not differ in the value they placed on handwashing to prevent the spread of infection. Unfortunately, non-compliance tends to be higher in ICUs, during procedures with a high risk of contamination, and when intensity of patient care is high (21). Association between non-compliance and intensity of care suggests that understaffing may decrease the quality of patient care.

Potential solutions to poor adherence with hand disinfection include earlier and more intensive education of medical and nursing students on the importance of hand hygiene. Continuing education of healthcare workers has demonstrated mixed results. In one intervention, the placement of warning labels on mechanical ventilators reminding "Wash Hands/Use Gloves" increased handwashing and glove use among respiratory therapy technicians from 45% to over 90% (25). One study concluded that nurses with better knowledge of infection control performed hand antisepsis more appropriately (26). Others have been unsuccessful in significantly improving handwashing compliance through education (27). Educating patients about the value of hand hygiene in preventing the transmission of infection may be valuable. In a prospective, controlled trial of patient handwashing education in four community hospitals, patients were provided an educational brochure and instructed to ask all health care workers who had direct contact with them, "Did you wash your hands?"(28) As a reminder patients were provided with signs that said, "Did you wash your hands?" This intervention resulted in a 34% increase in handwashing, calculated by soap usage.

Unfortunately, the time demands of total compliance with handwashing guidelines could interfere with patient care. Making hand disinfection easier with the use of topical antiseptics (e.g., alcoholic hand rubs) which take only 10 seconds to apply rather than the 30 to 60 seconds that it takes to walk to a sink, lather up with soap and water, rinse, and towel dry can improve compliance without sacrificing efficacy. One analysis estimated that in an ICU with 12 healthcare workers, 100% compliance with handwashing would consume 16 hours of nursing time per shift (or 17% of nursing time) whereas the use of an alcoholic hand disinfectant from bedside dispensers would require only 3 hours (or 3% of nursing time) (29). Topical antiseptics may also be more effective than soap and water handwashing in eradicating pathogens form the hands of caretakers, in part by providing residual bactericidal activity. Alcohol-based skin disinfectants have been shown to be more effective than soap and water in eradicating VRE and gram-negative bacilli from the hands of volunteers (14,30,31). Healthcare workers randomly assigned to use an alcoholic disinfectant handrub demonstrated an 88% reduction in bacterial microflora as compared to a 50% decrease with soap and water (32).

Providing hand emollients may help prevent dermatitis, allowing personnel to wash as frequently as necessary. In addition, dermatitis is associated with higher rates of colonization with gram negative rods providing additional support for the widespread use of skin moisturizers (33).

While the level of hand disinfection in most audits has been far from ideal, the level of compliance that might be considered a minimum goal is uncertain. In fact, the level of compliance necessary to effectively reduce the transmission of nosocomial pathogens may vary as a function of the endemic colonization rate. Austin and colleagues studied transmission dynamics of VRE in an ICU environment (34). They identified transmission of VRE via contact with the hands of contaminated healthcare workers as an important determinant of spread and persistence of VRE. The higher the endemic rates of VRE colonization, the higher the level of compliance with infection control necessary to prevent cross-transmission. Their analysis concluded that the high levels of VRE colonization in patients admitted to their ICU required handwashing compliance significantly in excess of reported levels, or cohorting of nursing staff, to control VRE transmission. This increased risk of VRE colonization as a result of VRE colonization prevalence in a unit has been called "colonization pressure" (35). In a Cox regression analysis, colonization pressure was the single most important risk factor for acquisition of VRE in their ICU. Perhaps the minimum level of hand disinfection compliance for a particular unit is a function of the prevalence of colonization with problem pathogens, which stresses the need for additional control measures, e.g., cohorting of colonized/

Table 1. Isolation Precautions

Precautions	When Used	Disease Examples	Instructions
Standard	All patients	All patients	Use barrier precautions as needed to prevent contact with blood, body fluids, excretions, secretions and contaminated items; disinfect hands after contact with blood or body fluids and after glove removal; disinfect or wash hands between patients
Airborne	Disease spread by small droplets (2–5 μm in diameter)	Tuberculosis, varicella, measles	Use private room with negative air pressure, 6–12 air exchanges per hour, and direct exhaust or filtration of air discharge; all persons entering room wear respiratory protection
Droplet	Disease spread by larger droplets (5 μm in diameter)	*Neisseria meningitidis, Haemophilus influenzae* influenza, streptococcal pharyngitis, drug-resistant pneumococcus	Use private room; wear mask when within 3 ft of patient
Contact	Disease spread by contact with body surfaces	Multidrug-resistant bacteria (MRSA, VRE) *Clostridium difficile*, Herpes zoster (localized in immuno-competent patients), Herpes simplex, cellulitis, conjunctivitis	Use private room; wear gloves when entering room; change gloves after contact with infective material; wear gown for substantial contact with patient or environmental surfaces

Adapted from Garner JS, HICPAC. Guideline for isolation precautions in hospitals. Infect Control Hosp Epidemiol 1996;17:53–80.

infected patients, when hand hygiene compliance remains inadequate to stem cross-infections.

ISOLATION AND BARRIER PRECAUTIONS

Routine isolation precautions are designed to prevent patient-to-patient spread of unrecognized pathogens and to protect healthcare workers from potential infection. Standard precautions combine universal precautions (barriers to prevent transmission of blood-borne pathogens) and isolation precautions (barriers to prevent transmission from body surfaces). Standard precautions are supplemented by transmission-based precautions when caring for patients with diseases spread by the particle or aerosol route or spread by direct contact (table 1)(36). Reinforcement of barrier precautions has been credited with control of outbreaks of infection caused by MRSA (37,38) and VRE (39). Other investigators have reported failure of usual barrier precautions to control similar outbreaks (40,41). The difficulty in identifying colonization with problem pathogens has prompted a recommendation by some authors for routine isolation of all patients whether known to be colonized or not

(38). The potential benefits of isolation must be weighed against the costs of procedures to limit cross-contamination (nursing, laboratory, use of disposables), reduction in contact with healthcare workers (42) and limited rehabilitation resulting from reduced access, prolonged hospitalization resulting from resistance to placement, and the effect on patient morale.

Private Rooms

The impact of private patient rooms, rather than open wards, on the risk of transmission of nosocomial pathogens has been variable. Conversion of a burn unit from an open ward to single bed isolation rooms decreased nosocomial gram-negative bacteremia rates from 31% to 12% (43). However, this study used an historical cohort for comparison. Mulin and coworkers reported a decrease in *Acinetobacter* infection from 28% to 5% after their ICU was converted from an open unit to all private rooms (44). Alternatively, conversion of a medical-surgical ICU from an open unit to isolation rooms had no apparent effect on the incidence of colonization and infection (45). The impact of private rooms on infection rates is uncertain, but they are generally desirable for many other reasons and necessary for certain types of isolation.

Gloves

Gloves have proven effective in reducing contamination of hands of hospital personnel by nosocomial pathogens. Glove use resulted in an 87% decrease in the incidence of gentamicin-resistant Enterobacteriaceae (46). A controlled trial of glove use for all body substance contact (prior to the institution of universal body substance precautions) was associated with a significant decrease in the incidence of *C. difficile* diarrhea and provided indirect evidence for hand carriage as a means of *C. difficile* spread (47). Like handwashing, glove use compliance is frequently less than 100% (48).

Gloves should not be washed and reused. A microbiologic study evaluating the effectiveness of three different types of cleansing agents for decontaminating gloved hands that had been inoculated with nosocomial pathogens showed that, in general, bacteria adhere to gloves and are not easily washed off, even in the best of handwashing circumstances (49). The importance of glove removal between patient contact was illustrated by an outbreak of *Acinetobacter* in a surgical ICU that was associated with failure to change gloves between patient contacts (50). From 13% to 50% of hands are contaminated after glove removal (51,49), emphasizing the importance of handwashing following glove removal. Badri and coworkers evaluated the efficacy of glove use in preventing VRE hand contamination in 50 healthcare workers caring for 10 VRE-colonized patients (52). Twenty (40%) personnel were colonized with VRE prior to patient contact and a similar number (39%) demonstrated glove contamination with VRE after contact. After glove removal, 29% of those with glove contamination by VRE had the same strain on their hands—a 71% reduction in potential for hand contamination. These findings suggest that routine glove use can decrease risk of hand contamination, but gloves should be changed between patients and hands should be washed after removing gloves.

Gowns

The role of gowns in preventing transmission of nosocomial pathogens apart from the use of patient isolation and gloves remains controversial. A prospective, controlled study showed a 50% reduction in the infection rate in a pediatric ICU associated with the use of disposable nonwoven polypropylene gowns and nonsterile gloves (53). Although the incidence of pneumonia was similar in the gown-and-glove and the standard care groups, there were nearly four times as many cases of tracheobronchitis in the standard care group. Extrapolation of these findings to the adult ICU may not be justified because of the much higher rate of viral infections in the pediatric setting. Data from a longitudinal pediatric intervention study over three respiratory syncytial virus (RSV) seasons showed that the adjusted relative risk of nosocomial RSV transmission decreased three-fold as the frequency of glove and gown use increased from 38.5% of contact to 81% (54). However, in both of these studies (53,54), gowns and gloves were used together, making it impossible to determine the relative benefit of each of these barrier precautions.

Boyce and colleagues were unable to control an outbreak of VRE with isolation of colonized patients in private rooms and glove use (55). The addition of gowns successfully controlled the outbreak. However, this was not a controlled trial. Slaughter and coworkers randomized 181 medical ICU patients to gloves and gowns or gloves alone and found no difference in the rate of acquisition of VRE colonization (56). However, the addition of gowns was associated with higher overall compliance (79% versus 62% for gloves alone). Perhaps a gown requirement serves to remind caretakers of the importance of glove use and hand disinfection and limits contact of colonized or infected patients with less motivated personnel. Other studies of the use of gowns in neonatal and pediatric ICUs, in the newborn nursery, and in caring for immunocompromised cancer patients have not shown a significant reduction in infection rates (57,58,59). As a result, the use of gowns for infection control cannot be recommended except in situations where soiling or splashing of body fluids is expected; in some ICUs, such as burn units, this risk may be high enough to recommend routine gowning.

Masks

Masks decrease the risk of airborne transmission of organisms spread by small ("airborne") or large ("droplet") airborne particles. Airborne diseases include *Mycobacterium tuberculosis*, varicella (chicken pox or disseminated varicella), and measles. These diseases are spread by small airborne droplets (<5 μm) suspended in the air or by dust particles containing the microorganism and. These pathogens are easily dispersed widely by air currents and may be inhaled by a susceptible host in the same room or in an area of shared air circulation. Susceptible persons entering the patient's room should wear respiratory protection (N95 particulate respirator or HEPA filtration mask). If the patient must be transported outside of respiratory isolation, they should wear a surgical mask.

Droplet transmission is a risk when large-particle droplets (>5 μm) from an infectious person are generated by talking, coughing, sneezing, and during procedures involving manipulation of the airway. Transmission via large droplets requires close contact (within 3 feet) between the source and the recipient. Infections spread by respiratory droplets include meningococcal meningitis, multidrug-resistant pneumococcal meningitis or pneumonia, pertussis, streptococcal pharyngitis or pneumonia, and influenza. Surgical masks should be worn when one is within 3 feet of a patient with one of these illnesses. The patient should leave the room only when necessary and should wear a surgical mask when doing so.

The use of surgical masks is routine during the performance of invasive procedures. ICU personnel with viral upper respiratory infections (especially RSV) and orolabial HSV who continue to work while infected can decrease the risk of transmission to susceptible patients by wearing surgical masks.

Cohorting

An alternative or supplemental approach to private rooms is patient cohorting. Cohorting of staff has been employed successfully in the control of outbreaks of infection caused by VRE, MRSA and multidrug-resistant gram-negative bacteria (18,59,61). A corollary of staff cohorting is staffing levels. Understaffing limits the time available to staff to comply with infection control measures. In addition, understaffing exposes more patients to an individual caretaker increasing the risk of cross-transmission. Low staffing levels in ICUs has contributed to infection outbreaks with MRSA and gram-negative bacilli (62,63). Equipment can also be cohorted—a stethoscope, electronic thermometer, or sphygmomanometer dedicated for use in a particular patient or patient cohort known to be colonized or infected with a particular pathogen.

Stethoscope Disinfection

The role of stethoscopes in the transmission of nosocomial pathogens is not well defined. In studies of stethoscope contamination, bacteria have been recovered from 66%–100% of stethoscopes and 9%–38% of stethoscopes carried potentially pathogenic bacteria (64,65,66). Bacteria can survive on stethoscopes long enough to result in transmission from one patient to the next. VRE have been documented to survive for 30 minutes on stethoscope diaphragms (23) and some bacteria (e.g., *S. aureus*) survived for up to 18 hours (66). Disinfection with an alcohol pledget reliably reduces bacterial contamination. Disinfection of stethoscope diaphragms even if just cleansing with an alcohol wipe after each use would seem to be a prudent step, but the effect of this approach on infection prevention is unproved.

ENVIRONMENTAL CONTROLS

The hospital environment contributes negligibly to the acquisition and spread of most endemic nosocomial infections. However, there are important exceptions.

Air

Mycobacterium tuberculosis is transmitted from person-to-person via airborne droplet nuclei. Maintenance of "negative pressure" rooms with 6–12 room exchanges per hour of unrecirculated air [or of recirculated air through high efficiency particulate air (HEPA) filters] provides protection against the transmission of droplet nuclei of *M. tuberculosis* (67). Rooms should be monitored to ensure the maintenance of negative pressure with respect to anteroom or corridor air. Invasive aspergillosis usually is acquired via the inhalation of *Aspergillus* conidia. Use of "positive pressure" rooms that receive air after HEPA filtration helps protect severely immunosuppressed patients from airborne *Aspergillus* spores. Routine monitoring of air samples for airborne contamination by fungal spores is not recommended but may be useful during hospital renovation to evaluate adequacy of environmental controls in areas housing patients at risk for invasive aspergillosis (68).

Water

Legionella pneumophila colonization of hospital water systems has been linked to nosocomial legionnaires' disease and may go unrecognized for many years (69). Routine environmental cultures for *Legionella* in hospital water distribution systems have been recommended even if the hospital has not previously recognized cases of hospital-acquired legionnaires' disease (70), but this issue remains controversial. Disinfection methods have been developed which effectively eradicate the organism from the water supply (71). Non-fermenting gram-negative bacilli including *Pseudomonas aeruginosa, Stenotrophomonas maltophilia, Burkholderia cepacia* and *Acinetobacter* species have been found in almost every moist environment in the hospital (72). Plausible circumstantial evidence has implicated a variety of contaminated items in the transmission of non-fermenting gram-negative bacilli to patients including water, food, antiseptics, and medical devices. Nevertheless, most nosocomial infections with non-fermenting gram-negative bacilli result from overgrowth of endogenous flora or transmission from person-to-person on the hands of healthcare workers.

Environmental surfaces

Acinetobacter has been found to contaminate environmental surfaces including patient charts, tabletops, telephone handsets, and coffeepot handles (73). Investigation demonstrated that *Acinetobacter* survived better on dry Formica surfaces than on skin (74) and survived on Formica surfaces up to 13 days (73).

VRE have been identified from environmental cultures (56) including doors, bed rails, blood pressure cuffs, electronic thermometers, stethoscopes, pulse oximeters, tables, floors, patient gowns, linens and urometers (75,55,76,77). In one study, 26 (28%) of 92 environmental cultures were positive. Conventional disinfection procedures may incompletely eliminate VRE from hospital rooms. One study demonstrated that 16% of hospital room surfaces remained colonized with VRE after routine terminal disinfection (78). Conventional cleaning required an average of 2.8 disinfections to eradicate VRE from a hospital room. An alternative method of soaking surfaces for 10 minutes in quaternary ammonium compound was effective.

Environmental contamination may play a role in the transmission of *Clostridium difficile*. *C. difficile* spores have been shown to persist for as long as 5 months on surfaces in close proximity to patients with *C. difficile* infection (79). In one study, 49% of environmental cultures were positive for *C. difficile* in the rooms of patients with *C. difficile* infection versus only 8% in uninfected patients (80). Surface contamination was detected on patient charts, bed rails, commodes, floors, call buttons, bedpans, and windowsills.

The role of environmental contamination in the transmission of MRSA is uncertain. The organism has been recovered from many environmental surfaces in hospitals, but only rarely have these sites been implicated in transmission of infection. One notable exception may be the heavy environmental contamination in burn units, which may constitute an important reservoir (81).

No studies have shown a decreased nosocomial infection rate as a result of changes in the physical environment of the ICU. Nevertheless, the use of non-porous surfaces and sealed, water-resistant surfaces around plumbing is advisable (82). Wet acoustic ceiling tile may serve as a reservoir for fungal spores so prompt identification and repair of water leaks and replacement of water-damaged tiles is also recommended. Carpeting can harbor *Aspergillus*, *Fusarium*, and *Clostridium difficile* spores, but carpeting has not been clearly linked to the transmission of nosocomial infection (83). Several reports have identified an increased risk of nosocomial infection and death during hospital renovation and construction (84,85) and particular attention should be paid to air and water quality maintenance during these periods.

ANTIBIOTIC CONTROL

Inadequate antimicrobial therapy is an important determinant of mortality in ICU patients (86). Unfortunately, excessive antimicrobial therapy carries with it an increased risk of selection of drug-resistance. In a one-day point prevalence study of 1417 European ICUs, 62% of 10,038 patients received antibiotics on the day of the study (1). The intensive antibiotic therapy given to ICU patients inevitably leads to the emergence of resistance. ICUs show the highest rates of antibiotic use and the highest rates of antibiotic resistance. Data from the National Nosocomial Infection Surveillance (NNIS) system show a significant stepwise increase in the frequency of resistance for all major nosocomial pathogens from outpatient to inpatient ward to ICU (87). Unfortunately, by the time resistance among clinical isolates becomes apparent, colonization with resistant microorganisms may well be endemic. At that time, even high compliance rates with basic infection control measures may no longer effectively reduce endemnicity.

In response to the spread of resistant bacteria from patient to patient, a number of measures have been proposed (88,89). The goal of these measures is to reduce the incidence of resistant infections and to prolong or restore the effectiveness of existing antibiotics. In addition to improvements in infection control procedures, suggested measures have included controls on antibiotic use and cycling of different antibiotics.

Formulary Management

There is evidence that a policy of restriction—or complete withdrawal—of certain antibiotics has been useful in dealing with the emergence of multiresistant microorganisms. An outbreak of multi-resistant *Klebsiella pneumoniae* in an ICU was associated with previous treatment with third-generation cephalosporins and aminoglycosides (90). Barrier precautions and a significant reduction in the use of third-generation cephalosporins controlled the outbreak. A hospital-wide outbreak of ceftazidime-resistant *Klebsiella* was controlled with barrier precautions and ceftazidime restriction (91). Restriction of third-generation cephalosporins and vancomycin and addition of β-lactamase inhibitors decreased the prevalence of fecal colonization with VRE from 47% to 15% (92). Clindamycin restriction successfully controlled two different outbreaks of *Clostridium difficile*, showing a reduction from 11.5 cases/month to 3.33 cases/month in one study (93) and a reduction from 15.8 infections/1000 discharges to 1.9 infections/1000 discharges in another (94). Strict guidelines for the use of vancomycin have been proposed to limit the emergence of vancomycin resistance in enterococci and staphylococci (95).

Antibiotic Rotation

Antibiotic cycling is the purposeful alternation of routinely used antimicrobials. Antibiotic cycling proposes to reduce the antibiotic pressure that favors the emergence of resistance in a specific environment. Initial attempts at antibiotic cycling have produced encouraging results, but skepticism is appropriate. Aminoglycoside substitution programs at Veterans' Affairs hospitals exploited the ability of amikacin to withstand modification by most known aminoglycoside-modifying enzymes as a rationale for substituting amikacin for gentamicin and tobramycin (96). Replacement of gentamicin and tobramycin by amikacin resulted in reduced gentamicin resistance and amikacin resistance remained near baseline levels during all cycles. Replacement of ceftazidime by ciprofloxacin for the empiric treatment of suspected gram-negative bacterial infections in patients undergoing cardiac surgery during consecutive 6-month periods was associated with a significant reduction in the incidence of nosocomial pneumonia caused by antibiotic-resistant gram-negative bacteria (4.0% versus 0.9%) (97). No second round of ceftazidime was employed so no cycle was completed, i.e., the decrease in gram-negative nosocomial pneumonia may have had less to do with a scheduled change in antibiotic class and more to do with differences in the antimicrobial activity and risk of superinfection for ceftazidime and ciprofloxacin. A pilot study of cycling 4 different antibiotic regimens among neutropenic cancer patients showed no increase in antimicrobial resistance during the course of the study (98). However, the duration of the study was limited to 19 months and no regimen was repeated. It has not yet been shown that transferable

Table 2. Recommended Conventional Infection Control Measures for ICUs

Targeted surveillance with outcome objectives

Hand disinfection
- — Educate and re-educate hospital personnel
- — Augment handwashing with bedside alcohol-based hand disinfectants
- — Incorporate moisturizers into skin care regimens

Barrier precautions
- — Use gloves for any patient infected or colonized with a resistant strain
- — Consider glove use for all ICU patient contact
- — Disinfect hands after glove removal
- — Reserve gowns for anticipated soiling or splashing by body fluids
- — Disinfect stethoscope diaphragms between patient contacts

Antibiotic control
- — Review antimicrobial agents and select a basic formulary
- — Establish prophylaxis, empiric, and therapeutic guidelines
- — Restrict agents that have special or limited indications, excess toxicity, or high cost
- — Release restricted agents for predetermined circumstances or after prospective approval
- — Coordinate susceptibility testing and reporting by the microbiology laboratory with antibiotics on the formulary
- — Monitor antibiotic susceptibility patterns and antibiotic usage trends, with periodic regular feedback to the medical staff
- — Audit use of specific antibiotics
- — Conduct ongoing educational programs
- — Regulate in-hospital promotional efforts of pharmaceutical companies

resistance elements are eliminated by the use of antibiotic cycling strategies (99). Mathematical modeling projected that when single drug antibiotic therapy was employed, the risk of development of a high level of resistance was independent of the pattern of drug use (100). Furthermore, when more than one antibiotic was employed, cycling was always inferior to treatment strategies where, at any given time, equal fractions of the population received different antibiotics. In summary, the data to support antibiotic cycling are limited and a test of this approach is needed before cycling can be recommended.

CONCLUSION

Recommended conventional infection control measures are listed in Table 2. Infection surveillance is a necessary component of any attempt to limit nosocomial infections. Targeted surveillance with identified outcome objectives provides for the most effective use of resources. Surveillance cultures may help to inform infection control measures in ICUs with epidemic (or hyperendemic) nosocomial infection rates. Hand disinfection should receive vigorous re-emphasis with the application of user-friendly approaches including bedside dispensers of alcohol-based hand disinfectants as an alternative to handwashing in busy ICUs where appropriate handwashing with soap and water may not always be practical. An approach that merits further investigation is universal gloving for all contact with ICU patients. Hand disinfection following glove removal should be emphasized. Except as a reminder as to the importance of glove use and hand disinfection, the role of gowns in prevention of transmission of nosocomial pathogens is unproven and should be limited to activities where soiling or splashing of body fluids is anticipated. Stethoscope disinfection between patients is not proven to reduce infection rates but seems to be a rather simple, low cost measure. Judicious and appropriate antibiotic use is an increasing challenge when caring for critically ill patients in the face of widespread antibiotic resistance. Restriction of overutilized antimicrobial agents has been successful in controlling outbreaks of some drug-resistant pathogens and may delay the emergence of resistance in selected microorganisms. Novel approaches, including the use of antibiotic cycling, deserve further study.

Traditional infection control measures in ICUs have focused on limiting person-to-person spread of infection. These often fail because they have little effect on patients' endogenous flora (101). Nosocomial infection rates correlate strongly with device use (102). Improvements in the design and aseptic care of invasive devices have helped to decrease the risk of progression from colonization to infection. Non-invasive and infection-resistant devices, discussed elsewhere in this book, may provide the best hope for significant reduction in nosocomial infection risk in the future (103,104). If you have a choice between trying to improve adherence to conventional measures or developing an infection-proof device, go for the device.

REFERENCES

1. Vincent JL, Bihari DJ, Suter PM, Bruining HA, White J, Nicolas-Chanoin MH, et al. The prevalence of nosocomial infection in intensive care units in Europe. JAMA 1995;274:639–644.
2. Woeltje KF, Fraser VJ. Preventing nosocomial infections in the intensive unit—lessons learned from outcomes research. New Horiz 1998;6:84–90.
3. Olson B, Weinstein RA, Nathan C, Chamberlin W, Kabins SA. Epidemiology of endemic *Pseudomonas aeruginosa*: why infection control efforts have failed. J Infect Dis 1984;150:808–816.
4. Bonten MJM, Slaughter S, Hayden MK, Nathan C, van Voorhis J, Weinstein RA. External sources of vancomycin-resistant enterococci for intensive care units. Crit Care Med 1998;26:2001–2004.
5. Bonten MJM, Hayden MK, Nathan C, van Voorhis J, Matushek M, Slaughter S, Rice T, Weinstein RA. Epidemiology of colonization of patients and environment with vancomycin-resistant enterococci. Lancet 1996;348:1615–1619.
6. Ostrowsky BE, Venkataraman L, D'Agata EMC, Gold HS, DeGirolami PC, Samore MH. Vancomycin-resistant enterococci in intensive care units. Arch Intern Med 1999;159:1467–1472.
7. D'Agata EMC, Venkataraman L, DeGirolami P, Burke P, Eliopoulos GM, Karchmer AW, Samore MH. Colonization with broad-spectrum cephalosporin-resistant Gram-negative bacilli in intensive care units during a nonoutbreak period: prevalence, risk factors, and rate of infection. Crit Care Med 1999;27:1090–1095.
8. Cosseron-Zerbib M, Roque Afonso AM, Naas T, Durand P, Meyer L, Costa Y, El Helai N, Huault G, Nordmann P. A control programme for MRSA (methicillin-resistant *Staphylococcus aureus*) containment in a paediatric intensive care unit: evaluation and impact on infections caused by other micro-organisms. J Hosp Infect 1998;40:225–235.
9. Girou E, Pujade G, Legrand P, Ciseau F, Brun-Buisson C. Selective screening of carriers for control of methicillin-resistant *Staphylococcus aureus* (MRSA) in high-risk hospital areas with a high level of endemic MRSA. Clin Infect Dis 1998;27:543–550.
10. Teare EL, Barrett SP. Stop the ritual of tracing colonized people. BMJ 1997;314:665–666.
11. Bauer TM, Ofner E, Just HM, Just H, Daschner FD. An epidemiological study assessing the relative importance of airborne and direct contact transmission of microorganisms in a medical intensive care unit. J Hosp Infect 1990;15:301–309.
12. Larson EL. Persistent carriage of gram-negative bacteria on hands. Am J Infect Control 1981;9:112–119.

13. Casewell M, Phillips I. Hands as route of transmission for Klebsiella species. BMJ 1977;2:1315–1317.
14. Wade JJ, Desai N, Casewell MW. Hygienic hand disinfection for the removal of epidemic vancomycin-resistant *Enterococcus faecium* and gentamicin-resistant *Enterobacter cloacae*. J Hosp Infect 1991;18:211–218.
15. Go ES, Burns J, Kreiswirth B, Eisner W, Mariano N, Mosinka-Snipas K, Rahal JJ. Clinical and molecular epidemiology of acinetobacter infections sensitive only to polymyxin B and sulbactam. Lancet 1994;344:1329–1332.
16. French GL, Shannon KP, Simmons N. Hospital outbreak of *Klebsiella pneumoniae* resistant to broad-spectrum cephalosporins and β-lactam-β-lactamase inhibitor combinations by hyperproduction of SHV-5 β-lactamase. J Clin Microbiol 1996;34:358–363.
17. Coello R, Jimenez J, Garcia M, Arroyo P, Minguez D, Fernondez C, Cruzet F, Gaspar C. Prospective study of infection, colonization and carriage of methicillin-resistant *Staphylococcus aureus* in an outbreak affecting 990 patients. Eur J Clin Microbiol Infect Dis 1994;13:74–81.
18. Handwerger S, Raucher B, Altarac D, Monka J, Marchione S, Singh KV, Murray BE, Wolff J, Walters B. Nosocomial outbreak due to *Enterococcus faecium* highly resistant to vancomycin, penicillin, and gentamicin. Clin Infect Dis 1993;16:750–755.
19. Conly JM, Hill S, Ross J, Lertzman J, Louie TJ. Handwashing practices in an intensive unit: the effects of an educational program and its relationship to infection rates. Am J Infect Control 1989;17:330–339.
20. Doebbeling BN, Stanley GL, Sheetz CT, Pfaller M, Houston AK, Annis L, Li N, Wenzel RP. Comparative efficacy of alternative hand-washing agents in reducing nosocomial infections in intensive care units. N Engl J Med 1992;327:88–93.
21. Pittet D, Mourouga P, Perneger TV. Compliance with handwashing in a teaching hospital. Ann Intern Med 1999;130:126–130.
22. Husni RN, Goldstein LS, Arroliga AC, Hall GS, Fatica C, Stoller JK, Gordon SM. Risk factors for an outbreak of multi-drug-resistant acinetobacter nosocomial pneumonia among intubated patients. Chest 1999;115:1378–1382.
23. Noskin GA, Stosor V, Cooper I, Peterson LR. Recovery of vancomycin-resistant enterococci on fingertips and environmental surfaces. Infect Control Hosp Epidemiol 1995;16:577–581.
24. Larson EL, Killien M. Factors influencing handwashing behavior of patient care personnel. Am J Infect Control 1982;10:93–99.
25. Khatib M, Jamaleddine G, Abdallah A, Ibrahim Y. Hand washing and use of gloves while managing patients receiving mechanical ventilation in the ICU. Chest 1999;116:172–175.
26. Gould D. Nurses' hand decontamination practice: results of a local study. J Hosp Infect 1994;28:15–30.
27. Mayer JA, Dubbert PM, Miller M, Burkett PA, Chapman SW. Increasing handwashing in an intensive care unit. Infect Control 1986;7:259–262.
28. McGuckin M, Waterman R, Porten L, Bello S, Caruso S, Juzaitis B, Krug E, Mazer S, Ostrawski S. Patient education model for increasing handwashing compliance. Am J Infect Control 1999;27:309–314.
29. Voss A, Widmer AF. No time for handwashing!? Handwashing versus alcoholic: can we afford 100% compliance? Infect Control Hosp Epidemiol 1997;18:205–208.
30. Cardoso CL, Pereira HH, Zequim JC, Guilhermetti M. Effectiveness of hand-cleansing agents for removing *Acinetobacter baumanii* strain from contaminated hands. Am J Infect Control 1999;27:327–331.
31. Paulson DS, Fendler EJ, Dolan MJ, Williams RA. A close look at alcohol gel as an antimicrobial sanitizing agent. Am J Infect Control 1999;27:332–338.
32. Zaragoza M, Salles M, Gomez J, Bayas JM, Trilla A. Handwashing with soap or alcoholic solutions? A randomized trial of its effectiveness. Am J Infect Control 1999;27:258–261.
33. Adams BG, Marrie TJ. Hand carriage of aerobic Gram-negative rods may not be transient. J Hyg (Camb)1982;89:33–46.
34. Austin DJ, Bonten MJM, Weinstein RA, Slaughter S, Anderson RM. Vancomycin-resistant enterococci: transmission dynamics, persistence, and the impact of infection control programs. Proc Natl Acad Sci 1999;96:6908–6913.
35. Bonten MJM, Slaughter S, Ambergen AW, Hayden MK, van Voorhis J, Nathan C, Weinstein RA. The role of "colonization pressure" in the spread of vancomycin-resistant enterococci. Arch Intern Med 1998;158:1127–1132.
36. Garner JS, HIPAC. Guideline for isolation precautions in hospitals. Infect Control Hosp Epidemiol 1996;17:53–80.

37. Guiguet M, Rekacewicz C, Leclercq, Brun Y, Escudier B, Andremont A. Effectiveness of simple measures to control an outbreak of nosocomial methicillin-resistant *Staphylococcus aureus* infections in an intensive care unit. Infect Control Hosp Epidemiol 1990;11:23–26.
38. Hartstein AI, Denny MA, Morthland VH, LeMonte AM, Pfaller MA. Control of methicillin-resistant *Staphylococcus aureus* in a hospital and an intensive care unit. Infect Control Hosp Epidemiol 1995;16:405–411.
39. Montecalvo MA, Jarvis WR, Uman J, Shay DK, Petrullo C, Rodney K, et al. Infection-control measures reduce transmission of vancomycin-resistant enterococci in an endemic setting. Ann Intern Med 1999;131:269–272.
40. Meier PA, Carter CD, Wallace SE, Hollis RJ, Pfaller MA, Herwaldt LA. A prolonged outbreak of methicillin-resistant *Staphylococcus aureus* in the burn unit of a tertiary medical center. Infect Control Hosp Epidemiol 1996;17:798–802.
41. Lai KK, Kelley AL, Melvin ZS, Belliveau PP, Fontecchio SA. Failure to eradicate vancomycin-resistant enterococci in a university hospital and the cost of barrier precautions. Infect Control Hosp Epidemiol 1998;19:647–652.
42. Kirkland KB, Weinstein JM. Adverse effects of contact isolation. Lancet 1999;354:117–118.
43. McManus AT, Mason AD, McManus WF, Pruitt BA. A decade of reduced gram-negative infections and mortality associated with improved isolation of burned patients. Arch Surg 1994;129:1306–1309.
44. Mulin B, Rouget C, Clement C, Bailly P, Julliot MC, Viel AFF, et al. Association of private isolation rooms with ventilator-associated *Acinetobacter baumanii* pneumonia in a surgical intensive care unit. Infect Control Hosp Epidemiol 1997;18:499–503.
45. Preston GA, Larson EL, Stamm WE. The effect of private isolation rooms on patient care practices, colonization and infection in an intensive care unit. Am J Med 1981;70:641–645.
46. Weinstein RA, Nathan C, Gruensfelder R, et al. Endemic aminoglycoside resistance in gram negative bacilli: epidemiology and mechanisms. J Infect Dis 1980;141:338–345.
47. Johnson S, Gerding DN, Olson MM, Weiler MD, Hughes RA, Clabots CR, Peterson LR. Prospective controlled study of vinyl glove use to interrupt Clostridium difficile nosocomial transmission. Am J Med 1990;88:137–140.
48. Lund S, Jackson J, Leggett J, Hales L, Dworkin R, Gilbert D. Reality of glove use and handwashing in a community hospital. Am J Infect Control 1994;22:352–357.
49. Doebbelling BN, Pfaller MA, Houston AK, Wenzel RP. Removal of nosocomial pathogens from the contaminated glove. Ann Intern Med 1988;109:394–398.
50. Patterson JE, Vecchio J, Pantelick EL, Farrel P, Mazon D, Zervos M, Heirholzer WJ. Association of contaminated gloves with transmission of *Acinetobacter calcoaceticus* var. *anitratus* in an intensive care unit. Am J Med 1991;91:479–483.
51. Olsen RJ, Lynch P, Coyle MB, Cummings J, Bokete T, Stamm WE. Examination gloves as barriers to hand contamination in clinical practice. JAMA 1993;270:350–353.
52. Badri SM, Sahgal NB, Tenorio AR, Law K, Hota B, Matushek M, Hayden MK, Trenholme GM, Weinstein RA. Effectiveness of gloves in preventing the transmission of vancomycin-resistant enterococcus (VRE) during patient care activities. 36th Annual Meeting of the Infectious Diseases Society of America, Denver;1998:abstract 599.
53. Klein BS, Perloff WH, Maki DG. Reduction of nosocomial infection during pediatric intensive care by protective isolation. N Engl J Med 1989;320:1714–1721.
54. Leclair JM, Freeman J, Sullivan BF, et al. Prevention of nosocomial respiratory syncytial virus infections through compliance with glove and gown isolation precautions. N Engl J Med 1987;317:329–334.
55. Boyce JM, Opal SM, Chow JW, Zervos MJ, Potter-Bynoe G, Sherman CB, et al. Outbreak of multidrug-resistant Enterococcus faecium with transferable *van*B class vancomycin resistance. J Clin Microbiol 1994;32:1148–1153.
56. Slaughter S, Hayden MK, Nathan C, Hu TC, Rice T, Van Voorhis J, et al. A comparison of the effect of universal use of gloves and gowns with that of glove use alone on acquisition of vancomycin-resistant enterococci in a medical intensive care unit. Ann Intern Med 1996;125:448–456.
57. Haque KN, Chagla AH. Do gowns prevent infection in neonatal intensive care units? J Hosp Infect 1989;14:159–162.
58. Donowitz LG. Failure of the overgown to prevent nosocomial infection in a pediatric intensive care unit. Pediatrics 1986;77:35–38.
59. Nauseef WM, Maki DG. A study of the value of simple protective isolation in patients with granulocytopenia. N Engl J Med 1981;304:448–453.

60. Matsumura H, Yoshizawa N, Narumi A, Harunari N, Sugamata A, Watanabe K. Effective control of methicillin-resistant *Staphylococcus aureus* in a burn unit. Burns 1996;22:283–286.
61. Acolet D, Ahmet Z, Houang E. Hurley R, Kaufmann ME. *Enterobacter cloacae* in a neonatal intensive care unit: account of an outbreak and its relationship to use of third generation cephalosporins. J Hosp Infect 1994;28:273.
62. Arnow PM, Allyn PA, Nichols EM, Hill DL, Pezzlo M, Bartlett RH. Control of MRSA in a burn unit: role of nurse staffing. J Trauma 1982;22:954–959.
63. Harbarth S, Sudre P, Dharan S, Cadenas M, Pittet D. Outbreak of *Enterobacter cloacae* related to understaffing, overcrowding, and poor hygiene practices. Infect Control Hosp Epidemiol 1999;20:598–603.
64. Smith MA, Mathewson JJ, Ulert A, Scerpella EG, Ericsson CD. Contaminated stethoscopes revisited. Arch Intern Med 1996;156:82–84.
65. Marinella MA, Pierson C, Chenoweth C. The stethoscope: a potential source of nosocomial infection? Arch Intern Med 1997;157:786–790.
66. Bernard L, Kereveur A, Durand D, Gonot J, Goldstein F, Mainardi JL, et al. Bacterial contamination of hospital physicians' stethoscopes. Infect Control Hosp Epidemiol 1999;20:626–628.
67. Centers for Disease Control. Guidelines for preventing the transmission of *Mycobacterium tuberculosis* in health-care facilities. MMWR 1994;43(RR-13):i–132.
68. Cornet M, Levy V, Fleury L, Lortholary J, Barquins S, Coureul MH, et al. Efficacy of prevention by high-efficiency particulate air filtration or laminar airflow against Aspergillus airborne contamination during hospital renovation. Infect Control Hosp Epidemiol 1999;20:508–513.
69. Kool JL, Fiore AE, Kioski CM, Brown EW, Benson RF, Pruckler JM, et al. More than 10 years of unrecognized nosocomial transmission of legionnaires' disease among transplant patients. Infect Control Hosp Epidemiol 1998;19:898–904.
70. Goetz AM, Stout JE, Jacobs, Fisher MA, Ponzer RE, Drenning S, Yu VL. Nosocomial legionnaires' disease discovered in community hospitals following cultures of the water system: seek and ye shall find. Am J Infect Control 1998;26:8–11.
71. Stout JE, Lin YE, Goetz AM, Muder RR. Controlling *Legionella* in hospital water systems: experience with superheat-and-flush method and copper-silver ionization. Infect Control Hosp Epidemiol 1998;19:911–914.
72. Arnow PM, Flaherty JP. Nonfermentative gram-negative bacilli. In; Hospital Epidemiology and Infection Control, 2nd edition. Mayhall CG, ed. Lippincott, Williams & Wilkins, Philadelphia, 1999.
73. Getchell-White SI, Donowitz LG, Groschel DHM. The inanimate environment of an intensive care unit as a potential source of nosocomial bacteria: evidence for long survival of *Acinetobacter calcoaceticus*. Infect Control Hosp Epidemiol 1989;10:402–407.
74. Musa EK, Desai N, Casewell MW. The survival of *Acinetobacter calcoaceticus* inoculate on fingertips and on formica. J Hosp Infect 1990;15:219–227.
75. Karanfil LV, Murphy M, Josephson A, Gaynes R, Mandel L, Hill BC, et al. A cluster of vancomycin-resistant *Enterococcus faecium* in an intensive care unit. Infect Control Hosp Epidemiol 1992; 13:195–200.
76. Livornese LL Jr, Dias S, Samel C, Romanoski B, Taylor S, May P, et al. Hospital-acquired infection with vancomycin-resistant *Enterococcus faecium* transmitted by electronic thermometers. Ann Intern Med 1992;117:112–116.
77. Porwancher R, Sheth A, Remphrey S, Taylor E, Hinkle C, Zervos M. Epidemiological study of hospital-acquired infection with vancomycin-resistant *Enterococcus faecium*: possible transmission by an electronic ear-probe thermometer. Infect Control Hosp Epidemiol 1997;18:771–773.
78. Byers KE, Durbin LJ, Simonton BM, Anglim A, Adal KA, Farr BM. Disinfection of hospital rooms contaminated with vancomycin-resistant *Enterococcus faecium*. Infect Control Hosp Epidemiol 1998;19:261–264.
79. Fekety R, Kim KH, Brown D, Batts DH, Cudmore M, Silva J Jr. Epidemiology of antibiotic-associated colitis. Isolation of *Clostridium difficile* from the hospital environment. Am J Med 1981;70:906–908.
80. McFarland LV, Mulligan ME, Kwok RYY, Stamm WE. Nosocomial acquisition of *Clostridium difficile* infection. N Engl J Med 1989;320:204–210.
81. Boyce JM, white RL, Causey WA, Lockwood WR. Burn units as a source of methicillin-resistant *Staphylococcus aureus* infections. JAMA 1983;249:2803–2807.
82. Harvey MA. Critical-care-unit bedside design and furnishings: impact on nosocomial infections. Infect Control Hosp Epidemiol 1998;19:597–601.

83. Skoutelis AT, Westenfelder GO, Beckerdite M, Phair JP. Hospital carpeting and epidemiology of *Clostridium difficile*. Am J Infect Control 1993;22:212–217.
84. Weems JJ Jr, Davis BJ, Tablan OC, Kaufman L, Martone WJ. Construction activity: an independent risk factor for invasive aspergillosis and zygomycosis in patients with hematologic malignancy. Infect Control 1987;8:71–75.
85. Mermel LA, Josephson SL, Giorgio CH, Dempsey J, Parenteau S. Association of legionnaires' disease with construction: contamination of potable water. Infect Control Hosp Epidemiol 1995;16:76–81.
86. Kollef MH, Sherman G, Ward, Fraser VJ. Inadequate antimicrobial treatment of infections; a risk factor for hospital mortality among critically ill patients. Chest 1999;115:462–474.
87. Archibald L, Phillips L, Monnet D, McGowan JE, Tenover F, Gaynes R. Antimicrobial resistance in isolates from inpatients and outpatients in the United States: increasing importance of the intensive care unit. Clin Infect Dis 1997;24:211–215.
88. Shlaes DM, Gerding DN, John JF, Craig WA, Bornstein DL, Duncan RA, et al. Society for Healthcare Epidemiology of America and Infectious Diseases Society of America Joint Committee on the Prevention of Antimicrobial Resistance: guidelines for the prevention of antimicrobial resistance in hospitals. Clin Infect Dis 1997;25:584–599.
89. Flaherty JP, Weinstein RA. Nosocomial infection caused by antibiotic-resistant organism in the intensive-care unit. Infect Control Hosp Epidemiol 1996;17:236–248.
90. Asensio A, Oliver A, Gonzalez-Diego P, Baquero F, Perez-Diaz JC, Ros P, et al. Outbreak of a multiresistant *Klebsiella pneumoniae* strain in an intensive care unit: antibiotic use as risk factor for colonization and infection. Clin Infect Dis 2000;30:55–60.
91. Meyer KS, Urban C, Eagan JA, Berger BJ, Rahal JJ. Nosocomial outbreak of *Klebsiella* infection resistant to late-generation cephalsporins. Ann Intern Med 1993;119:353–358.
92. Quale J, Landman, Saurina G, Atwood E, DiTore V, Patel K. Manipulation of a hospital formulary to control an outbreak of vancomycin-resistant enterococci. Clin Infect Dis 1996;23:1020–1025.
93. Climo MW, Israel DS, Wong ES, Williams D, Coudron P, Markowitz SM. Hospital-wide restriction of clindamycin: effect on the incidence of *Clostridium difficile*-associated diarrhea and cost. Ann Intern Med 998;128:989–995.
94. Pear SM, Williamson TH, Bettin KM, Gerding DN, Galgiani JN. Decrease in nosocomial *Clostridium difficile*-associated diarrhea by restricting clindamycin use. Ann Intern Med 1994;120:272–277.
95. Centers for Disease Control and Prevention. Recommendations for preventing the spread of vancomycin resistance: recommendations of the Hospital Infection Control Practices Advisory Committee (HICPAC). MMWR 1995;44 (RR-12):1–12.
96. Gerding DN. Antimicrobial cycling: lessons learned from the aminoglycoside experience. Infect Control Hosp Epidemiol 2000;21(Suppl):S12–S17.
97. Kollef MN, Vlasnik J, Sharpless L, Pasque C, Murphy D, Fraser V. Scheduled change of antibiotic classes: a strategy to decrease the incidence of ventilator-associated pneumonia. Am J Resp Crit Care Med 1997;156:1040–1048.
98. Dominguez EA, Smith TL, Reed E, Sanders CC, Sanders WE. A pilot study of antibiotic cycling in a hematology-oncology unit. Infect Control Hosp Epidemiol 2000;21(Suppl):S4–S8.
99. John JF, Rice LB. The microbial genetics of antibiotic cycling. Infect Control Hosp Epidemiol 2000;21(Suppl):S22–S31.
100. Bonhoeffer S, Lipsitch M, Levin B. Evaluating treatment protocols to prevent antibiotic resistance. Proc Natl Acad Sci USA 1997;94:12106–12111.
101. Weinstein RA. Epidemiology and control of nosocomial infections in adult intensive care units. Am J Med 1991;91(Suppl 3B):179S–184S.
102. Richards MJ, Edwards JR, Culver DH, Gaynes RP, and the NNIS system. Nosocomial infections in medical intensive care units in the United States. Crit Care Med 1999;27:887–892.
103. Nourdine K, Combes P, Carton MJ, Beuret P, Cannamela A, Ducreux JC. Does noninvasive ventilation reduce the ICU nosocomial infection risk? A prospective clinical survey. Intensive Care Med 1999;25:567–573.
104. Darouiche RO. Anti-infective efficacy of silver-coated medical prostheses. Clin Infect Dis 1999;29:1371–1377.

17. CONVENTIONAL INFECTION CONTROL MEASURES: VALUE OR RITUAL?

C.A.M. SCHURINK M.D., M.J.M. BONTEN M.D.

Department of Internal Medicine, Division of Aids and Infectious Diseases, University Hospital Utrecht, PO Box 85000, 3508 GA Utrecht, the Netherlands

INTRODUCTION

Patients admitted to intensive care units (ICU) are prone to develop nosocomial (or hospital acquired) infections (1). Besides immunosuppression as a result of underlying disease, infections are facilitated by the necessary exposure to life-saving procedures (e.g. use of ventilation tubes, urine catheters and central venous lines) which break the first lines of defense against microorganisms. Nosocomial infections are associated with increased morbidity and mortality and generate high costs. Infections usually develop after preceding colonization on the skin or in the respiratory, gastrointestinal or urogenital tract.

Colonization may be facilitated via different routes. On admission, patients are frequently colonized by small (even non-detectable) numbers of bacteria, such as e.g. *Pseudomonas aeruginosa* (2) and Enterobacter species (3) in the gut and methicillin-resistant coagulase-negative staphylococci on the skin (4). Under the selective pressure of antibiotics these bacteria proliferate to become major components of the patients flora, sometimes developing resistance to multiple antibiotics (5). This route of colonization is called endogenous colonization.

In addition, ICU-patients may acquire colonization after an event of "cross-acquisition", when pathogens are transmitted from one patient, via health care worker (HCW) or via contaminated materials to another patient. The purpose of hand hygiene is to prevent hand-associated microbial transfer from one patient to another via the hands of HCW. In the mid-1800s Semmelweis already demonstrated,

R.A. Weinstein and M.J.M. Bonten (eds.). INFECTION CONTROL IN THE ICU ENVIRONMENT.

by means of a natural experiment, the importance of disinfection of the hands in reducing infection and mortality in the Obstetric University Clinic in Vienna (6).

The different routes of colonization indicate the need of different approaches for infection control. When cross-transmission is involved, the possibilities for transmission should be limited. This can be achieved by adequate handwashing or by using gloves. Another way of limiting transmission possibilities is by reducing the number of contacts between a single HCW and different patients, by cohorting nursing staff. In contrast, when endogenous colonization is the most important route of acquisition, adequate hand-washing and cohorting will not influence colonization rates. In these circumstances restriction of antibiotic use may reduce the risk of colonization and infection (7).

In theory, handwashing and cohorting of nursing staff are very effective infection control measures. However, little is known about the quantitative effects of these measures. In optimal circumstances compliance with handwashing would be 100%, and with 100% efficacy of handwashing there would be no cross-contamination. However, multiple studies have demonstrated that compliance with handwashing is usually low, and far less is known about the efficacy of different substances that are used for handwashing. When evaluating these variables, one should know the normal flora of hands and the different techniques to culture hand contamination.

Cohorting of nursing staff to single patients may even be a more efficient method of infection prevention. If each HCW would only contact one single patient, there would be no cross- contamination. Although a one-to-one patient-nurse ratio is pursued during day shifts in many ICUs, there is considerable mixing in practice. When colonization or infection with multiple resistant pathogens occurs sporadically, individual patients can be strictly isolated. However, this is not possible if colonization with these pathogens is endemic. Little is known about the level of cohorting of nurses in ICU and about its effects on spread of pathogens. Moreover, physicians are, by definition, not cohorted to single patients, and thus represent an important vector for bacterial spread. In this chapter we will discuss the different aspects of handwashing and cohorting with regard to cross-transmission in ICU.

MICROBIAL FLORA OF THE HANDS

The microbial flora of hands can be divided in three groups: organisms that reside on the skin (resident flora), organisms that contaminate hands for a short period of time (transient flora) and pathogens that cause infections on the hands (infectious flora).

Resident Flora

The common skin flora contains aerobic and anaerobic bacteria which colonize the stratum corneum (the most superficial layer of the skin). These bacteria multiply in the upper regions of hair follicles. Examples of these bacteria are Staphylococcal species (coagulase negative staphylococci and *S. aureus*), micrococci and Diphteroids like Corynebacteria species (*e.g. C. jeikeii*) and *Propionibacterium acnes*. Gram-negative bacteria like Acinetobacter species, Enterobacter species and Pseudomonas species and yeasts like Candida species are also considered natural habitants of the skin (8).

The ducts of sebaceous glands are frequently colonized with anaerobic propionibacteria, whereas ducts of eccrine and apocrine glands and deeper regions are usually sterile. Composition of the skin flora varies qualitatively and quantitatively with body site, sex, age, health condition, length of hospitalization and season (9). Unless introduced into body tissues by trauma or with foreign bodies, the pathogenic potential of the resident flora is usually regarded as low.

The population density of resident skin bacteria on hands ranges from 10^2 to 10^3 colony-forming units (cfu)/cm^2 (9) and may differ significantly in separate areas. Highest densities of microorganisms (especially fungi and Gram-negative bacteria) have been found on the subungal region (10). Resident flora is difficult to remove (9). The purpose of extensive handwashing before surgery is to diminish the quantity of resident flora in order to reduce contamination in case of punctured or thorn gloves during surgery.

Transient Flora

The transient flora is characterized by bacteria which can not multiply on the skin. These bacteria, usually Gram-negative bacteria, are regarded as skin contaminants, which may be pathogenic. This flora is easily removed by mechanical means like handwashing (9), which is the purpose of routine hand cleansing in ICU to prevent transmission of pathogens to other patients.

Infectious Flora

Usually *S. aureus* and β-hemolytic group streptococci are the etiologic agents of infections, such as abscesses, panaritium or paronychia. Needless to say that in case of infection of the hand, a HCW should refrain from working with patients, food and pharmaceuticals.

METHODS OF CULTURING HANDS

There are several methods to culture the microbial flora of hands. Imprints of fingertips can be made on selective agar plates, and numbers of colonies can be counted after incubation for 24 or 48 hours. Another method is to rub hands in a plastic bag or glove filled with water, and to pipet a defined amount of fluid on agar plates for incubation. Finally, a moistened cotton swab or spatula can be used to culture or scrub the skin. Wet swabs have been demonstrated to yield equal results on culturing surface and subsurface flora as compared to the scrub method (11).

Cleansing the Hands with Water and Soap or Anti-Septic Ingredients?

Although rubbing the hands with plain or antiseptic soap and water is assumed to remove transient flora (12), some studies have shown that frequent hand-washing

Table 1. Reduction of the Release of Test Bacteria from Artificially Contaminated Hands by Washingwith Soap and Water (9)

Duration	Mean $\log_{10}$ Reduction
15 sec	0.6–1.1
30 sec	1.8–2.8
1 minute	2.7–3.0
2 minutes	3.3
4 minutes	3.7

with soap and water only results in a minimal reduction or even increase in bacterial contamination. The increase may result from increased shedding of bacteria in desquamating epithelium during the washing procedure (12). The efficacy of hand-washing with water and soap is time-dependent (Table 1). Hands are usually washed for no longer than 15–30 seconds, during which time bacterial clearance is far from optimal.

For removal of transient flora, anti-septic solutions are at least as good as washing with water and soap, as long as the period of washing with water and soap is 15 to 30 seconds (13,14).

Recent studies have demonstrated superiority of using hand antiseptic solutions over water and soap. For example, hand cleansing with unmedicated soap and water after patient care was associated with significantly higher bacterial counts than hand cleansing with an antiseptic agent (15). And in an experimental study, hand washing did not prevent transfer of Gram-negative bacteria from hands from HCW to urine catheters in 12 out of 12 experiments, whereas transfer occurred in only 2 of 12 experiments when alcohol was used for disinfection (16).

The Fulkerson Scale (17,18) (Table 2) can be used to distinguish activities for which either alcohol rub or handwash with water and soap is adviced. In this scale, nursing activities are ranked from "clean" to "dirty" activities. Activities ranked from 1 to 7 are considered 'clean' and activities ranging from 8 to 15 are considered dirty.

Although it has been demonstrated that vigorous hand-washing could disperse highly pathogenic organism such as *Salmonella typhi* in the environment and onto the person who was washing (9), this is very seldom the case, so it should be advised that activities ranked on the Fulkerson Scale as very dirty (ranks 13–15) or dirty (ranks 8–12) are followed by a disinfection rub. When the hands are visibly soiled hand-washing with water and soap should be performed.

The guidelines of the Association for Professionals in Infection Control and Epidemiology (APIC) for hand-washing also advice to wash hands with water and soap only when they are visibly soiled (see table 3). In all other situations, the use of anti-septic hand rubs is recommended (12).

Washing the Hands Manual or by Hand-Washing Machine?

Hand-washing machines have been designed to improve compliance of washing, but in fact reduced compliance as they proved to be more time consuming and less

Table 2. Fulkerson Scale Ranking Contacts of Nursing Personnel from Clean to Dirty (9)

Rank	Contact with
1	Sterile or autoclaved materials
2	Thoroughly cleaned or washed materials
3	Materials not necessary cleaned but free from patient contact (e.g. papers)
4	Objects contacted by patients either infrequently or not expected to be contaminated (e.g. patient furniture)
5	Objects intimately associated with patients, but not known to be contaminated (e.g. patient gowns, linens, dishes, bedside rails)
6	Patient, but minimal and limited (e.g. shaking hands, taking pulse)
7	Objects in contact with patient secretions
8	Patient secretions or mouth, nose, genitoanal area, etc
9	Materials contaminated by patient urine
10	Patient urine
11	Materials contaminated with feces
12	Feces
13	Materials contaminated with feces
14	Secretions or excretions from infected sites
15	Infected patient sites (e.g. wounds, tracheotomy)

"clean" = activities 1–7
"dirty" = activities 8–15

Table 3. Association for professionals in infection Control and Epidemiology (APIC) guidelines for Handwashing and Hand antisepsis in Health Care Settings (12)

A. Health care personell handwashing and handantisepsis.

1. Hands must be washed thoroughly with soap and water when visibly soiled.

2. Hands must be cared for by handwashing with soap and water or by hand antisepsis with alcohol-based handrubs (if hands are not visibly soiled):
   a. Before and after patient contact.
   b. After contact with a source of microorganisms (body fluids and substances, mucous membranes, non intact skin, inanimate objects that are likely to be contaminated).
   c. After removing gloves.

3. Wet hands with running water. Apply hand-washing agent and thoroughly distribute over hands. Vigorously rub hands together for 10 to 15 seconds, covering all surfaces of the hands and fingers.

4. For general patient care, a plain, nonantimicrobial soap is recommended in any convenient form (bar, leaflets, liquid, powder). Such detergent-based products may contain very low concentrations of antimicrobial agents that are used as preservatives to prevent microbial contamination. If bar soap is used, small bars that can be changed frequently and soap racks that promote drainage should be used.

5. Hand antisepsis, achieved by handwashing or surgical scrub with antimicrobial-containing soaps or detergents or by use of alcohol-based antiseptic handrubs, is recommended in the following instances:
   a. Before the performance of invasive procedures such as surgery or the placement of intravascular catheters, indwelling urinary catheters, or other invasive devices.
   b. When persistent antimicrobial activity on the hands is desired.
   c. When it is important to reduce numbers of resident skin flora in addition to transient microorganisms.

6. In settings where handwashing facilities are inadequate or inaccessible and hands are not soiled with dirt or heavily contaminated with blood or other organic material, alcohol-based handrubs are recommended for use. In situations where soilage occurs, detergent-containing towelettes should be used to cleanse the hands; alcohol-based handrubs can then be used to achieve hand antisepsis.

Table 3. (Continued)

7. In the event of interruption of water supply, alternative agents such as detergent-containing towelettes and alcohol-based hand-rubs should be available.
8. Products used for handwashing, surgical scrubs, and hand care should be chosen by persons knowledgeable about the purpose of use, the advantages and disadvantages, cost, and acceptance of the product by users.
9. Routine use of hexachlorophene is not recommended.

B. Personnel hand preparation for operative procedures

1. The procedure for surgical hand scrub should include the following steps:
   a. Wash hands and forearms thoroughly.
   b. Clean under nails with a nail cleaner.
   c. Rinse thoroughly.
   d. Apply antimicrobial agent to wet hands and forearm with friction for at least 120 seconds.
2. If an alcohol-based preparation is selected for use, wash hands and arms, clean fingernails thoroughly, dry completely, and follow manufacturer's recommendations for application. Generally, application should last for at least 20 seconds.

C. Other aspects of hand care and protection.

1. Glove use
   a. Gloves should be used as an adjunct to, not a substitute for, handwashing.
   b. Gloves should be used for hand-contaminating activities. Gloves should be removed and hands washed when such activity is completed, when the integrity of the gloves is in doubt, and between patients. Gloves may need to be changed during the care of a single patient, for example when moving from one procedure to another.
   c. Disposable gloves should be used only once and should not be washed for reuse.
   d. Gloves made of other materials should be available for personnel with sensitivity to usual glove material (such as latex).
2. Condition of nails and hands
   a. Nails should be short enough to allow the individual to thoroughly clean underneath them and not cause glove tears.
   b. The hands, including the nails and surrounding tissue, should be inflammation free.
3. Lotion
   a. Lotions may be used to prevent skin dryness associated with handwashing.
   b. If used, lotion should be supplied in small, individual-use or pump dispenser containers that are not refilled.
   c. Compatibility between lotion and antiseptic products and the effect of petroleum or other oil emollients on the integrity of gloves should be considered at the time of product selection.
4. Storage and dispensing of hand care products
   a. Liquid products should be stored in closed containers.
   b. Disposable containers should be used. If disposable containers cannot be used, routine maintenance schedules for cleaning and refilling should be followed. Reusable containers should be thoroughly washed and dried before refilling.
   c. There should be a routine mechanism to ensure that soap and towel dispensers function properly and are adequately supplied.
   d. Containers of alcohol should be stored in cabinets or areas approved for flammables.
5. Drying of hands
   a. Cloth towels, hanging or roll type, are not recommended for use in health care facilities.
   b. Paper towels or hand blowers should be within easy reach of the sink but beyond splash contamination.
   c. Lever-operated towel dispensers should be activated before beginning hand-washing. Hand blowers should be activated with the elbow.
6. Behavior and compliance. Efforts to improve handwashing practice should be multifaceted and should include continuing education and feedback to staff on behavior or infection surveillance data. Unit clinical and administrative staff should be involved in the planning and implementation of strategies to improve compliance and handwashing.

Table 4. Hygienic handwash: efficacy of various antiseptic detergents in reducing the release of test bacteria from artificially contaminated hands (9)

Detergent	Conc (%)	Mean log reduction
Povidone-iodine	0.75*	3.5#
Chlorhexidine gluconate	4.0*	3.1
Triclosan	0.1$	2.8
2-Biphenylol	2.0$	2.6
Octenidine	0.5$	2.5
Soft soap	20.0*	2.7

Duration of treatment: 1 minute
* weight/volume
$ weight/weight
# significantly better than soap

effective than washing hands manually (19). Moreover, these machines may become contaminated, for example with *coagulase negative staphylococci* (20).

Effect on Hands by Washing

Handwashing induces changes in pH and reduces the amount of fatty acids on the skin. These changes are usually transient, but when performed frequently, handwashing may lead to contact-dermatitis and eczema. This disadvantage of handwashing can be an important reason of non-compliance by HCW. Moreover, damaged skin is prone to become colonized with potential pathogens, washing at these sites is less effective in reducing bacteria and pathogens will be shed more easily than from healthy skin flora (21). Washing hands with water and unmedicated soap gave more skin irritation than using alcoholic handgels, as was demonstrated in a recently published article (22).

CHARACTERISTICS OF SELECTED ANTI-SEPTIC INGREDIENTS

1. Alcohol

Alcohol probably derives its antimicrobial effect by denaturation of proteins (tables 4 en 5). It has excellent bactericidal activity against most Gram-positive and Gram-negative microorganisms, and is also active against many fungi and viruses. In appropriate concentrations, alcohol provides the most rapid and greatest reduction in microbial counts on the skin. Alcohol applications as short as 15 seconds in duration have been effective in preventing hand-transmission of Gram-negative bacteria (16). Three alcoholic substances are most appropriate for use on skin: ethyl (ethanol), normal-propyl (η-propyl), and isopropyl. There are slight differences in antimicrobial efficacy, but for clinical practice the concentration of alcohol is much more important. Alcohol concentrations between 60% to 90% by weight are most effective.

The major disadvantage of alcohol for skin antisepsis is its drying effect. Therefore, maximum concentrations of 70% are generally used. Some marketed prepara-

Table 5. Characteristics of topical antimicrobial ingredients (24)

	Alcohols	Chlorhexidine	Iodine/iodophors	Triclosan (Irgasan DP-300)
Mode of action	Denaturation of protein	Cell wall disruption	Oxidation/ substitution by free iodine	Cell wall disruption
Rapidity of action	Most rapid	Intermediate	Intermediate	Intermediate
Residual activity	None	Excellent	Minimal	Excellent
Usual concentration (%)	70–92	4.2 detergent base 0.5 in alcohol	0.5–2.0–7.5–10	0.3–1.0
Spectrum of activity:				
Gram-positive bacteria	Excellent	Excellent	Excellent	Good
Gram-negative bacteria	Excellent	Good	Good	Good (Fair for Pseudomonas species)
Mycobacterium Tuberculosis	Good	Poor	Good	Fair
Fungi	Good	Fair	Good	Poor
Viruses	Good	Good	Good	Unknown

tions contain 60% to 70% alcohol in combination with emollients to minimize skin drying and to decrease skin irritation (12).

2. Chlorhexidine Gluconate

Chlorhexidine gluconate (CHG) causes disruption of microbial cell membranes and precipitation of cell contents. It is more effective against Gram-positive than Gram-negative bacteria. Although the antibacterial activity of CHG is not as rapid as that of alcohol, several studies report excellent reduction of the transient flora after hand-washing for 15 seconds. Importantly, CHG remains chemically active on the skin for at least 6 hours, which is an advantage for surgeons, wearing gloves for a period of time. Moreover, as compared to alcohol, CHG has a relatively low skin irritation potential. In some countries, CHG is also available as an alcohol-based hand rinse (0,5%CHG), which combines the rapid effect of alcohol and the persistent activity of CHG (12).

3. Triclosan

Triclosan, chlorinated dioxy-diphenylether, disrupts the cell wall. As compared to chlorhexidine, triclosan is less active against Gram-negative bacteria (such as *Pseudomonas aeruginosa*), but may be more active against methicillin-resistant *S. aureus*; 1% triclosan eliminated methicillin-resistant *S. aureus*, whereas 4% chlorhexidine failed to do so (23).

4. Iodophors

The main mechanism of microbicidal activity is based on the oxidizing potential of iodine. The strongest antimicrobial effect occurs with diluted rather than strong solutions. The spectrum is wide, but the sustained effect is small and short. As iodine is absorbed through the intact skin, its use may be associated with side effects such as hypothyroidism (12).

COMPLIANCE

Although hand washing is generally regarded as a very important preventive measure against nosocomial infections, compliance rates with hand washing are unacceptably low. "Experts in infection control coax, cajole, threaten and plead, but still their colleagues neglect to wash their hands" (25).

In the last decade several intervention studies have been performed to increase compliance rates, most of them with disappointing results (table 6). Among the interventions introduced were education and feedback programs, introduction of new soap or alcohol dispensers and automated sinks. Since these studies varied widely in their design and execution strict comparison of the results is impossible, but some common trends can be observed.

Monitoring of compliance is usually performed by observation of daily activities in the ward, and these observations can be performed visible or invisible. As can be expected, visible observations of compliance rates, in the periods before intervention, resulted in higher handwash compliance rates (varying from 38 to 81%) than invisible observations (varying from 10 to 32%). There were two outliners, where compliance rates of 60% and 63% were monitored with invisible observations (27,26).

Interestingly, compliance rates are usually better *after* a defined critical procedure (such as contacts with mucous membranes, non-intact skin, secretions or excretions and manipulations of patient's vascular lines and other tubes) (12–28) than *before* contact with patients. After these procedures compliance rates were 12–28%, as compared to 10–14% before.

In general there was a moderate effect of education and feedback on compliance rates. The increase in compliance rates ranged from 5 to 22%, with 53% in one study (28). Moreover introduction of alcohol dispensers also resulted in variable outcomes. In one study, dispensers were placed next to every ICU door which resulted in a decrease of compliance of 8% (27). Placement of dispensers in the ICU, with 1 dispenser for every 4 beds increased compliance by 16% (29) and increasing the number of dispensers, in the same ward, to 1 for each bed increased compliance by 23% (29). In only 3 of 10 studies (26,28,30)a follow-up period was included. In one study (26) compliance rates, as monitored by invisible observations, decreased during follow-up to rates that were even lower than before intervention. In the second study (28), also with invisible observation, compliance rates were 23% in 1982, after these rates had been 81% during an intervention in 1978. In the third study (30) no differences in compliance rates between the experimental and control

Table 6. Intervention studies on handwash compliance and nosocomial infections on ICU's

Reference	Setting	Type of evaluation	Design	Hand wash compliance rates	Infection rates	Conclusion
Mayer, 1986 (26)	Nurses in 2 ICUs	Invisible observation of handwash compliance	A. Baseline observation (5 weeks) B. Introduction of new emollient soap in ICU-1 (5 weeks) C. Daily feedback on hand wash compliance in ICU-1(3 weeks) D. Follow-up	A. 63% vs 63% (ICU-1 vs ICU-2) B. 59% vs 58% C. 92% vs 73% D. 50% vs 57%	NA	No increase in HWC after introduction of new soap; Increase in handwashing when feedback phase began
Conly, 1989 (28)	All staff in 1 ICU	1. Invisible observation of handwash compliance before and after contact 2. Nosocomial infection rate	A. Baseline observation (1978) B. Education and feedback (1978) C. Baseline observation (1982) D. Education and feedback (1982)	A. 14% (before contact); 28% (after contact); B. 73% and 81%; C. 26% and 23%; D. 38% and 60%;	A. 33% B. 12% C. 33% D. 0%	Big increase in HWC in '78; decrease in nosocomial infections
Simmons, 1990 (45)	All staff in 2 ICUs	1. Invisible observation of handwash compliance 2. Nosocomial infection rate	A. Baseline observation (4.5 months) B. Single lecture with handouts (2 months) C. Button campaign (3 months) D. Direct feedback of hand wash compliance (2 weeks)	A. 22% B/C/D 30%	A. 50 B. 53	No significant increase in handwash compliance
Dubbert, 1990 (46)	All staff in 1 ICU	Visible observation of handwash compliance after all patient contacts and defined critical procedures	A. Baseline observation (6 weeks) B. Education (4 weeks) C. Observation with direct feedback (4 weeks)	A. 81% (after all contacts) and 70% (after critical procedures) B. 86% and 66% C. 92% and 92%	NA	High handwash compliance in baseline period with visible observation; highest rise in frequency due to direct feedback
Graham, 1990 (47)	All staff, 1 ICU	Invisible observation of handwash compliance	A. Baseline observation (2 weeks) B. Introduction of handrub solution at each bed (4 weeks)	A. 32% B. 45%	NA	Significant rise in handwash compliance

Larson, 1991 (48)	All staff in recovery room and neonatal ICU	Visible observation of handwash compliance	Cross-over model comparing introduction of automated sink with normal sink (2 times 5 weeks)	Handwashing frequency was measured as Frequency washes on automated sink (per site): 1.21 number of washes/hour/staff member and 0.85 compared with washes on manual sink: 1.69 and 2.11.	NA	The handwash compliance decreased significantly due to automated sink, but the duration of handwashing improved.
Doebbeling, 1992 (49)	All staff in 3 ICUs	1. Visible observation of handwash compliance 2. Nosocomial infection rate	A. Baseline observation nosocomial infection rate B. Chlorhexidine gluconate vs isopropyl-alcohol and soap in monthly cross-over model (8 months)	A. 42% (chlorhexidine) vs 38% (alcohol)	A. not mentioned B. Chlorhexidine: 152 vs alcohol and soap 202	During use of chlorhexidine the handwash compliance increased significantly. The nosocomial infection rate decreased, but not significantly.
Larson, 1997 (30)	Nurses in 2 ICUs	Visible observation of handwash compliance before and after contact	A. Baseline observation (4 months) B. In ICU1: Education and feedback and installation of automated sinks 1. at random mode (3 months) 2. in automatic mode 3. in sequenced mode C. Follow-up (3 months)	A. 56% (ICU1) vs 55% B1. 70% vs 69%, B2. 76% vs 65%, B3. 83% vs 48%, C. 76% vs 65%,	NA	Increase in handwash compliance during intervention, after several months no difference between units.
Bischoff, 2000 (29)	All staff in 3 ICUs	Invisible observation of handwash compliance before and after contact	A. Baseline observation (6 weeks) B. Education and feedback (6 weeks) C. Alcohol-dispensers (dispenser-bed ratio) 1. ratio 1:4 (6 weeks) 2. ratio 1:1 (6 weeks)	A. 10% (before contacts) and 12% (after) B. 16% and 25% C1. 19% and 41% C2. 23% and 48%	NA	Little change of hand-wash compliance during education and feedback; significant increase while using alcohol dispensers
Muto, 2000 (27)	All staff in 1 ICU and medium care	Invisible observation of handwash compliance before and after contact	A. Baseline observation B. Education and feedback and introduction alcohol dispensers (placed next to every door)	A. 60% B. 52%	NA	Intervention did not effect handwash compliance

unit could be demonstrated in the follow-up period. So the long-term effects of interventions to increase compliance with handwashing seem to be very disappointing.

Pittet (31) and coworkers investigated factors associated with poor handwash compliance. In this observational study, performed in ICU's and non-ICU's, overall compliance with handwashing was 48%. The lowest compliance rate (36%), however, was found in ICU's. Compliance differed significantly among HCW (physicians scored worst with 30%) and was lowest in morning-shifts and on weekdays. Interestingly, compliance was lower for procedures carrying a high risk for transmission of pathogens from HCW to patient (before intravenous care (39%), before respiratory care (18%) and care between a dirty and a clean body site (11%)) than activities that are more likely to contaminate HCW such as contact with body fluid (63%) and woundcare (58%). It seems as if HCW are more considered about protecting themselves against bacteria from patients than protecting patients for their own bacteria. Another important observation was that compliance was worse when the activity index was high.

The latter observations underscore the importance of the time aspect of handwashing. Voss et al. (32) calculated time consumption for handwashing and alcoholic hand disinfection, based on different compliance levels (40%, 60% and 100%), and different duration's of handwashing with water and soap (40–80 seconds) and alcoholic hand disinfection (20 seconds). They concluded that 100% compliance with handwashing might interfere with patient care, but that alcoholic hand disinfection allowed 100% compliance without interfering with patient care. This finding was confirmed in a recent study by Bischoff et al. (29) in which a program of educational feedback and improved patient awareness failed to improve handwashing compliance. However, introduction of easily accessible dispensers with alcohol based waterless handwashing antiseptics significantly increased handwashing rates among HCW.

Skin damage due to frequent washing or rubbing with disinfectants is another important reason for poor compliance. This may be prevented by moisturizers, as they prevent dehydration by restoring the water-holding capacity of the keratin layer and increase the width of corneocytes. There is growing interest in the use of barrier creams and lotions that not only shield damaged skin but also restore its structure and/or function. In a Swedish single-blind study, a moisturizing cream was found to accelerate the rate of recovery of surfactant-damaged skin (33). In a recently published trial the effect on skin irritation and dryness during use of soap and water was compared with an alcoholic hand gel (22). Skin irritation and dryness of hands increased significantly when nurses washed their hands with water and soap as compared with alcoholic handgel.

Disinfectants seem to be more widely used in Europe than in the US. One explanantion for this difference has been formulated recently by an American physician: "This could probably be explained in part by the fact that much of the research has come from Europe, and we seem to be more familiar with and take more seriously research done in this country" (21). Therefor alcoholic rubs reduce bacterial load on hands, decrease skin irritation and dryness and consequently increase compliance in handcleansing (34).

COHORTING AND ISOLATION

Cohorting

Limitation of the number of contacts between individual HCW and different patients is another measure to prevent cross-transmission. In theory, direct transmission would be impossible if a HCW would only contact a single patient in the ward. This is pursued with one-on-one nursing. In a theoretical framework of cross-transmission in ICU, the level of cohorting seemed to be more effective than increasing HCW (35). However, little is known about the level of cohorting of nurses and physicians in ICUs. Moreover, there are no studies evaluating infection rates in situations of one-on-one or one-on-two nurse to patient ratios.

There is, however, circumstantial evidence that cohorting does influence infection rates in ICUs. The level of cohorting decreases in situations of understaffing. Furthermore, understaffing will increase the workload, which will be accompanied by a decrease in compliance with hand-washing (31).

At least five studies have described increased infection rates during periods of understaffing (36,37,38,39,40).

Haley et al. (41) described a relationship between the incidence of staphylococcal infections in neonates and the number of nurses working on night shifts. In periods of severe understaffing (more than 7 infants per nurse), the rate of clustered infections was 16 times higher than in periods of adequate staffing.

In another period, Haley et al. (42) again demonstrated that periods with high MRSA infection rates were associated with understaffing, which was defined as nurse/child ratio lower than 1.

Fridkin et al. (37) showed an increase in central venous catheter-bloodstream infections during nursing staff reductions below a critical level. A patient-to-nurse ratio of 1 gave an adjusted odds ratio of 1. The odds ratio rose from 3.9, 15.6 to 61.5, when the patient-to-nurse ratio increased from 1.2 to 1.5 and 2.0, respectively.

In another study (38), MRSA-infections in ICU were correlated with periods with reduced nurse/patient ratios in the unit. Finally understaffing was one of the risk factors in an outbreak with *E. cloacae* in a neonatal ICU (39).

Besides understaffing the architecture of the ICU may interfere with cohorting levels. One can imagine that HCW will contact individual patients more frequently when all patients are tended in one open patient-care room. The number of these, more or less, random contacts will probably decrease when patients are treated in individual boxes. Although this has never been studied prospectively, there is some circumstantial evidence to support this hypothesis. In one study the incidence of *Acinetobacter baumanii* infections in mechanically ventilated patients decreased from 28.1% to 5%, after moving from a unit with both enclosed and open patient-care areas to an ICU with all private rooms (43). Similarly, Shirani (33) reported a decrease from 58.1% to 30.4% in infection rates in a burn unit after moving from an open unit to one with all private rooms.

Patient Isolation

Isolation is an another way to avoid transmission of pathogens from one patient to another. The principle of isolation is to separate a patient from healthy persons.

The Centres for Disease Control (CDC) have developed isolation-guidelines, in which six forms of isolation are distinguished:

1. *Strict isolation*: to prevent transmission of highly contagious or virulent infections that may be spread by aerosol and contact transmission. For example pharyngeal diphteria, hemorrhagic fevers, pneumonic plague, varicella and disseminated herpes zoster. Specifications include: a private room with appropriate air flow, masks, gowns and gloves for all persons entering the room, special treatment of contaminated material.

2. *Contact Isolation*: to prevent transmission of highly transmissible or epidemiologically important infections that do not need strict isolation and are not transported by aerosol. For example pediatric patients with certain acute respiratory infections, pharyngitis, or pneumonia; newborns with gonococcal conjunctivitis, herpes simplex infections; patients colonized with significant multiple drug-resistant bacteria, major staphylococcal infections, pediculosis, scabies. Specifications include: a private room, a mask to prevent large droplet transmission, gowns, gloves.

3. *Respiratory isolation*: to prevent transmission of infectious diseases by aerosol. For example children with *H. influenza* epiglottis, meningitis or pneumonia, meningococcal disease, mumps, pertussis. Specifications include: a private room, or sharing the room with a patient infected with the same micro-organism, masks for those who come close to the patient, good handwashing after touching the patient.

4. *Tuberculosis Isolation*: to prevent infectious tuberculosis. Specifications include: private room, dilution and removal of airborn contaminants, better-fitting and filtering masks.

5. *Enteric Precautions*: to prevent infections that are transmitted by fecal material. For example: known or suspected infectious diarrhea. Specifications include: gowns, gloves for touching infectious material, good hand washing after taking care of patient.

6. *Drainage/Secretion Precautions*: to prevent infections transmitted by contact of purulent material. Specifications include: gowns, gloves, good hand washing after taking care of patient (40).

Within ICU's, isolation of a single or a few patients has been demonstrated to be an effective preventive strategy to control outbreaks of multiple resistant (44). The Dutch strategy isolating patients colonized with MRSA is a good example of a successful way of controlling MRSA-outbreaks and prevention of MRSA becoming endemic in the Netherlands (50).

CONCLUSION

With a world-wide emergence of antibiotic resistance among nosocomial pathogens, effective infection control procedures will become more and more important. Although dedicated physicians and researchers have demonstrated the failures of current infection control practices for decades, daily practice seems not to have significantly. Although all HCW will be acquainted with the concept of hand-washing before and after patient contacts, strikingly little is known about quantitative effects of infection control procedures. Future studies should focus on these aspects in order to design appropriate and achievable infection control practices.

As for now, hand disinfection remains the cornerstone of infection prevention, and disinfectants with either alcohol or chlorhexidine are superior to hand washing with water and soap. Only when hands are visibly soiled they should be washed with water and soap. Studies evaluating compliance rates with infection control procedures and investigating the (long-term) effects of different interventions hereon are also warranted.

REFERENCES

1. Vincent JL, Bihari DJ, Suter PM, Bruining HA, White J, Nicolas-Chanoin MH, Wolff M, Spencer RC, Hemmer M. The prevalence of nosocomial infection in intensive care units in Europe. Results of the European Prevalence of Infection in Intensive Care (EPIC) Study. EPIC International Advisory Committee. *JAMA.* 1995;274(8):639–644.
2. Olson B, Weinstein RA, Nathan C, Chamberlin W, Kabins SA. Occult aminoglycoside resistance in Pseudomonas aeruginosa: epidemiology and implications for therapy and control. *J.Infect.Dis.* 1985;152(4):769–774.
3. Flynn DM, Weinstein RA, Nathan C, Gaston MA, Kabins SA. Patients' endogenous flora as the source of "nosocomial" Enterobacter in cardiac surgery. *J.Infect.Dis.* 1987;156(2):363–368.
4. Kernodle DS, Barg NL, Kaiser AB. Low-level colonization of hospitalized patients with methicillin-resistant coagulase-negative staphylococci and emergence of the organisms during surgical antimicrobial prophylaxis. *Antimicrob. Agents. Chemother.* 1988;32(2):202–208.
5. Goldmann DA. The role of barrier precautions in infection control. *J.Hosp.Infect.* 1991;18 Suppl A:515–523.
6. Rotter ML. Hygienic hand disinfection. *Infect.Control.* 1984;5(1):18–22.
7. Man P, de, Verhoeven BAN, Verbrugh HA, Vos MC, Anker JN van den. An antibiotic policy to prevent emergence of resistant bacilli. *Lancet* 2000;355:973–978.
8. Tramont EC. General or nonspecific host defense mechanisms. In: *Principles and practice of infectious diseases*, edited by Mandell GL, Gordon D, and Bennett JE, 1990, pp. 33–41.
9. Rotter ML. Handwashing and hand disinfection. In: *Hospital epidemiology and infection control*, edited by Mayhall CG, 1996, pp. 1052–1068.
10. McGinley KJ, Larson EL, Leyden JJ. Composition and density of microflora in the subungual space of the hand. *J.Clin.Microbiol.* 1988;26(5):950–953.
11. Evans A, Stevens RJ. Differential quantitation of surface and subsurface bacteria of normal skin by the combined use of the cotton swab and the scrub methods. *J.Clin.Microbiol.* 1976;3(6):576–581.
12. Larson EL. APIC guideline for handwashing and hand antisepsis in health care settings. *Am.J.Infect.Control.* 1995;23(4):251–269.
13. Huang Y, Oie S, Kamiya A. Comparative effectiveness of hand-cleansing agents for removing methicillin-resistant Staphylococcus aureus from experimentally contaminated fingertips. *Am.J.Infect.Control.* 1994;22(4):224–227.
14. Noskin GA, Stosor V, Cooper I, Peterson LR. Recovery of vancomycin-resistant enterococci on fingertips and environmental surfaces. *Infect.Control.Hosp.Epidemiol.* 1995;16(10):577–581.
15. Pittet D, Dharan S, Touveneau SS, Sauvan V, Perneger TV. Bacterial contamination of the hands of hospital staff during routine patient care. *Arch.Intern.Med.* 1999;159(8):821–826.
16. Ehrenkranz NJ, Alfonso BC. Failure of bland soap handwash to prevent hand transfer of patient bacteria to urethral catheters. *Infect.Control.Hosp.Epidemiol.* 1991;12(11):654–662.
17. Fox MK, Langner SB, Wells RW. How good are hand washing practices? *Am.J.Nurs.* 1974;74(9):1676–1678.
18. Larson E, Lusk E. Evaluating handwashing technique. *J.Adv.Nurs.* 1985;10(6):547–552.
19. Turner JG, Gauthier DK, Roby JR, Larson E, Gauthier JJ. Use of image analysis to measure handwashing effectiveness. *Am.J.Infect.Control.* 1994;22(4):218–223.

20. Wurtz R, Moye G, Jovanovič B. Handwashing machines, handwashing compliance, and potential for cross-contamination. *Am.J.Infect.Control.* 1994;22(4):228–230.
21. Larson E. Skin Hygiene and Infection Prevention: More of the same or different approaches? *Clinical.Infectious.Diseases.* 1999;29:1287–1294.
22. Boyce JM, Kelliher S, Vallande N. Skin irritation and dryness associated with two hand-hygiene regimens: soap-and-water hand washing versus hand antisepsis with an alcoholic hand gel. *Infect.Control.Hosp.Epidemiol.* 2000;21:442–448.
23. Faoagali JL, George N, Fong J, Davy J, Dowser M. Comparison of the antibacterial efficacy of 4% chlorhexidine gluconate and 1% triclosan handwash products in an acute clinical ward. *Am.J.Infect.Control.* 1999;27:320–326.
24. Larson E. Skin cleasing. In: Prevention and control of nosocomial infection. Wenzel RP, editor. P. 450–459. Baltimore: William and Wilkens; 1993.
25. Goldmann D, E. Larson. E. Hand-washing and nosocomial infections. *N.Engl.J.Med.* 1992;327(2):120–122.
26. Mayer JA, Dubbert PM, Miller M, Burkett PA, Chapman SW. Increasing handwashing in an intensive care unit. *Infect.Control.* 1986;7(5):259–262.
27. Muto CA, Sistrom MG, Farr BM. Hand hygiene rates unaffected by installation of dispensers of a rapidly acting hand antisepsis. *Am.J.Infect.Control.* 2000;28:273–276.
28. Conly JM, Hill S, Ross J, Lertzman J, Louie TJ. Handwashing practices in an intensive care unit: the effects of an educational program and its relationship to infection rates. *Am.J.Infect.Control.* 1989;17(6):330–339.
29. Bischoff WE, Reynolds TM, Sessler CN, Edmond MB, Wenzel RP. Handwashing compliance by healthcare workers: the impact of introducing an accessible, alcohol-based hand antiseptic. *Arch.Intern.Med.* 2000;160(7):1017–1021.
30. Larson EL, Bryan JL, L, Adler M, Blane C. Amultifaceted approach to changing handwashing behavior. *Am.J.Infect.Control.* 1997;25(1):3–10.
31. Pittet D, Mourouga M, Perneger TV. Compliance with handwashing in a teaching hospital. *Ann.Intern.Med.* 1999;130:126–130.
32. Voss A, Widmer AF. No time for handwashing!? Handwashing versus alcoholic rub: can we afford 100% compliance? *Infect.Control.Hosp.Epidemiol.* 1997;18(3):205–208.
33. Loden M. Barrier recovery and influence of irritant stimuli in skin treatment with a moisturizing cream. *Contact.Dermatitis.* 1997;36;256–260.
34. Boyce JM. Using alcohol for hand antisepsis: dispelling old myths. *Infect.Control.Hosp.Epidemiol.* 2000;21:438–441.
35. Austin J, Bonten MJ, Weinstein RA, Slaughter S, Anderson RM. Vancomycin-resistant enterococci in intensive-care hospital settings: transmission dynamics, persistence, and the impact of infection control programs. *Proc.Natl.Acad.Sci.* 1999;96(12):6908–6913.
36. Fridkin SK, Pear SM, Williamson TH, Galgiani JN, Jarvis WR. The role of understaffing in central venous catheter-associated bloodstream infections. *Infect.Control.Hosp.Epidemiol.* 1996;17(3):150–158.
37. Vicca AF. Nursing staff workload as a determinant of methicillin-resistant staphylococcus aureus spread in an adult intensive care unit. *J.hosp.Infect.* 1999;43(2):109–113.
38. Harbath S, Sudre P, Dharan S, Cadenad M, Pittet D. Outbreak of *Enterobacter cloacae* related to understaffing, overcrowding, and poor hygiene practices. *Inf.Control.Hosp.Epidem.* 1999;20(9):598–603.
39. Garner JS, Hierholzer WJ. Controversies in isolation policies and practices. In: Wenzel RP, editor. Prevention and control of nosocomial infections. Baltimore: William and Wilkens; 1993, pp. 70–81.
40. Lynch P, Jackson MM, Cummings MJ, Stamm WE. Rethinking the role of isolation practices in the prevention of nosocomial infections. *Annals.Intern.Med.* 1987;107:243–246.
41. Haley RW, Cushion NB, Tenover FC, Bannerman TL, Dryer D, Ross J, Sanchez PJ, Siegel JD. Eradication of endemic methicillin-resistant Staphylococcus aureus infections from a neonatal intensive care unit. *J.Infect.Dis.* 1995;171(3):614–624.
42. Haley RW, Bregman DA. The role of understaffing and overcrowding in recurrent outbreaks of staphylococcal infection in a neonatal special-care unit. *J.Infect.Dis.* 1982;145(6):875–885.
43. Mullin C, Rougetc, Clement C, Baily P. Association of private rooms with ventilator-associated Acinetobacter baumanii pneumonia in a surgical intensive-care unit. *Infect.Control.Hosp.Epidemiol.* 1977;18:499–503.
44. Shirani KZ, McManus AT, Vaughan GM, McManus WF, Jr Pruitt BA, Jr Mason AD. Effects of environment on infection in burn patients. *Arch.Surg.* 1986;121(1):31–36.
45. Simmons B, Bryant J, Neiman K, Spencer L, Arheart K. The role of handwashing in prevention of endemic intensive care unit infections. *Infect.Control.Hosp.Epidemiol.* 1990;11(11):589–594.

46. Dubbert PM, Dolce J, Richter W, Miller M, Chapman SW. Increasing ICU staff handwashing: effects of education and group feedback. *Infect.Control.Hosp.Epidemiol.* 1990;11(4):191–193.
47. Graham M. Frequency and duration of handwashing in an intensive care unit. *Am.J.Infect.Control.* 1990;18(2):77–81.
48. Larson E, McGeer A, Quraishi ZA, Krenzischek D, Parsons BJ, Holdford J, Hierholzer WJ. Effect of an automated sink on handwashing practices and attitudes in high-risk units. *Infect.Control.Hosp. Epidemiol.* 1991;12(7):422–428.
49. Doebbeling BN, Stanley GL, Sheetz CT, Pfaller MA, Houston AK, Annis L, Li N, Wenzel RP. Comparative efficacy of alternative hand-washing agents in reducing nosocomial infections in intensive care units. *N.Engl.J.Med.* 1992;327(2):88–93.
50. Vandenbroucke-Grauls CM. Methicillin-resistant Staphylococcus aureus control in hospitals: the Dutch experience. *Infect.Control.Hosp.Epidemiol.* 1996 Aug;17(8):512–513.

18. MODELING OF ANTIBIOTIC RESISTANCE IN THE ICU

MARC LIPSITCH, D.PHIL.

Department of Epidemiology, Harvard School of Public Health, 677 Huntington Avenue, Boston, MA 02115, lipsitch@epinet.harvard.edu

CARL T. BERGSTROM, PH.D.

Department of Zoology, University of Washington, Box 351800, Seattle, WA 98195-1800

Mathematical models are valuable tools with which to predict and explain the epidemiology of nosocomial infection. As such, modeling will play a crucial role in the effort to control the growing threat posed in hospitals by antibiotic-resistant bacteria. In this chapter, we illustrate the utility of the model-based approach, using a simple mathematical model of colonization and infection by antibiotic-sensitive and resistant bacteria in a hospital setting. The model explains a number of otherwise counterintuitive observations regarding the spread of nosocomial resistance: (1) nonspecific infection control measures such as hand-washing will disproportionately reduce the prevalence of resistant bacteria within the hospital; (2) resistance-control interventions should generate reductions in resistance much more rapidly in hospitals than in communities as a whole; (3) treatment with one antibiotic may be an individual risk factor for acquisition of resistance to another antibiotic, even in the absence of genetically linked resistance mechanisms.

WHY MATHEMATICAL MODELS?

Mathematical models have made substantial contributions to our understanding of the within-host population dynamics of microorganisms and the epidemiological dynamics of infections (1,2). Such models underlie our present understanding of phenomena as diverse as the multi-year cycles of measles incidence and their changes following vaccination (1), the dynamic state of viral replication during the "latent" period in HIV infection (3,4), and the maintenance of immune memory

R.A. Weinstein and M.J.M. Bonten (eds.). INFECTION CONTROL IN THE ICU ENVIRONMENT.

(5,6). Recently, such models have been used with particularly promising results to evaluate the relationship between antimicrobial use and antimicrobial resistance, both at the level of individual patients and at the hospital or community level (7,8,9,10,11,12,13,14,15,16,17).

In the context of those infections that are acquired in a hospital or ICU, models will be valuable for answering three sets of questions of particular interest:

- How fast will resistance to a particular antibiotic rise in response to increased use? Will it appear rapidly in a large fraction of treated hosts, as in monotherapy of tuberculosis (18); will it take several decades but then spread rapidly in some institutions, as with vancomycin resistance in enterococci (19); or will it appear rapidly but remain rare, except in immunocompromised patients, as in the case of acyclovir resistance in herpes simplex viruses (20,21)?
- How fast is resistance expected to decline if use of an antibiotic is reduced (8,9,13,22,23)? Will dramatic changes be seen within weeks to months (24,25,26,27,28), or will it take several years to see a substantial change (9,29)?
- When an individual receives antimicrobial treatment, what is the effect on resistance in the bacteria in that individual, in other individuals in the same hospital or ward, and in other individuals in the community at large (30)? What are the relationships among these different effects, and which ones are most important to measure?

Despite the success of mathematical models in beginning to address these and other questions about antimicrobial resistance, the use of population biological modeling in this domain is sometimes greeted with a degree of skepticism. The concerns are essentially twofold.

Some critics suggest that mathematical models are too complicated to be useful, that models are merely complicated (and often confusing) restatements of results already well-known through clinical experience. Such a skeptic might wryly point out, for example, that it does not take a rocket scientist, let alone a mathematical epidemiologist, to realize that increasing the use of an antibiotic is likely to increase the level of resistance to that antibiotic. There is indeed a valid point here. It is certainly appropriate to ask, "What do I know, or understand, after seeing the results of this mathematical model, that I did not know, or did not understand, before seeing them?" The answer to this question determines—to a large extent—the value of the model to users, such as clinicians, epidemiologists, and public health planners. However, it is essential to realize that even when the models do not yield results that are qualitatively surprising, quantitative description of epidemiological phenomena is crucial to the design and evaluation of interventions to control resistance. To evaluate whether an intervention might be worthwhile (or whether one has been successful), it is necessary to know how large an effect the intervention should have and how quickly its benefits should accrue. Indeed, the work described in this chapter will illustrate the utility of models for these purposes.

A second set of skeptics argue essentially the opposite, asserting that mathematical models are too simple to be useful in the complex world of hospital epidemiology. This group points out that the transmission dynamics of antimicrobial-resistant organisms, especially in the hospital, are extremely complicated, and that mathematical models are far too idealized to capture this complexity; therefore, it is asserted, the models cannot hope to be of any help. Such skeptics might go on to argue that since the goal is to reduce the effect of resistance on morbidity and mortality, the important thing is to figure out what works in the real world.

Certainly, we do not dispute the complexities inherent to the biology and epidemiology of resistance. Rather, we acknowledge a number of particularly thorny complexities associated with hospital epidemiology. These include

- The tremendous diversity in the genetic bases, biochemical properties, drug specificities, and fitness consequences of resistance mechanisms.
- Difficulties in pinpointing the routes and causes of transmission of susceptible and resistant organisms when a carrier state typically precedes disease, as is the case in most nosocomial infections. This process is further complicated by the roles of health care workers as vectors of transmission (8) and the manner in which the hospital environment serves as a reservoir of microorganisms.
- Ignorance about the role of the normal flora in modulating an individual's susceptibility to colonization by bacteria from the environment or to over-growth of endogenous bacteria (31,32).
- The probable importance of rare, "random," and unpredictable events that can have major consequences for the epidemiology of resistance. These events occur on a global scale, as when resistance to a particular drug first appears in a species of clinical significance, and they are then repeated locally, in a particular community or hospital, when a resistant organism or a new set of resistance genes is introduced from outside.

Despite these complexities, carefully constructed models that incorporate key features of hospital epidemiology can provide useful answers to questions about the relationships among antibiotic use, infection control, and antibiotic resistance. The models will indeed be simplifications, and an important step in the modeling process is to check whether the predictions of the models are robust, or whether they are artifacts introduced by the simplifications themselves. Because of these complexities, we are not enthusiastic about the abilities of models to "fit" precisely and quantitatively the time course of particular epidemics of resistant pathogens. Rather, we think that models can be valuable for the study of antimicrobial resistance in general, and in the ICU in particular, in three ways:

- by making testable, quantitative predictions about the epidemiology of a particular pathogen that were not apparent to intuition alone,
- by suggesting explanations for epidemiological phenomena that have been observed but whose mechanisms were not understood, and

- by aiding in the design and justification of standards for judging the success of interventions that are intended to control resistance in a specific context.

In this chapter, we describe a simple mathematical model of the transmission dynamics of antibiotic-resistant and -susceptible bacteria in a hospital or a unit of a hospital. We hope that this model and its predictions will exemplify all three of these uses for models.

A MODEL FOR HOSPITAL-ACQUIRED INFECTIONS

Several fundamental differences—with important epidemiological consequences—distinguish hospital-acquired infections from their community-acquired counterparts. First, for most of the important nosocomial pathogens, asymptomatic colonization of the skin, upper respiratory tract, or gut by the bacteria normally precedes infection (33). As a consequence, transmission of the bacteria typically proceeds from carrier to carrier, rather than from infected case to infected case. Second, a hospital or intensive care unit has highly fluid human and microbial populations, unlike most other communities in which resistance is studied. The average patient in many hospital units stays only about a week (34,26,30) and therefore the hospital population turns over rapidly, bringing in bacteria from outside and discharging them, with the patients, back into the community. This flow of patients and bacteria between community and hospital can be seen in Figure 1.

The model in Figure 1 is designed to reflect the transmission dynamics of a single bacterial species, which is transmitted among individuals within the hospital (or ICU). Within the hospital, the model considers three populations of patients: those not carrying the bacterial species of interest (hereafter, the bacteria), those carrying bacteria susceptible to a particular drug ("drug 1"), and those carrying bacteria resistant to drug 1. The number of individuals in each group is given by X, S, and R respectively. Patients may enter the hospital in any of these categories. For mathematical simplicity, we will describe the model for the special case in which patients carrying resistant bacteria enter only very rarely; most newly admitted patients are either uncolonized by the bacteria or are carrying susceptible bacteria. We describe elsewhere (13) how the model changes if large numbers of patients enter the hospital carrying resistant bacteria.

Once in the hospital, patients may be treated with either of two drugs. If they are treated with drug 1, patients carrying susceptible bacteria will be cleared (S patients will be converted into X patients). By contrast, patients treated with a second, unrelated drug (drug 2) will be cleared of their bacteria, regardless of which kind of bacteria they carry; we assume for this basic model that all bacteria are susceptible to drug 2. Patients not carrying either kind of bacteria can be colonized, either by susceptible or resistant bacteria, at rates proportional to the current prevalence of that kind of bacteria. Patients already carrying susceptible bacteria may be colonized with resistant bacteria, and vice versa, but this "super-colonization" process occurs at a rate lower than the colonization of uncolonized patients. Patients may

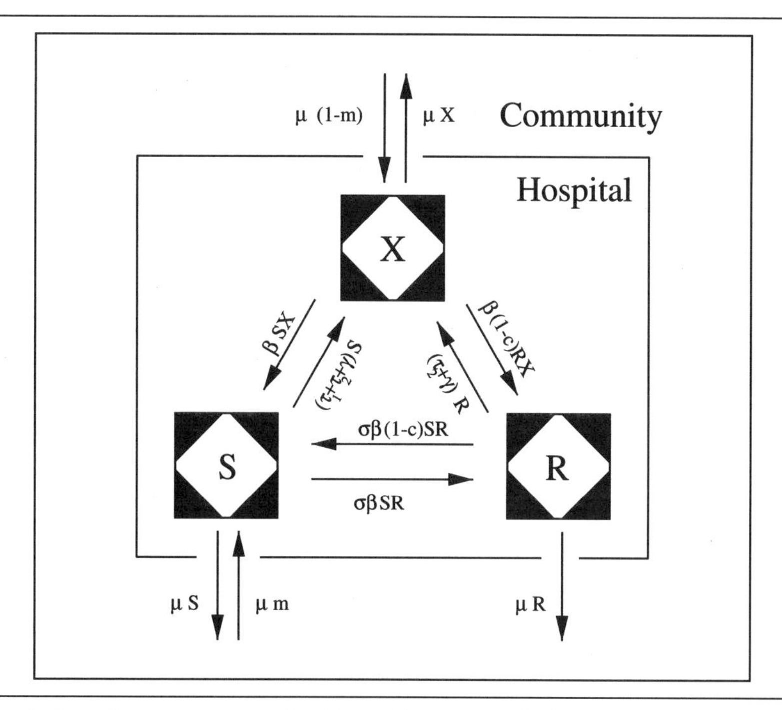

Figure 1. A simple compartment model of bacterial tranmission dynamics in a hospital setting. Patients may be uncolonized (X), colonized with sensitive bacteria (S), or colonized with bacteria resistant to drug 1 (R). Patients enter (and leave) the hospital at rate μ per day; of the newly-admitted patients, a fraction m are colonized with sensitive bacteria and $1 - m$ are uncolonized. Colonization of the uncolonized patients occurs by mass action with transmission rate parameter β; resistant bacteria suffer a proportional reduction in transmission rate of c. Superinfection—the infection and conversion of already-colonized individuals—occurs at a rate σ relative to infection of uncolonized individuals. Patients are treated with drug 1 and drug 2 at rates τ_1 and τ_2 per day, respectively, and patients spontaneously clear bacterial colonization at a rate γ per day. The model is fully specified by three ordinary differential equations: $dS/dt = m\mu + \beta SX - (\tau_1 + \tau_2 + \gamma + \mu)S + \sigma\beta cSR$; $dR/dt = \beta(1 - c)RX - (\tau_2 + \gamma + \mu)R - \sigma\beta cSR$; $dX/dt = (1 - m)\mu + (\tau_1 + \tau_2 + \gamma)S + (\tau_2 + \gamma)R - \beta SX - \beta(1 - c)RX - \mu X$.

spontaneously clear carriage of bacteria of either sort, at a low rate. Patients from each category leave the hospital at a fixed rate.

The mathematical details of this model have been given elsewhere (13). Rather than recapitulate them here, we instead summarize some of the clinically important predictions of the model, and compare these predictions with data from the literature on nosocomial infections and resistance.

MODEL PREDICTIONS, EMPIRICAL DATA, AND CLINICAL IMPLICATIONS

The model defines the conditions under which resistant bacteria can persist in the hospital, and conversely defines the conditions under which endemic resistant bacteria can be eradicated. Endemic transmission of resistant bacteria can persist in the hospital if the trans-

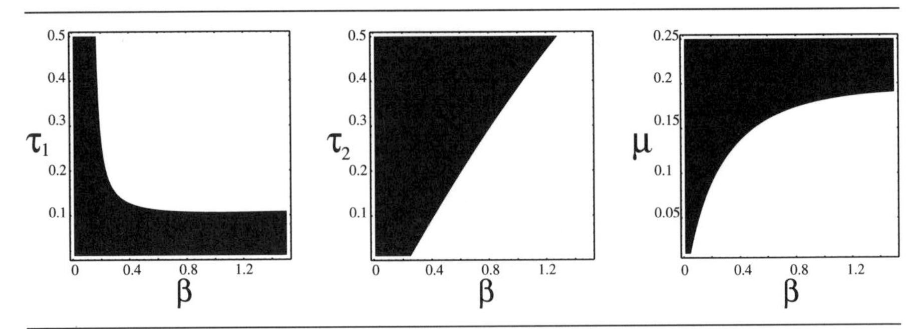

Figure 2. Parameters for which resistant bacteria can persist (white) and cannot persist (black) in the hospital (see text). Parameters (except when varied on *x* or *y* axes): $c = 0.05$, $\gamma = 1/30$, $m = 0.75$, $\tau_1 = 0.2$, $\tau_2 = 0$, $\mu = 0.1$, $\sigma = 0.25$.

mission rate of bacteria in the hospital is sufficiently high, if use of drug 1 is sufficiently common, if use of drug 2 is sufficiently rare, and if the average length of stay is sufficiently long. Figure 2 shows how these parameters trade off with one another. If within-hospital transmission rates β are high (Fig. 2a), then resistant bacteria can persist despite relatively low rates τ_1 of drug 1 use. If within-hospital transmission rates are reduced, then a higher level of drug 1 use is required to maintain endemic transmission of bacteria resistant to drug 1. As the rate τ_2 of use of drugs for which resistance is not present increases (Fig. 2b), higher rates of transmission β (or higher rates of drug 1 use) are required for endemic persistence of resistant bacteria. In hospitals (or units) where the average length of stay $1/\mu$ is longer, endemic transmission of resistant bacteria is more easily maintained (Fig. 2c).

These predictions have several implications for the control of resistance in a hospital. As Figure 2 demonstrates, different interventions—reduction in the use of the drug to which resistance is observed, increased use of other antimicrobials, and infection control measures aimed at generally reducing within-hospital cross-colonization of patients—can achieve the goal of reducing or eliminating resistant bacteria. In some cases two partially successful measures can in concert result in elimination of endemic transmission, although neither would have sufficed alone.

Even without the model, it is clear that one way to approach this goal is to reduce use of the antibiotic to which the bacteria are resistant; this intuition is confirmed by the model. Less clear is how the use of other antimicrobial agents, to which bacteria are not resistant, affects the transmission of bacteria resistant to a particular drug (drug 1 in our model). Clinical studies and clinical practice give conflicting evidence on this point. On one hand, many studies show that antimicrobial use in general is a risk factor for colonization or infection with bacteria resistant to a particular drug (35,36,37,38,39,40,41) (the model's predictions for such studies are discussed below). Presumably following this logic, one response to problems of

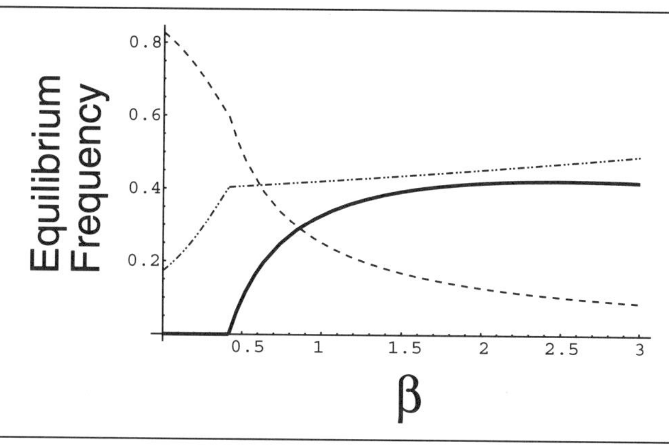

Figure 3. Equilibrium frequency of uncolonized individuals (dashed line), individuals colonized with sensitive bacteria (dash-dotted line), and individuals colonized with resistant bacteria (solid line). When resistant bacteria are endemic, decreases in transmission rate typically reduce disproportionately the frequency of resistance. Parameters are as in Figure 19.2, except $\tau_2 = 0.1$.

resistance has been to curtail use of all antibiotics in a hospital or unit (26,42). On the other hand, the use of antimicrobial prophylaxis to reduce resistance (34), or the implementation of antimicrobial cycling programs (43,44) both rely on the intuition that the use of some drugs, for which resistance is not observed, can help control the level of resistance to other drugs, for which resistance is a problem.

The model's prediction supports the latter intuition, that increased use of one antimicrobial agent (drug 2) can help reduce the prevalence of resistance to another drug (drug 1). A key caveat to this prediction is that the bacteria resistant to drug 1 are not cross-resistant to drug 2. Thus, the prediction would not be appropriate for closely related drugs sharing the same resistance mechanism, or for drugs for which resistance genes are linked on a plasmid.

The model predicts that infection control measures such as hand-washing and barrier precautions, which are directed nonspecifically at reducing transmission of all bacteria, will disproportionately help to reduce the prevalence of resistant bacteria. Figure 3 shows the predicted prevalence of colonization with susceptible and resistant bacteria at equilibrium in the model, as a function of the rate of within-hospital transmission β. For a wide range of transmission rates β (given that resistance can persist in an endemic state), decreases in the transmission rates decrease the equilibrium prevalence of resistance more than they affect the equilibrium prevalence of susceptible bacteria. Notice that this prediction provides a further rationale for the importance of infection control in the hospital as a measure for reducing antimicrobial resistance.

Though counterintuitive at first glance, this observation can be explained from the structure of the model shown in Figure 1. Patients enter the hospital either carrying sensitive bacteria or none, but only very rarely carrying resistant bacteria.

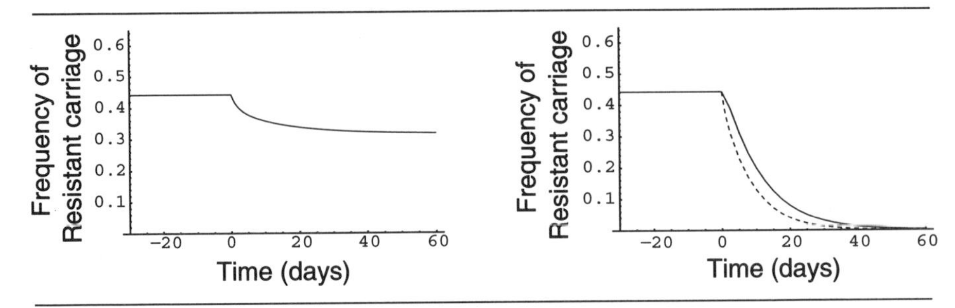

Figure 4. Response to resistance control interventions: frequency of resistance carriage after (a) reduction of transmission rate by 50%; (b) cessation of drug 1 use with (dashed line) and without (solid line) replacement by use of drug 2. Parameters are as in Figure 2.

Thus, resistant bacteria depend for their survival solely on transmission within the hospital, while sensitive bacteria are maintained both by transmission in the hospital and by "immigration" with newly admitted patients. Reductions in transmission therefore do disproportionate harm to resistant bacteria.

The model predicts that successful interventions will reduce resistance in a very short time, within weeks or a few months. Figure 4 shows the change in the prevalence of colonization with resistant bacteria, starting from an equilibrium level, following various interventions. As the figure demonstrates, different interventions will have different effects, but in each case noticeable change is apparent within a very short time period. Such rapid changes are observed for very wide ranges of parameters, as long as the average stay of a patient in the hospital is assumed to be days or weeks.

The reason for the rapid changes in prevalence of resistant and sensitive bacteria is the rapid "flow" of patients through the hospital, and the fact that some of the newly entering patients bring susceptible bacteria with them. Thanks to this constant influx of susceptible bacteria, which compete with resistants to colonize patients, resistant bacteria cannot persist in the hospital for long if conditions are unfavorable for their transmission. Interestingly, in contrast to other models of the transmission dynamics of antimicrobial resistant bacteria, this process does not depend on a difference in Darwinian fitness (transmissibility, ability to colonize, or ability to persist within a patient) between susceptible and resistant bacteria. In a hospital (under our assumptions), the entry of patients already carrying susceptible bacteria will replenish the sensitive population rapidly, allowing them to outcompete resistant bacteria whenever conditions are no longer favorable for the resistant strains (due to reduced transmission, reduced use of the drug to which they are resistant, etc.).

This prediction is consistent with the observed consequences of interventions designed to reduce resistance in hospitals. Many of these interventions result in substantial changes in the prevalence of resistance within a very short time (25,26,27,28). The prediction is specific to nosocomial infections, because it depends on the entry into the system of individuals (from outside) who carry susceptible

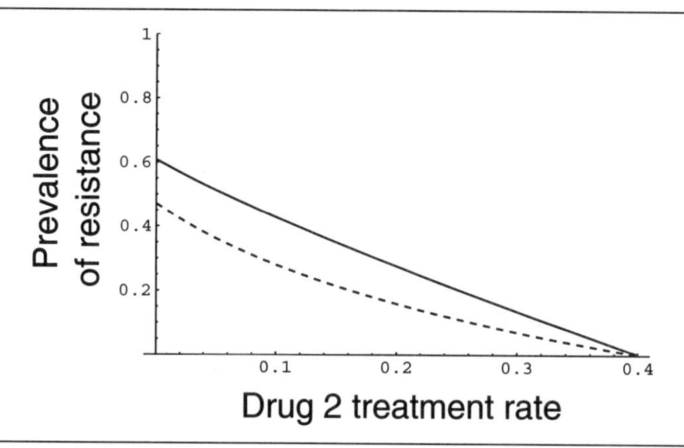

Figure 5. Equilibrium frequency of drug 1 resistance carriage in individuals treated with drug 2 (solid line), and untreated with drug 2 (dashed line). Increasing drug 2 usage decreases the overall frequency of resistance in the hospital, but individuals treated with drug 2 are always more likely to be infected by bacteria resistant to drug 1. For numerical tractability, an example with no superinfection is shown (parameter values are $c = 0.05$, $\gamma = 1/30$, $m = 0.75$, $\tau_1 = 0.2$, $\tau_2 = 0$, $\mu = 0.1$, $\sigma = 0$). Qualitatively similar results obtain when superinfection is present.

bacteria. Thus, it would not be expected to hold for most community-acquired infections, and indeed it does not. In the rare cases where interventions intended to limit resistance in community-acquired pathogens have been reported, their success has occurred on a time scale of years (9,29). The model thus suggests that when interventions to reduce resistance in hospitals do not produce rapid results, it is appropriate to seek a specific explanation for the failure: perhaps, a longer average duration of stay than in most hospitals, or the existence of a reservoir—an environmental source or a long-term colonized patient or health care worker—which could be slowing the "wash-out" of resistant bacteria.

The model predicts that, measured at the individual level, use of one antibiotic (drug 2) will be a risk factor for colonization with bacteria resistant to another antibiotic (drug 1). This result is paradoxical because, as we have just seen, the use of drug 2 can help to reduce the prevalence of bacteria resistant to drug 1 in the hospital as a whole. Thus, there is a positive association between drug 2 use and drug 1 resistance for individuals, but a negative association between drug 2 use and the total prevalence of resistance to drug 1 (at the population level). These relationships are shown in Figure 5.

Like some of the previous predictions, this opposition between individual risk and population-wide effects is a consequence of the entry of individuals already carrying drug-sensitive bacteria into the hospital, and is therefore not expected to appear in community-acquired infections. We see this result in hospitals because treatment with drug 2 has two opposing effects on bacteria resistant to drug 1: (a) If a patient already carries susceptible bacteria, drug 2 clears bacterial carriage and increases the chance that the individual will be colonized by bacteria resistant to

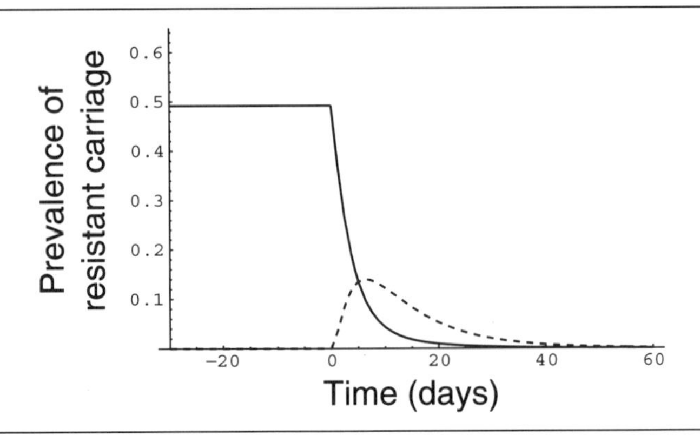

Figure 6. Dynamics of resistance after switching from using drug 1 exclusively to using drug 2 exclusively, at time 0. The frequency of resistance declines rapidly as a consequence, even though individuals treated with drug 2 (dashed line) are temporarily at greater risk of acquiring bacteria resistant to drug 1 than are individuals who remain untreated with drug 2 (solid line). Parameters are as in Figure 5.

drug 1, which are circulating in the hospital; (b) if an individual already carries bacteria resistant to drug 1, drug 2 clears their carriage of these resistant bacteria. At the individual level, the effect (a) is more powerful, while at the level of the population, effect (b) is stronger.

This prediction of the model is consistent with published studies of antimicrobial use and resistance in hospitals. Such studies often find an association at the individual level between prior use of one antibiotic and infection or colonization with bacteria resistant to another drug (45,38,41). Sometimes, this association has a trivial explanation; for example, the same gene, or two genes located on the same plasmid, might determine resistance to both drugs. However, in several cases no such explanation is available; for example, quinolones (for which resistance is chromosomal) have been detected as a risk factor for carriage of enterobacteria carrying plasmid-mediated cephalosporin resistance (45,41).

In highlighting the opposition between individual and population-level consequences of intervention, the model shows that information about individual risk factors cannot be extrapolated to predict the effects of interventions at a population level (46). This distinction means that it is crucial to measure the right quantities when assessing the effects of interventions. For example, if a hospital chose to switch its formulary from empiric therapy with one drug (for which resistance had become a problem) to therapy with another drug (for which resistance was rare) (43), the model predicts that the use of the new drug would help to bring down resistance to the first, but that as resistance to the first declines, patients treated with the second drug would be at increased risk of carrying resistance to the first. If only individual risk factors were measured in this hospital, one might erroneously conclude that the new drug was responsible for maintaining resistance to the old drug, whereas in fact it was contributing to the decline of that resistance. Such a situation is illustrated in Figure 6.

CONCLUSIONS, CAVEATS, AND FUTURE DIRECTIONS

In this chapter, we have illustrated the way in which a simple mathematical model can be applied to the problem of antibiotic resistance in hospitals and ICUs. Of course, several caveats must be noted. While the model suggests that in the short term, resistance to one drug can be controlled by the use of a second drug, it would be a mistake to treat this prediction as a prescription, without considering several additional factors. First, the model assumes that there is no resistance to drug 2; when resistance to drug 2 is present in the population as well, more complicated models (and perhaps consideration of drug-cycling strategies) will be required. Second, even in the absence of resistance to drug 2, the use of this drug will presumably select for the generation of resistance to it and therefore broad use may be undesirable. Third, use of drug 2 in order to control resistance to drug 1 may accelerate the evolution of multiply-resistant strains of bacteria, which could in turn pose a far more grave threat than either singly-resistant strain.

Despite these limitations, our results illustrate all three of the general applications of modeling that were mentioned in the introduction. First, the model makes testable predictions that were not intuitively obvious. For example, the model predicts that in hospitals, resistance-control interventions should take effect rapidly, within a matter of weeks to months and that if change does not occur on this time scale, specific explanations (e.g. environmental reservoirs) should be sought. Second, the model allows us to explain mechanistically a series of puzzling observations about hospital-acquired infections. By taking into account the constant flow of patients between hospital and community and the commensal nature of many bacterial species responsible for nosocomial infections (including the fact that individuals entering the hospital may already be colonized), the model explains why (1) reducing transmission disproportionately affects the prevalence of resistant bacteria; (2) microbial populations in hospitals can respond to interventions within a very short time span compared to community acquired infections; (3) treatment with one antibiotic can be a risk factor for bacteria that are resistant to another antibiotic. Third, and perhaps most importantly, the model provides insight for designing standards by which to judge the success of interventions. In particular, our analysis illustrates the way in which static epidemiologic measures of association (individual risk factors) can be misleading predictors of the effects of intervention.

REFERENCES

1. Anderson RM, May RM. *Infectious Diseases of Humans: Dynamics and Control.* Oxford University Press, Oxford, 1991.
2. Levin BR, Lipsitch M, Bonhoeffer S. Population biology, evolution, and infectious disease: Convergence and synthesis. *Science*, 283(5403):806–809, 1999.
3. Ho DD, Neumann AU, Perelson AS, Chen W, Leonard JM, Markowitz M. Rapid turnover of plasma virions and CD4 lymphocytes in HIV-1 infection. *Nature*, 373:123–126, 1995.
4. Wei X, Ghosh SK, Taylor ME, Johnson VA, Emini EA, Deutsch P, Lifson JD, Bonhoeffer S, Nowak MA, Hahn BH. Viral dynamics in human immunodeficiency virus type 1 infection. *Nature*, 373(6510):117–122, 1995.
5. Michie CA, McLean A, Alcock C, Beverley PC. Lifespan of human lymphocyte subsets defined by CD45 isoforms. *Nature*, 60(6401):264–265, 1992.

6. Slifka MK, Antia R, Whitmire JK, Ahmed R. Humoral immunity due to long-lived plasma cells. *Immunity*, 8:363–372, 1998.
7. Austin DJ, Anderson RM. Transmission dynamics of epidemic methicillin-resistant Staphylococcus aureus and vancomycin-resistant enterococci in England and Wales. *J Infect Dis*, 179(4):883–891, 1999.
8. Austin DJ, Bonten MJ, Weinstein RA, Slaughter S, Anderson RM. Vancomycin-resistant enterococci in intensive-care hospital settings: Transmission dynamics, persistence, and the impact of infection control programs. *Proc Nat Acad Sci USA*, 96(12):6908–6913, 1999.
9. Austin DJ, Kristinsson KG, Anderson RM. The relationship between the volume of antimicrobial consumption in human communities and the frequency of resistance. *Proc Natl Acad Sci USA*, 96(3):1152–1156, 1999.
10. Blower SM, Porco TC, Darby G. Predicting and preventing the emergence of antiviral drug resistance in HSV-2. *Nature Medicine*, 4:673–678, 1998.
11. Blower SM, Small PM, Hopewell PC. Control strategies for tuberculosis epidemics: New models for old problems. *Science*, 273(5274):497–500, 1996.
12. Kepler TB, Perelson AS. Drug concentration heterogeneity facilitates the evolution of drug resistance. *Proc Nat Acad Sci USA*, 95(20):11514–11519, 1998.
13. Lipsitch M, Bergstrom CT, Levin BR. Antibiotic resistance in hospitals: Paradoxes and prescriptions, Submitted, 1999.
14. Lipsitch M, Levin BR. The population dynamics of antimicrobial chemotherapy. *Antimicrobial Agents and Chemotherapy*, 41(2):363–373, 1997.
15. Lipsitch M, Levin BR. Population dynamics of tuberculosis treatment: Mathematical models of the roles of non-compliance and bacterial heterogeneity in the evolution of drug resistance. *International Journal of Tuberculosis and Lung Disease*, 2(3):187–199, 1998.
16. Ribeiro RM, Bonhoeffer S. A stochastic model for primary HIV infection: optimal timing of therapy. *AIDS*, 13(3):351–357, 1999.
17. Stilianakis NI, Perelson AS, Hayden FG. Emergence of drug resistance during an influenza epidemic: Insights from a mathematical model. *J Infect Dis*, 177(4):863–873, 1998.
18. Rist N. Nature and development of resistance of tubercle bacilli to chemotheraputic agents. In Barry VC, etitor, *Chemotherapy of Tuberculosis*, pages 192–227, Butterworths, Ldonon, 1964.
19. Leclerq R, Derlot E, Duval J, Courvalin P. Plasmid-mediated resistance to vancomycin and teicoplanin in *Enterococcus faecium*. *New England Journal of Medicine*, 319:157–161, 1988.
20. Christophers J, Clayton J, Craske J, Ward R, Collins P, Trowbridge M, Darby G. Survey of resistance of herpes simplex virus to acyclovir in northwest England. *Antimicrobial Agents and Chemotherapy*, 42:868–872, 1998.
21. Corey L. Herpes simplex virus infections during the decade since the licensure of acyclovir. *Journal of Medical Virology*, Suppl. 1:7–12, 1993.
22. Schrag SJ, Perrot V, Levin BR. Adaptation to the fitness costs of antibiotic resistance in Escherichia coli. *Proceedings of the Royal Society of London, Ser. B*, 264:1287–1291, 1997.
23. Stewart FM, Antia R, Levin BR, Lipsitch M, Mittler JE. The population genetics of antibiotic resistance. II: Analytic theory for sustained populations of bacteria in a community of hosts. *Theor Popul Biol*, 53(2):152–165, 1998.
24. Boyce JM, Landry M, Deetz TR, DuPont HL. Epidemiologic studies of an outbreak of nosocomial methicillin-resistant Staphylococcus aureus infections. *Infect Control*, 2(2):110–116, 1981.
25. Cosseron-Zerbib M, Roque Afonso AM, Naas T, Durand P, Meyer L, Costa Y, el Helali N, Huault G, Nordmann P. A control programme for MRSA (methicillin-resistant Staphylococcus aureus) containment in a paediatric intensive care unit: Evaluation and impact on infections caused by other micro-organisms. *J Hosp Infect*, 40(3):225–235, 1998.
26. Dunkle LM, Naqvi SH, McCallum R, Lofgren JP. Eradication of epidemic methicillin-gentamicin-resistant Staphylococcus aureus in an intensive care nursery. *Am J Med*, 70(2):455–458, 1981.
27. Franco JA, Eitzman DV, Baer H. Antibiotic usage and microbial resistance in an intensive care nursery. *Am J Dis Child*, 126(3):318–321, 1973.
28. Lilly HA, Lowbury EJ. Antibiotic resistance of Staphylococcus aureus in a burns unit after stopping routine prophylaxis with erythromycin. *J Antimicrob Chemother*, 4(6):545–550, 1978.
29. Seppala H, Klaukka T, Vuopio-Varkila J, Muotiala A, Helenius H, Lager K, Huovinen P. The effect of changes in the consumption of macrolide antibiotics on erythromycin resistance in group A streptococci in Finland. *N Engl J Med*, 337(7):441–446, 1997.
30. Garber AM. A discrete-time model of the acquisition of antibiotic-resistant infections in hospitalized patients. *Biometrics*, 45(3):797–816, 1989.

31. Freter R, Stauffer E, Cleven D, Holdeman LV, Moore WE. Continuous-flow cultures as in vitro models of the ecology of large intestinal flora. *Infect Immun*, 39(2):666–675, 1983.
32. van der Waaij D. *Antibiotic choice: The importance of colonisation resistance*. Research Studies Press, Chichester, 1983.
33. Bonten MJ, Weinstein RA. The role of colonization in the pathogenesis of nosocomial infections. *Infection Control and Hospital Epidemiology*, 17:193–200, 1996.
34. Brun-Buisson C, Legrand P, Rauss A, Richard C, Montravers F, Besbes M, Meakins JL, Soussy CJ, Lemaire F. Intestinal decontamination for control of nosocomial multiresistant gram-negative bacilli. Study of an outbreak in an intensive care unit. *Ann Intern Med*, 110(11):873–881, 1989.
35. Gaynes R, Monnet D. The contribution of antibiotic use on the frequency of antibiotic resistance in hospitals. *Ciba Found Symp*, 207:47–56, 1997.
36. Lucet JC, Chevret S, Decre D, Vanjak D, Macrez A, Bedos JP, Wolff M, Regnier B. Outbreak of multiply resistant enterobacteriaceae in an intensive care unit: Epidemiology and risk factors for acquisition. *Clin Infect Dis*, 22(3):430–436, 1996.
37. McGowan, Jr. JE. Is antimicrobial resistance in hospital microorganisms related to antibiotic use? *Bull NY Acad Med*, 63(3):253–268, 1987.
38. Morris, Jr. JG, Shay DK, Hebden JN, McCarter Jr. RJ, Perdue BE, Jarvis W, Johnson JA, Dowling TC, Polish LB, Schwalbe RS. Enterococci resistant to multiple antimicrobial agents, including vancomycin. Establishment of endemicity in a university medical center. *Ann Intern Med*, 123(4):250–259, 1995.
39. Rao GG. Risk factors for the spread of antibiotic-resistant bacteria. *Drugs*, 55(3):323–330, 1998.
40. Rao GG, Ojo F, Kolokithas D. Vancomycin-resistant gram-positive cocci: Risk factors for faecal carriage. *J Hosp Infect*, 35(1):63–69, 1997.
41. Wiener J, Quinn JP, Bradford PA, Goering RV, Nathan C, Bush K, Weinstein RA. Multiple antibiotic-resistant Klebsiella and Escherichia coli in nursing homes. *JAMA*, 281(6):517–523, 1999.
42. Price DJ, Sleigh JD. Control of infection due to Klebsiella aerogenes in a neurosurgical unit by withdrawal of all antibiotics. *Lancet*, 2(7685):1213–1215, 1970.
43. Kollef MH, Vlasnik J, Sharpless L, Pasque C, Murphy D, Fraser V. Scheduled change of antibiotic classes: a strategy to decrease the incidence of ventilator-associated pneumonia. *Am J Respir Crit Care Med*, 156(4 Pt 1):1040–1048, 1997.
44. McGowan, Jr. JE. Minimizing antimicrobial resistance in hospital bacteria: Can switching or cycling drugs help? *Infect Control*, 7:573–576, 1986.
45. De Champs C, Rouby D, Guelon D, Sirot J, Sirot D, Beytout D, Gourgand JM. A case-control study of an outbreak of infections caused by Klebsiella pneumoniae strains producing CTX-1 (TEM-3) beta-lactamase. *J Hosp Infect*, 18(1):5–13, 1991.
46. Koopman JS, Longini, Jr. IM. The ecological effects of individual exposures and nonlinear disease dynamics in populations. *Am J Public Health*, 84(5):836–842, 1994.

19. MATHEMATICAL MODELS IN THE ICU: DYNAMICS, INFECTION CONTROL AND ANTIBIOTIC RESISTANCE

DAREN J. AUSTIN, PH.D.

Imperial College School of Medicine, Norfolk Place, London W2 1PG, United Kingdom

INTRODUCTION

The rise in antibiotic resistant pathogens presents a considerable challenge to human health. Nowhere has this challenge been greater felt than in the hospital setting (1). Nosocomial infections caused by both gram negative organisms such as *Klebsiella* or gram-positives such as methicillin-resistant *Staphylococcus aureus* (MRSA) and vancomycin-resistant enterococci (VRE), are becoming ever more difficult to treat. With the decreasing treatment options comes an ever-increasing reliance on control. To date, infection control practices such as hand washing and the cohorting of patients into distinct segregated Health Care Worker (HCW)-patient sub-units have tended to provide the cornerstone of control measures (2–9,10–23). Hand disinfection whether via the use of sinks or portable gel disinfectants is the focus of considerable attention, as the primary improvement in patient care. Cohorting has to a lesser extent also come under scrutiny, with a number of studies attempting to estimate the effectiveness of segregating infected patients and their carers from susceptible patients.

There has been only limited success in understanding to what extent infection control practices effectively control the spread of nosocomial pathogens in the ICU (24). The reasons for the lack of progress lie in part in a lack of understanding of the very nature of nosocomial outbreaks and a lack of controls in intervention studies. Typically during an outbreak an intervention will be implemented (e.g., improved hand-washing compliance or "cohorting") and any success ascribed to infection control. Although there have been a large number of studies of hand-washing practice (2–9) and several reports of cohorting, there have been limited quantitative measures of their practical efficacy (8,11).

Nosocomial outbreaks are characterised by the small populations involved, and the opportunities provided by close contact for rapid spread. In the ICU the hands of HCWs serve as vectors for the patient-patient spread (25–28), and the role of hand washing is self-evident. The small populations, typically less than 20 patients, mean that random chance will play a very important part in the overall course of an outbreak (24). For example, in an 8-bed ICU a single case can contribute 12.5% to the overall prevalence of infection. The role of chance cannot therefore be overlooked. A single outbreak, complete with intervention (if any) represents a single sample from a larger family of (hopefully) unobserved outbreaks. Consecutive outbreaks in the same institution may permit greater characterisation, although in most instances the numbers will be small. It is therefore reasonable to assume the characteristics of an "average" outbreak are unknown. Moreover, the average characteristics of infection control practices are equally unknown.

Traditional infectious disease epidemiology has centred on the identification and description of factors which are able to differentiate between cases and controls (i.e., risk factors) in order that some inferences be drawn. Without sufficient patient numbers the power of such studies can be low. In any event the statistical models are descriptive and cannot account for changes in practice (e.g., an increase in hand-washing compliance). More recent developments have adopted a "population ecology" approach to epidemiology in which mathematical descriptions of the processes are formulated into a population model (29). For example, distinct compartments can be used to describe a disease, with individuals being assigned according to their status. The rates with which individuals move between compartments (via processes such as birth, death, infection, recovery) are then modelled. These models, which owe much to the physical sciences, are necessarily simplistic—not all processes can be incorporated into a model. The art is to distil only those most relevant (e.g., transmission via patient-patient contact) from those of limited importance. Once parameterised, the models are descriptive in nature, and more importantly, when validated by data, are predictive of interventions. Particular successes in this field include the description of childhood infections such as measles and the impact of control via vaccination (29).

In the hospital setting, population models are very much in their infancy (24). The enormous impact that chance plays, combined with multifarious patient factors (e.g., as severity of illness), means that deterministic population models do not accurately account for typical behaviour—unlike large populations. Instead they must enter the world of "micro simulation", where multiple realisations of the model are invoked and chance inherent. It is via these techniques that mathematical models are able to access the unobserved superset of nosocomial outbreaks to make comparison between observation and model and make predictions regarding the outcome of control strategies.

Table 1. Potential sources of new cases by route

	Endogenous	Cross-transmission	Environment
Clonality	Polyclonal	Clonal	Clonal/ Polyclonal
Control strategy	Screening Ab restriction	Hand, washing Cohorting	Improved cleaning
Impact of fluctuations	Small	Large	Small/Med
Probability of new case	Constant	*f*(cases)	Constant/ *f*(cases)
References	(31–38)	(25–28)	(31,39–41)

MODEL FORMULATION AND PATHOGEN ACQUISITION ROUTES

The first stage in mode formulation is to gauge the important epidemiological processes. In the ICU the demographic processes of patient admission and discharge play an important role. The enormous resources required maintaining ICU beds mean that bed occupancy is high. Patient length of stay (LOS) is normally measured in days rather than weeks producing very rapid patient turnover. There is therefore only a relatively short window of opportunity for pathogen spread. The fact that pathogens can be readily passed from patient to patient in some settings is testament to the high contact levels between patients and HCWs. For bacterial pathogens, diseased patients may represent the tip of an iceberg of cases. Without routine daily surveillance at multiple patient sites and environmental cultures, the magnitude of the pathogen exposure to patients is often never known (30). Clinical cultures provide measures of disease, but it is the patients who harbour pathogens asymptomatically who stabilise an outbreak and maintain transmission.

Three routes of pathogen acquisition are routinely implicated (Table 1). Endogenous sources, in which patients harbour organisms on admission, often at sub-detectable levels have been implicated for both gram-negative and gram-positive organisms (31–36). If the host organisms are causing colonisation and infection, only the number of patients limits the clonality of the outbreak. Control should be aimed at early detection of carriers; followed by attempts to minimise the risk that colonisation progresses to infection. Since the patients already harbour the pathogen, the incidence of progressing to detectable colonisation/clinical infection is independent of the number of other patients harbouring the organism. Once a pathogen is identified, interventions aimed at reducing spread will also have some a role. Because colonised patients often enter the ICU undetected, the continuous trickle of new pathogens means that such outbreaks are inherently stable, and not subject to boom-bust epidemic.

Many outbreaks have implicated pathogen cross-transmission from patient to patient via the hands of transiently contaminated HCWs (25–28). Hand washing and grouping together of patients and HCWs (cohorting) are the primary methods of limiting opportunities for spread. Bacteria have been shown to persist on the hands of HCWs for periods of an hour or more—a process exacerbated when HCWs have infected nails (37). In other instances HCWs may become long-term carries of organisms such as *Pseudomonas aeruginosa* and MRSA (37,38) and induce outbreaks during periods of increased shedding (e.g., during the winter months). Opportunities for spread are related directly to the number of patients already colonised/infected. Therefore the incidence of new cases must be a function of the number of current cases, with some additional factor to account for the role of HCW intermediaries. Outbreaks of this nature are subject to the boom and bust epidemic cycle. Evidently when there are no cases there can be no cross-transmission. As the number of cases increase, so too does the number of opportunities for spread. Furthermore, fluctuations play a considerable role in the dynamics of such outbreaks.

Environmental sources have been implicated in a number outbreaks (39–41). The risks posed by airborne pathogens such as *Aspergillus*, particularly during building work, mean that without careful monitoring, many (if not all) patients can be exposed at once. If the pathogen is from a point source (e.g. food) then outbreaks will be clonal. Other outbreaks appear polyclonal, perhaps attributable to the underlying environmental flora. For the gram-positive organisms such as VRE, environmental contamination was held up as a primary source of transmission. Other studies using PFGE typing of isolates has called this role into question by demonstrating that environmental contamination is frequently sporadic and maintained only in the presence of colonised/infected patients (29,42). Where the pathogen source is common to all patients, the incidence of new cases is related only to exposure to the source. The primary risk factor for exposure will be exposure time (LOS). Where exposure is high (e.g., air contamination), the majority of patients can be colonised/infected at once. The outbreak will then persist endemically only until the source is identified (e.g., contaminated ducting), limited only by patient turnover. In rare circumstances, a contaminated patient environment may lead to spread to other patients, perhaps via an intermediate HCW or fomites (40). Such cases can, however, be indistinguishable from patient-HCW-patient transmission unless the environmental strain was different from the colonising strains.

ENDOGENOUS PATHOGEN MODELS

Consider an outbreak of endogenously acquired *Pseudomonas aeruginosa*, in which a fraction of patient enters the ICU carrying the organism (perhaps at undetectable levels). Following intubation, some patients may progress to develop infections such as ventilator-acquired pneumonia (VAP) (43,44). Subdividing patients into two classes, uncolonised and colonised, a total of five epidemiological events are of interest; admission and discharge of uncolonised/colonised patients and the detection of colonisation/infection from either surveillance or clinical specimens (Figure 1).

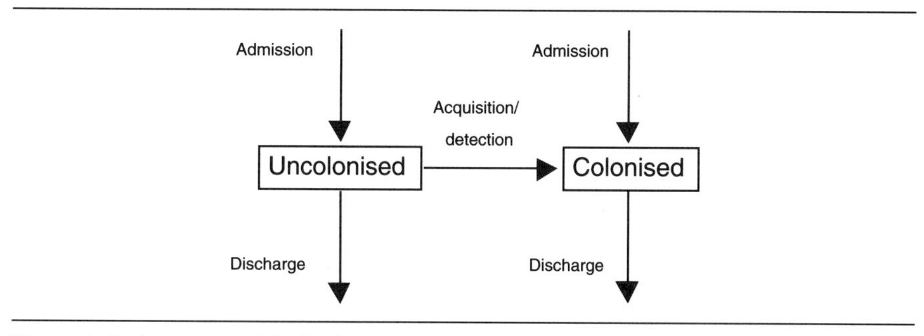

Figure 1. Endogenous model of pathogen acquisition.

The system can be described using two compartments each with a corresponding differential equation describing the rate of change of that population with time. Supposed there are B beds in the ICU. Let $X(t)$ denote the number of uncolonised patients at time, t, and $Y(t)$ the number colonised, then the equations describing the rates of change of X and Y are respectively

$$\frac{dX(t)}{dt} = \lambda(1-\phi\chi)(B-X-Y)-\mu X-\phi\sigma X$$
$$\frac{dY(t)}{dt} = \lambda\phi\chi(B-X-Y)-\mu' Y+\phi\sigma X \tag{1}$$

The first term in each equation is the admission rate, which is assumed to be bed-dependent at a rate λ/bed/day, with a maximum rate λB/day when empty and zero when full. A fraction of patients, ϕ, are assumed to be colonised at admission, although only some fraction, χ, are detected. The second term in each equation is the patient discharge rate. Patients are discharged at a per-capita rate μ/day if uncolonised, with average LOS = $1/\mu$ days (distributed exponentially), and μ'/day otherwise. Only patients already harbouring the pathogen are assumed to develop colonisation/infection, and once colonised, patients are assumed to remain so for the rest of their stay (there is no transition from Y to X). The final term describes the rate of endogenous acquisition/detection. Patients harbouring the pathogen (a fraction ϕ) are assumed to develop signs of detectable colonisation at a per-capita rate σ/day, with an average acquisition time, $T_a = 1/\sigma$ days.

Equation 1 is a deterministic formulation, in which the populations are counted using real numbers (i.e., it is perfectly acceptable to have 2.3 colonised patients). Patients of course come in integer quantities, and the usual interpretation of Equation 1 is that of the *average* number of colonised/uncolonised patients. For large populations, the difference between real numbers and integers is of no consequence. However in small populations there will be considerable differences between average behaviour predicted by Equation 1 and the course of any single outbreak.

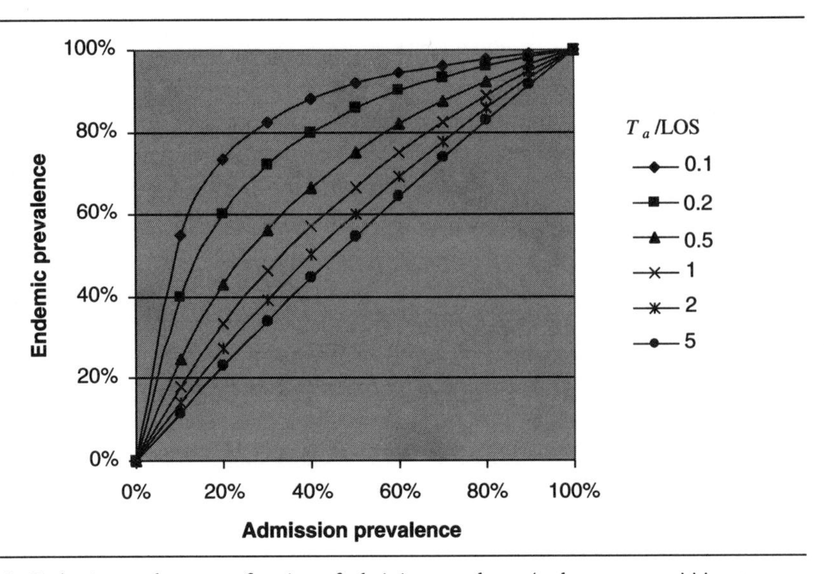

Figure 2. Endemic prevalence as a function of admission prevalence (endogenous acquisition χ = 100% detection).

In the complete absence of pathogen (zero admission prevalence, $\phi = 0$), the steady-state (equilibrium) occupancy is given by $X(t) = N = \lambda B/(\lambda + \mu)$, which is Binomially distributed with mean occupancy $\lambda/(\lambda + \mu)$, and $Y(t) = 0$. Since the model is linear (i.e., it does not involve terms of the form X^2, Y^2 or XY), given a starting condition, it can be solved exactly for all times. Moreover the stochastic form of the model can also be solved exactly and the mean uncolonised and colonised patient numbers are identical to the deterministic solution. The stochastic solution also permits estimation of the corresponding variances, which turn out to be less than the mean values (so-called under-dispersion). If colonised patients are admitted, whether detected or undetected, and colonisation does not increase patient LOS, then the endemic steady-state solution (no variation with time) is given by

$$X = \frac{(1-\chi\phi)}{1-\phi\sigma}N, \qquad Y = \frac{\phi(\sigma+\chi\mu)}{\mu+\phi\sigma}N$$

$$\text{Prevalence} = Y/N = \frac{\phi(1+\chi T_a/LOS)}{\phi+T_a/LOS} \tag{2}$$

where N is the average patient numbers, $\lambda B/(\lambda + \mu)$, and $T_a = 1/\sigma$, the acquisition time. Where detection rates are high and spontaneous progression low ($\chi \cong 1$, $\sigma \cong 0$), the endemic prevalence is approximately equal to the admission prevalence. Once the average acquisition time is short compared with the LOS ($\mu/\sigma = T_a/LOS < 1$) the prevalence increase disproportionately (Figure 2).

A) 16 beds, LOS = 7d, no endogenous acqusition

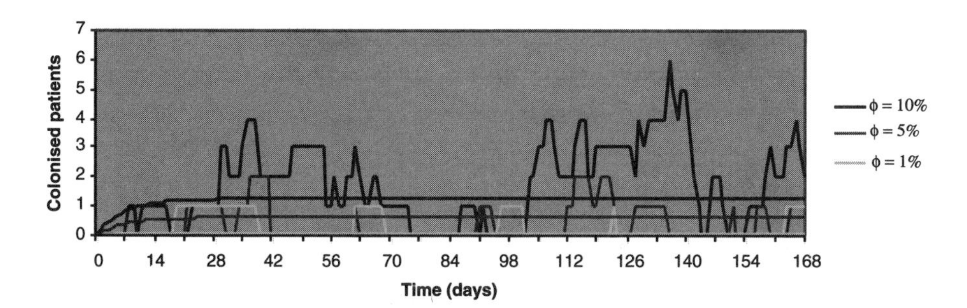

B) 16 beds, LOS = 7d, admission prevalence = 5%

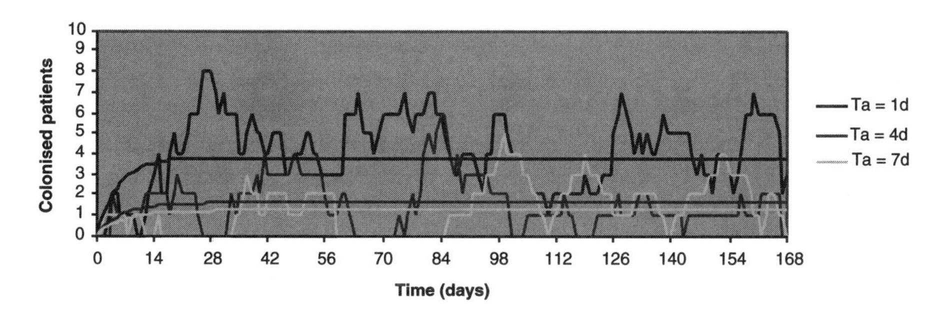

Figure 3. Simulations of endogenous acquisition.

Stochastic simulation of the model is straightforward. The deterministic model (Equation 1) represents the rates with which the five epidemiological processes of admission, discharge and acquisition occur. Treating $X(t)$ and $Y(t)$ as integer random variables, in some small time interval, dt, the numbers of each event can be simulated as a Poisson random number with mean: $dt \times$ rate. For example, the number of uncolonised new admissions in the time interval t to $t + dt$ will be approximately: Poisson$[dt \times \lambda(1 - \vartheta\chi)(B - X(t) - Y(t))]$. If sufficiently small time steps are taken, at most only one event will occur in any time step. Figure 3 shows three such stochastic realisations of the model (complete with deterministic solutions of Equation 1) for a 16-bed ICU (80% occupancy, LOS = 7 days) with A) increasing admission prevalence and B) increasing acquisition time, T_a. When the admission prevalence is low, cases are sporadic with considerable periods of "fade-out" (i.e., no affected patients). Notice that when the admission prevalence is only 10% the pathogen can become endemic for long periods. Without active surveillance only clinical cases are recognised. If the burden of colonisation: infection is 10:1 then the *observed* number of cases will be considerably lower.

It is important to note that endogenous cases represent the lowest achievable background, and reductions below this level will necessitate changes in surveillance. Cross-transmission is a threat that lies on top of this background. The limitation of patient-patient spread from an endogenously colonised case to another patient is the preserve of infection control. Without admission surveillance, it is however apparent that the stabilising influence of admissions will lead to rapid reintroduction.

MODELS OF PATHOGEN CROSS-TRANSMISSION

The Basic Reproductive Number R_0

A central foundation in infectious disease dynamics is the concept of a reproductive number. The basic reproductive number, R_0, is defined as the average number of secondary cases generated by an index case in a wholly susceptible population (29). For a pathogen to persist, each case must generate (on average) at least one new case. The magnitude of the reproductive number is a measure of the intensity of cross-transmission. If $R_0 > 1$ an epidemic is predicted, whereas if $R_0 < 1$, although secondary cases are possible the ultimate outcome will be extinction. Typically in large populations the endemic prevalence will be approximately $1 - 1/R_0$, implying that when $R_0 = 2$, half of the population will be colonised.

When patients are colonised on admission, the endemic prevalence is increased accordingly. In the ICU the situation is further complicate by two issues. First, the number of patients is small, which means that unless R_0 is much greater than one, outbreaks are still likely to fade out due to chance. Secondly, infection control reduces R_0 to an "effective" reproductive number, R, equal to the basic reproductive number multiplied by some reduction factor accounting for mixing and hand-washing practice. For directly transmitted infections such as childhood diseases, R_0 consists of a contact rate, a probability of infection and the duration of infectiousness.

For indirect transmission in via HCWs the basic reproductive number has two components: HCW-to-patient and patient-to-HCW. Typically HCWs will be contaminated transiently (hours), whereas patients will be colonised for much of their stay (days). Therefore colonised patients contaminate HCWs on many occasions, but contaminated HCWs colonise patients infrequently. For an outbreak to occur, only the product $R_0 = R_{\text{HCW-patient}} \times R_{\text{patient-HCW}}$ need be greater than unity. One consequence of this difference in magnitude is that the endemic prevalence of HCW contamination will be very low, and HCW surveillance via hand cultures may prove ineffectual in identifying sources of spread (27).

The Ross-Macdonald Model of Cross-transmission

Advances in molecular typing have clearly implicated the role of cross-transmission via the hands of HCWs in many outbreaks (25–28). We proposed a quantitative description of this process using mathematical models motivated by earlier work in vector-borne infections such as malaria (24,29). Using the Ross-Macdonald model

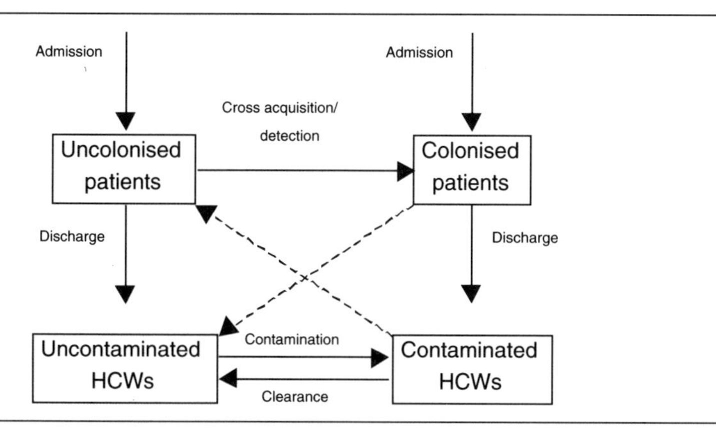

Figure 4. Ross-Macdonald model of cross-transmission.

of malaria (29), in which HCWs are identified as vectors, we were able to identify the key parameters necessary to characterise nosocomial cross-transmission.

The model of nosocomial cross-transmission requires four compartments to describe both uncolonised/colonised patients and HCWs in the ICU (Figure 4).

Using the same demographic assumptions as the endogenous model, and assuming that that detection at admission is complete ($\chi = 1$), the deterministic model of cross-transmission can be described by the following equations:

$$
\begin{aligned}
\frac{dX_p(t)}{dt} &= \lambda(1-\phi)(B - X_p - Y_p) - \mu X_p - ab_p Y_h X_p \\
\frac{dY_p(t)}{dt} &= \lambda\phi(B - X_p - Y_p) - \mu' Y_p + ab_p Y_h X_p \\
\frac{dX_h(t)}{dt} &= -ab_h Y_p X_h + \gamma Y_h \\
\frac{dY_h(t)}{dt} &= ab_h Y_p X_h - \gamma Y_h
\end{aligned} \tag{3}
$$

where X(t) denotes uncolonised/uncontaminated and $Y(t)$ colonised/contaminated. A subscript p implies patients and h HCWs. The parameter a is the per-capita contact rate/patient/HCW/day. Each susceptible patient receives aY_h infectious contacts with HCWs/day and has a probability b_p of subsequently developing colonisation. Likewise, Each uncolonised HCW has aY_p contacts with colonised patients/day and has a probability b_h of becoming contaminated. Once contaminated, the pathogen is cleared from the hands of HCWs at a rate γ/hour (i.e., they remain infectious for an average duration, $D_h = 1/\gamma$ hours). There are two underlying assumptions of the model. First, the number of HCWs is constant (note that $dN_h/dt = dX_h/dt + dY_h/dt = 0$). Secondly, there is "random mixing" in which all HCWs interact with all patients and vice versa. In the absence of cohorting this is a reasonable approximation, particularly for the movements of physicians. For nurses, however, cohorting plays an essential role and will be dealt with in the next section.

The basic reproductive number, R_0, for the model of Equation 3 can be shown to take the form;

$$R_0 = a^2 b_p b_h N_p N_h D_p D_h \tag{4}$$

where N_p is the number of patients, N_h the number of HCWs, D_p the colonised patient LOS and D_h the duration of HCW contamination. Notice that R_0 is a function of the contact rate squared because two contacts are required for transmission from patient to patient: patient-HCW and HCW-patient. A full analysis of the model is beyond the scope of the text, and being non-linear (i.e., there are terms involving $X_p Y_h$ and $Y_p X_h$), no exact solution is possible. It can however be shown that when no admissions are already colonised, the endemic prevalence of colonisation and contamination are respectively

$$\frac{Y_p}{N_p} = \frac{R_0 - 1}{R_0 + ab_p N_p D_h}, \quad \frac{Y_h}{N_h} = \frac{R_0 - 1}{R_0 + ab_h N_h D_p} \tag{5}$$

Since D_h is much less than D_p, the endemic patient prevalence will be approximately $1 - 1/R_0$ and the endemic HCW prevalence $(R_0 - 1)/ab_h N_h D_p$. When colonised patients are also admitted, admissions, provides a lower bound on endemic prevalence (Figure 4). Where colonisation confers an increase in LOS, the endemic prevalence will be more than proportional to admissions.

A Model Simplification: The Quasi Steady-State Approximation

The pronounced difference in time scale between HCW contamination (hours) and patient colonisation (days) means that on the time scale of days the dynamics of HCW contamination are effectively always at steady-state (i.e., $dX_h/dt = dY_h/dt = 0$). Therefore the number of contaminated HCWs at time t will be approximately

$$Y_h(t) = \frac{ab_h N_h}{\gamma + ab_h Y_p(t)} Y_p(t) \tag{6}$$

When this is substituted back into Equation 3 the two HCW equations can be omitted giving just two equations. Including endogenous acquisition, the full model can be approximated by;

$$\begin{aligned}
\frac{dX_p(t)}{dt} &= \lambda(1-\chi\phi)(B - X_p - Y_p) - \mu X_p - \phi\sigma X_p - R_0 \mu'(Y_p/N_p)X_p \\
\frac{dY_p(t)}{dt} &= \lambda\chi\phi(B - X_p - Y_p) - \mu' Y(t) + \phi\sigma X_p + R_0 \mu'(Y_p/N_p)X_p
\end{aligned} \tag{7}$$

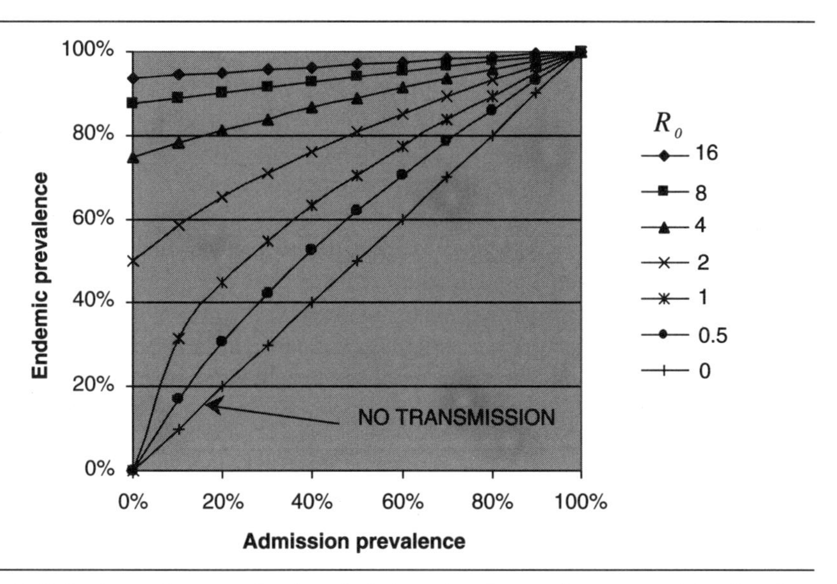

Figure 5. Endemic prevalence as a function of admission Prevalence and cross-transmission intensity (no excess LOS).

When formulated in this way, many of the difficult to estimate parameters, such as contacts rates, transmission probabilities and duration of HCW contamination can be "collapsed" into the basic reproductive number, R_0. Exact solution Equation 7 is possible provided colonisation confers no additional LOS (i.e., $\mu = \mu'$) and the steady-state endemic prevalence is given by

$$\text{Prevalence} = \frac{(R_0 - 1 - \phi T_a/LOS) + \sqrt{(R_0 - 1 - \phi T_a/LOS)^2 + 4R_0\phi(\chi + T_a/LOS)}}{2R_0} \tag{8}$$

Plotting this function produces a combination of Figures 2. and 5. (not shown).

Of greater interest is a stochastic realisation of the model, in which a total of six epidemiological events must be considered: uncolonised/colonised admissions and discharges, endogenous and cross-acquisition. Figure 6. Shows the effect of increasing basic reproductive number, R_0, on ten simulated outbreaks in a 16-bed ICU with demographics as before. As expected, the random fluctuations dominate, and it is only for relatively large values of R_0 that pathogens become endemically stable—albeit in a minority of outbreaks.

For ICUs with 16 beds or fewer, the deterministic solution is not a good approximation to the average behaviour because of the number of fade-outs; even when $R_0 > 1$. In the first example ($R_0 = 0.5$), no endemic state is possible and the model predicts that 95% of outbreaks will finish within 30 days. If $R_0 = 2$, where typically

A) R_0 = 0.5, no colonised admissions, no endogenous acquisition

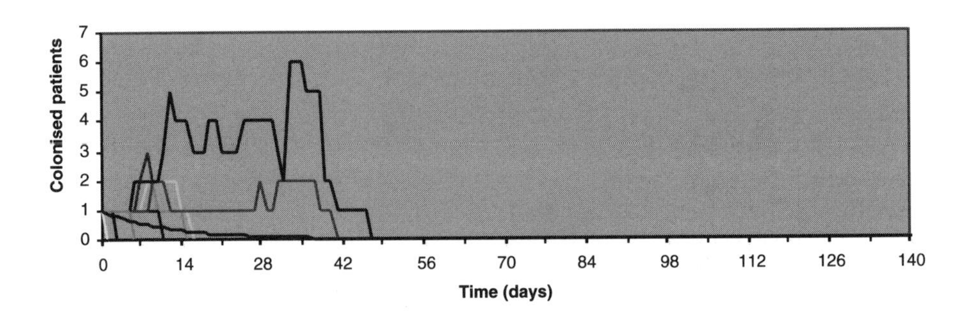

B) R_0 = 2, no colonised admissions, no endogenous acquisition

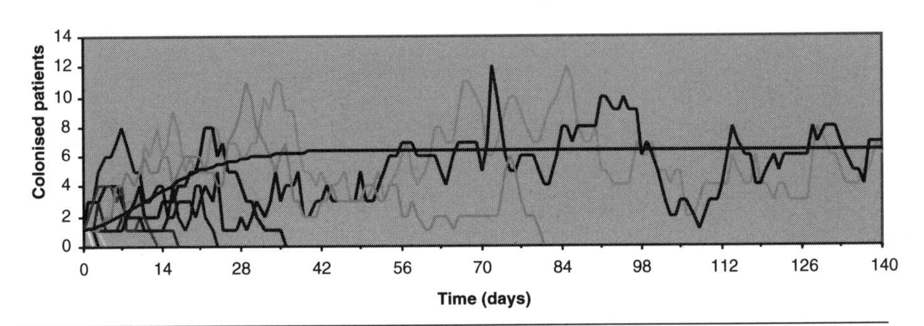

Figure 6. Stochastic realisation of the QSSA model, with deterministic solution, for a 16-bed ICU with LOS = 7 days.

50% of patients would be expected to be endemically colonised, the model predicts that 95% of outbreaks would fade out after 37 weeks. With as few as 1% of colonised admissions, the model predicts that reintroduction can easily stabilise endemicity.

ENVIRONMENTAL SOURCES

For completeness, environmental routes can be treated as analogous to either endogenous or cross-transmission, depending on nature. Where a point source is implicated, the incidence term will have a linear form similar to the endogenous case, although the acquisition rate, σ, will be independent of admission prevalence because all patients are potentially susceptible. With the exception of airborne pathogens, such outbreaks are fortunately rare and easily controlled once identified. Where a patient contaminates their environment, there is little to distinguish between patient-HCW-patient, environment-HCW-patient, or indeed environment-HCW-environment transmission. Typing studies are only now beginning to determine whether a patient contaminates their environment or vice versa. For the sake of the model the incidence term and basic reproductive number, R_0, can be thought of as encompassing both routes.

THE IMPACT OF INFECTION CONTROL

Infection control practices are aimed primarily at limiting opportunities for pathogen spread from patient to patient. Although the transmission process itself appears unable to sustain persistent outbreaks, the use of infection control practices will help shorten the outbreak and limit the number of cases. The practice of hand disinfection and barrier precautions act directly to reduce the basic reproductive number, R_0, to an effective reproductive number, R, which is be estimable from observation. Once infection control practices are quantified, extrapolation from the effective reproductive number, R, to the true reproductive number, R_0, provides an estimate of the efficacy of infection control.

Hand Washing and Disinfection

Where hand washing is practised either before *or* after patient after patient contact, there will be corresponding reductions in *one* of the two acquisition probabilities; b_p and b_h. Where hand washing is conducted before *and* after contact, the effect is multiplied. If p denotes the compliance with hand-washing guidelines, and hand washing is assumed 100% effective, then the effective reproductive number will be

$$R(p) = R_0(1-p)^{1 \text{ or } 2} \tag{9}$$

Since the efficacy of hand washing soaps is typically evaluated for a 30-second wash, the true efficacy is likely to be less than 100% (5). The compliance, p, should therefore be reduced accordingly, such that $p \equiv$ compliance $\times$ efficacy. Control of transmission is possible once the effective reproductive number reaches unity.

Observed compliance with hand washing practice have frequently proven disappointing, with compliance seldom greater than 50%, and reduced by factors such as profession, workload, and facility (7). Even in a best-case scenario Equation 9 suggests that control of transmission is only likely where R_0 lies is at most 2–3, perhaps considerably less when efficacy is factored into the equation. Early studies of gloving have shown contamination levels of up to 40% for VRE (47) and at least 15% for MRSA following glove removal (H. Grundmann, private communication). The use of hand disinfection is gaining considerable favour in Europe, both for reasons of improved convenience (i.e., compliance) and efficacy (9). In such circumstances, a two-fold reduction in the basic reproductive number seems feasible, with equally respectable reductions in prevalence (Figure 5).

HealthCare Worker—Patient Mixing

The Ross-Macdonald transmission model (Equation 3) assumes random mixing between HCWs and patients. For some professions this will be valid, although for nursing staff, where cohorting with patients is often practised, the assumption may be violated. Mixing enters the expression for R_0 (Equation 4) in several ways such that the precise effects of staffing levels may vary between settings. Where the number of patient contacts is the limiting factor (i.e., patients require a *fixed* number of contacts, aN_h/day), increasing the number of HCWs will lower the per-capita contact rate, a, and subsequently R_0 (because it is squared). Doubling the number of staff halves transmission. Conversely where the HCWs are working at full capacity the per-capita contact rate, a, remains constant, and the introduction of additional staff *increases* transmission. Doubling the number of HCWs doubles the number of contacts and hence transmission. In the ICU setting the former scenario appears more likely (20,46,47).

The grouping of patients and HCWs into cohorts provides a powerful method of restricting transmission—provided the cohort is not broken (10–23). Colonised patients may be physically grouped together (e.g., multiple occupancy isolation rooms) or nurses assigned to specific patients. In either event, provided HCWs do not move between colonised and uncolonised patients their role in cross-transmission will be minimal. Unlike hand washing, there have been no attempts to quantify cohorting rates. We defined a cohorting probability as the probability that a HCW returns to the same patients for the following contact (24). Evidently if all HCWs move randomly from patient to patient this probability has a lower value of $1/N_p$, the number of patients. If HCWs only see the same patient then the probability must be unity. In fact an upper bound on the cohorting probability is provided by the staff-patient ratio.

Observational studies of mixing have yet to be published, although preliminary work suggests that the cohorting probability may be as high as 80% for nursing staff in ICU settings (24). The overall impact on cohorting is to reduces the effective number of HCWs contributing to transmission, such that if q is the cohorting probability, then the effective reproductive number is

$$R(q) = R_0 \frac{(1-q)}{1-1/N_p} \tag{10}$$

Where the denominator is a small correction factor accounting for the limited patient numbers. Where physical cohorts are implemented, the cohorting probability can be viewed as the probability that a contact is from within the same cohort. Sub-models of Equation 3 can be used to describe each patient cohort, with mixing between cohorts at a rate reduced by a factor $(1 - q)$. The fact that the cohorting probability appears much higher than hand-washing compliance is of considerable importance. Equation 10 suggests that protection against cross-transmission can be afforded when is as large as $R_0 = 5$ with 1:1 nursing.

Combined Infection Control Practices

The fact that hand washing alone may not afford complete control of transmission means that a combined infection control strategy is needed. Combining the prac-

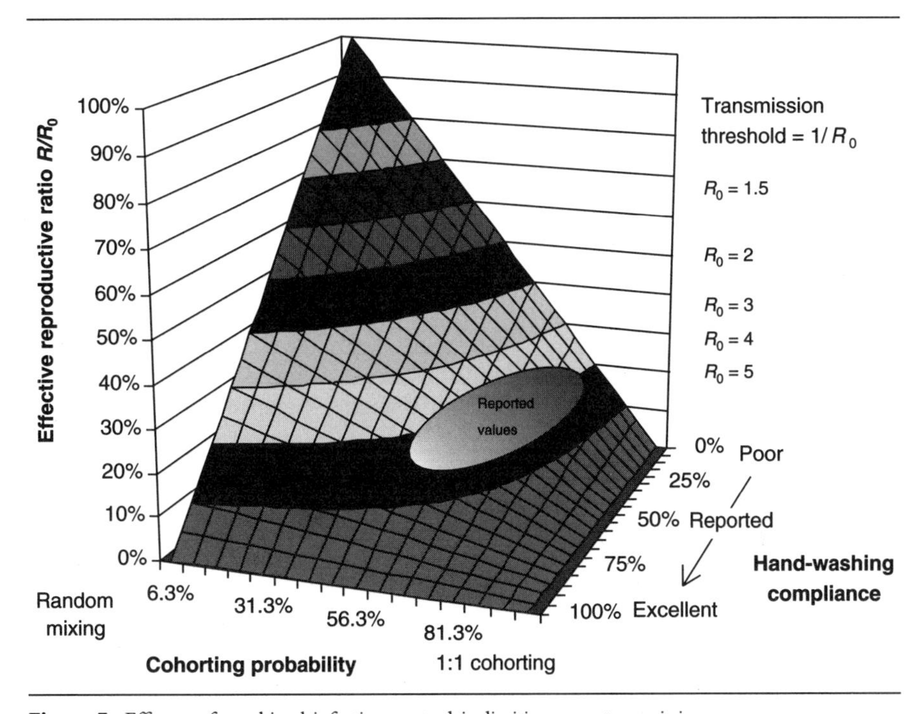

Figure 7. Efficacy of combined infection control in limiting cross-transmission.

tices of hand washing and cohorting produces an effective reproductive number that is a function of both hand-washing compliance and cohorting probability;

$$R(p,q) = R_0 \frac{(1-p)(1-q)}{1-1/N_p} \tag{11}$$

Figure 7 shows the effect of combined infection control measures on reducing the intensity of transmission assuming that hands are washed only once between contacts. Control is possible provided the effective reproductive ratio, R/R_0, is greater than $1/R_0$. Reported hand-washing compliance and suggested cohorting probabilities indicate that control is be possible for $R_0 < 5$. In settings where pathogens persist despite such measures, other sources of colonisation should be considered; reintroduction, endogenous routes and environmental contamination.

Intervention studies of infection control have shown mixed results (e.g., reference 11). One explanation for the apparent discrepancies in outcome is the stochastic nature of outbreaks. Using a stochastic formulation of Equation 7. In which the basic reproductive number, R_0 is replaced by its effective counterpart, $R(p,q)$, numerical experiments are possible. Consider a 16-bed ICU in which hand-washing compliance is 50% and cohorting 80%, the basic reproductive number will be reduced by a factor $(1 - 0.5) \times (1 - 0.8) = 0.1$. Contrast this with an intervention that raises hand-washing compliance to an (unlikely) 75%, giving a reduction factor of 0.05. If the basic reproductive number, $R_0 = 10$ then the effective reproductive numbers will be 1 and 0.5 respectively. We can pose the question how often will things be "worse" (defined as higher prevalence in the intervention ICU) by chance? Surprisingly, the model predicts that unless R_0 is large (e.g., 16), only 1/2–3/4 of outbreaks will end faster with intervention. The low power of such intervention trials is of obvious concern.

ANTIBIOTIC USE

Patients in the ICU are subject to relatively high antibiotic pressure either for therapeutic or prophylactic reasons. This antibiotic use exerts considerable selection on the patient host flora, generating de novo antibiotic-resistant mutants, which subsequently grow up under selection to cause endogenous resistant colonisation. Furthermore, the use of broad-spectrum antibiotics can effectively reduce the patient host flora, increasing their susceptibility to subsequent colonisation via cross-transmission by pathogens such as VRE and MRSA.

Endogenous Colonisation

The use of antibiotics give resistant a selective growth advantage (43,44). If patients already harbour resistant strains (or sensitive strains where other flora are reduced) the rate of acquisition (σ/day in Equation 1) will become a function of antibiotic use. Suppose that antibiotic pressure is measured as the fraction of the patient LOS, α, for which antibiotics are prescribed, and that whilst on antibiotic therapy there is an increased relative risk, r, of endogenous acquisition. Then the rate of acquisition will be approximately

$$\sigma(\alpha, r) = (1-\alpha)\sigma + r\alpha\sigma = \sigma(1+\alpha(r-1)) \tag{12}$$

Substituting this expression into the formula for endemic prevalence (Equation 2) gives the prevalence as a function of antibiotic pressure. Figure 8 shows the endemic prevalence when there is a relative risk of two of endogenous selection and the average acquisition time is half the LOS. Because the endogenous model does not account for de novo selection, the endemic prevalence depends only weakly on antibiotic pressure and such a relationship is unlikely to seen in situ.

If de novo selection is also included in the model, then an additional endogenous term must be added to Equation 1 of the form; $\alpha\varepsilon\sigma X(t)$, where ε is the probability of selecting resistant strains (i.e., the strains of interest) from the host flora during the course of therapy. The endemic steady-state prevalence will be

$$\text{Prevalence} = \frac{\phi(1+T_a(\alpha,r)/LOS)+\alpha\varepsilon}{\phi+T_a(\alpha,r)/LOS+\alpha\varepsilon} \tag{13}$$

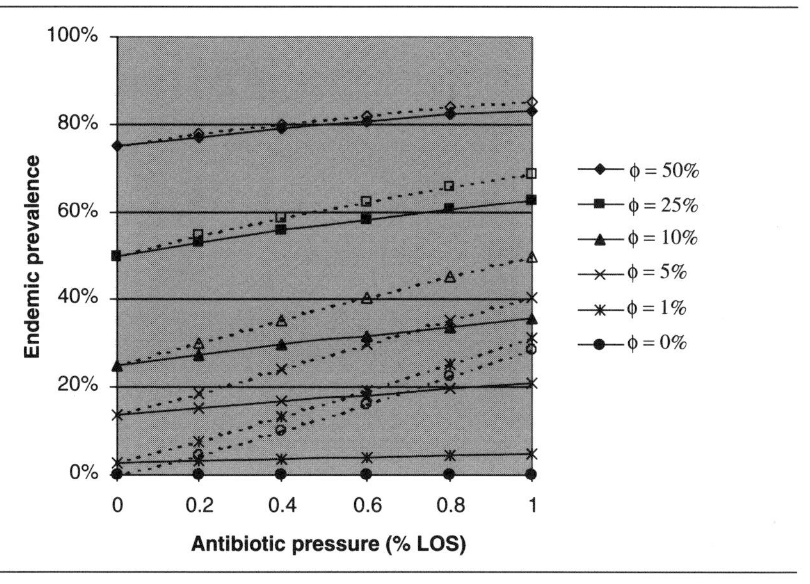

Figure 8. Effect of antibiotic pressure on endogenous acquisition (T_a/LOS = 0.5, relative risk of acquisition = 2/day, ε = 10%).

shown as the dashed lines in Figure 8 Where the prevalence of carriage is high (e.g., commensal organisms), the endemic colonisation prevalence is equivalent to the frequency of resistance. The form of Equation 13. implies that antibiotic selection can maintain resistance even in the absence of colonised admissions at an approximate frequency $\alpha\varepsilon\mathrm{LOS}/T_a(\alpha,r)$—the effect being most evident when colonisation is rare on admission.

Cross-transmission

Antibiotic use also has implications for cross-transmission. The use of selective digestive decontamination (SDD) for prophylaxis presents potential antibiotic resistant pathogens with an open colonisation site. Recall that the basic reproductive number, R_0, is proportional to the probability of colonisation, b_p, following an infectious contact with a contaminated HCW (Equation 4). If antibiotic selection confers an additional risk of colonisation, then the effective reproductive number, R, becomes an increasing function of antibiotic pressure. By analogy with the endogenous case, the effective reproductive number will be

$$R(\alpha,r) = R_0(1+\alpha(r-1)) \tag{14}$$

Where r is now a measure of the increased relative risk of colonisation via cross-transmission. The QSSA endemic prevalence under antibiotic selection will be

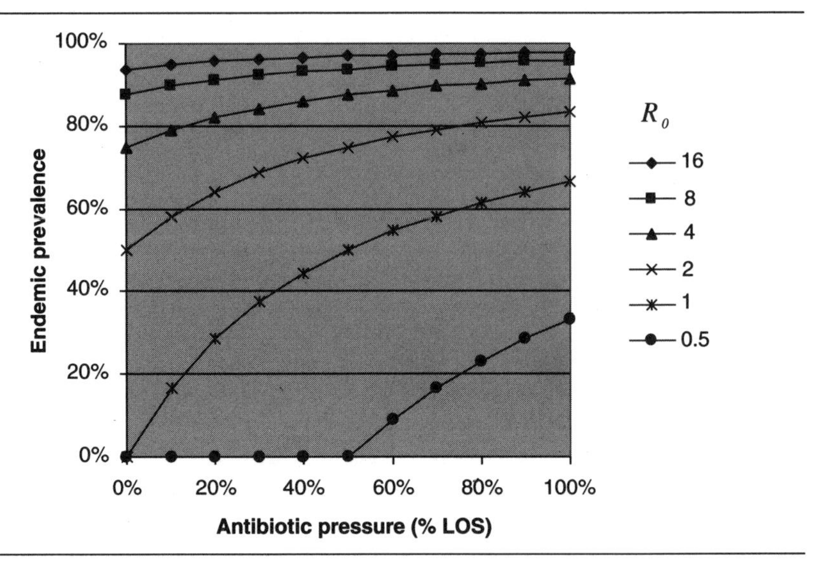

Figure 9. Effect of antibiotic pressure on cross-acquisition (relative colonisation risk/day = 2).

$$\text{Prevalence}(\alpha, r) = 1 - 1/R(\alpha, r) \tag{15}$$

as shown in Figure 9 for a relative colonisation risk, r = 2. Although the precise additional risk is not known for many pathogens, the model clearly shows that the greatest effect on transmission is to be found when the basic reproductive number is close to the transmission threshold R_0 = 1. In fact, it can be shown that when R_0 is below the cross-transmission threshold, if the relative risk exceeds $1/R_0$, antibiotic selection can force the effective reproductive number $R(\alpha,r)$ to be greater than unity. Combining this effect with those of endogenous selection means that antibiotic resistant pathogens can easily become endemic under antibiotic pressure.

CASE STUDY: VRE

Our original study of VRE transmission was based on a 16-bed surgical/medical ICU at the Cook County Hospital, Chicago, IL (8,24,28). During the course of a 133-day study, 189 patients were admitted to the ICU, 15% of whom were already colonised with VRE. A further 45 patients acquired VRE during their stay. Bed occupancy averaged 87% and the endemic prevalence of colonisation was 36%. The deterministic steady-state solution suggests that the effective reproductive number, R was 0.69, with a basic reproductive number $R_0 \cong 4$ after accounting for infection control practices. Using these numbers, infection control practices were estimated to have reduced the endemic prevalence from a predicted 76% to the observed 36%. Parameters were estimated by fitting 10^5 stochastic realisations of the

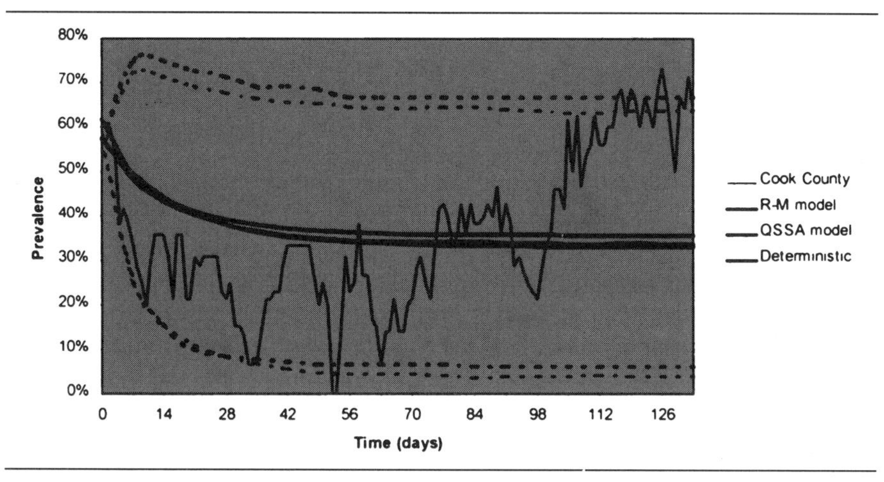

Figure 10. Prevalence of VRE at Cook County 16-bed surgical/medical ICU. LOS = 9d (14d for VRE cases), $R(p,q) = 0.69$, $\phi = 15\%$, $\chi = 1$, $\sigma = 0$.

Ross-Macdonald model (Equation 3) to observation, and good agreement was found, both qualitatively and quantitatively.

Figure 10 shows: A) the observed endemic prevalence of VRE colonisation during the study, B) the predicted mean (solid lines) and 95% confidence intervals (dotted lines) calculated from 10^5 simulations of the Ross-Macdonald model, C) the predicted mean and 95% confidence intervals from 10^5 simulations of the QSSA model where the confidence intervals are estimated as mean $\pm$ 1.96 $\times$ standard deviation, and D) the deterministic QSSA solution. There is excellent between the mean behaviour of the two simulation methods and the deterministic solution, although there is slight bias in the QSSA estimate of the 95% confidence intervals because the assumption of normality is violated.

The QSSA model clearly has advantages; namely that parameter estimation is minimal. From the endemic prevalence an estimate of the effective reproductive number is found and simulation possible. Moreover, by incorporating the endogenous acquisition term, it is equally possible to fit other aspects of the data such as fade-out probabilities and time between cases in non-endemic settings using $R(p,q)$, admission prevalence and endogenous acquisition time as variables to be fitted.

SUMMARY

Understanding the dynamics of nosocomial outbreaks in the ICU setting is of considerable importance if the threat of antibiotic resistance is to be countered. Pathogens are typically acquired by any of three routes; endogenous carriage, cross-transmission via the hands of HCWs and environmental contamination. Identification of the primary acquisition route is of key importance in understanding how best to tackle outbreaks. Typically only a small fraction of the total pathogen burden is manifest in clinical disease. The remaining colonisation pressure, however, plays the dominant role in maintaining endemic pathogens in the ICU. The use of mathematical models to quantitatively describe the colonisation processes is a new field. The small populations involved mean that identifying the signal of persistence from the noise of random fluctuations is very difficult. Nevertheless models show that the cross-transmission process is inherently unstable and endemic pathogens are unlikely to be maintained solely by such a route.

Cross-transmission is characterised by the number of secondary cases produced by the index case, termed the basic reproductive number, R_0. Endemicity requires that the basic reproductive number be greater than unity, although without readmission or endogenous pathways, eventual fade-out is the likely outcome. The Ross-Macdonald model of malaria transmission provides an accurate description of the patient-HCW-patient spread in ICUs, with predicted basic reproductive numbers of at least four. Infection control reduces R_0 to values typically less than unity, whereas antibiotic pressure increases it. The model predicts that limitations in hand-washing compliance mean that control of spread is unlikely without further measures such as patient-HCW cohorting. Antibiotic restriction is predicted to play an important role when close to the transmission threshold but will have only limited impact in highly endemic settings.

ACKNOWLEDGEMENT

This work was supported in part by a grant from The Wellcome Trust, and by *Glaxo Wellcome*.

REFERENCES

1. Weinstein RA. Nosocomial infection update. *Emerging Infectious Diseases* 1998;4:416–419.
2. Albert RK, Condie F. Hand washing patterns in medical intensive care units. *New England Journal of Medicine* 1981;304:1465–1468.
3. Larson E. Compliance with isolation technique. *American Journal of Infection Control* 1983;11:221–225.
4. Simmons B, Bryant J, Neiman K, Spencer L, Arheart K. The role of hand washing in the prevention of endemic intensive care unit infections. *Infection Control and Hospital Epidemiology* 1992;11:589–594.
5. Doebbelling BN, Stanley GL, Sheetz CT, Pfaller MA, Houston AK, Li N, Wenzel RP. Comparative efficacy of alternative hand-washing agents in reducing nosocomial infections in intensive care units. *New England Journal of Medicine* 1992;327:88–93.
6. Watanakunakorn C, Wong CJH. An observational study of hand washing and infection control practices by healthcare workers. *Infection Control and Hospital Epidemiology* 1998;19:858–860.
7. Pittet D, Mourouga P, Perneger TV. Compliance with hand washing in a teaching hospital. *Annals of Internal Medicine* 1999;130:126–130.
8. Slaughter S, Hayden MK, Nathan C, Hu TC, Rice T, Van Voortis J, Matusheka M, Franklin C, Weinstein RA. A comparison of the effect of universal use of gloves and gowns with that of glove use alone on the acquisition of vancomycin-resistant enterococci in a medical intensive care unit. *Annals of Internal Medicine* 1996;125:448–456.
9. Boyce JM. Is it time for action: Improving hand hygiene in hospitals. *Annals of Internal Medicine* 1999;130:153–154.
10. Doherty JA, Brookfield DS, Gray J, McEwan RA. Cohorting of infants with respiratory syncytial virus. *Journal of Hospital Infection* 1998;38:203–206.
11. Ehrenkranz NJ, Sanders CC, Eckert-Schollenberger D, Hufcut RM, MacDonald N, Stone J, Sander Jr WE. Lack of efficacy of cohorting nursing personnel in a neonatal intensive care unit to prevent

contact spread of bacteria: an experimental study. *Paediatric Infectious Diseases Journal* 1992;11:105–113.

12. Garcia R, Raad I, Abi-Said D, Bodey G, Champlin R, Tarrand J, Hill LA, Umphrey J, Neumann J, Englund J, Whimbey E. Nosocomial respiratory syncytial virus infections: prevention and control in bone marrow transplant patients. *Infection Control and Hospital Epidemiology* 1997;18:412–416.
13. Gerding DN, Johnson S, Peterson LR, Mulligan ME, Silva Jr. J. *Clostridium difficile*-associated diarrhea and colitis. *Infection Control and Hospital Epidemiology* 1995;16:459–477.
14. Isaacs D, Dickson H, O'Callaghan C, Sheaves R, Winter A, Moxon ER. Hand washing and cohorting in prevention of hospital acquired infections with respiratory syncytial virus. *Archives of Diseases in Children* 1991;66:227–231.
15. Mayall B, Martin R, Keenan AM, Irving L, Leeson P, Lamb K. Blanket use of intranasal mupriocin for outbreak control and long-term prophylaxis of endemic methicillin-resistant *Staphylococcus aureus* in an open ward. *Journal of Hospital Infection* 1996;32:257–266.
16. Moisiuk SE, Robson D, Klass L, Kliewer G, Wasliuk W, Davi M, Plourde P. Outbreak of parainfluenza virus type 3 in an intermediate care neonatal nursery. *Paediatric Infectious Diseases Journal* 1998;17:49–53.
17. Struelens MJ, Maas A, Nonhoff C, Deplano A, Rost F, Serruys E, Delmee M. Control of nosocomial transmission of *Clostridium difficile* based on sporadic case surveillance. *American Journal of Medicine* 1991;16:138S–144S.
18. Cohen SH, Morita MM, Bradford M. A seven-year experience with methicillin-resistant *Staphylococcus aureus*. *American Journal of Medicine* 1991;91:233S–237S.
19. CDC. Recommendations for preventing the spread of vancomycin resistance. *MMWR* 1995;44((RR12)):1–13.
20. Haley RW, Cushion NB, Tenover FC, Bannerman TL, Dryer D, Ross J, Sanchez PJ, Siegel JD. Eradication of endemic methicillin-resistant *Staphylococcus aureus* from a neonatal intensive care unit. *Journal of Infectious Diseases* 1995;171:614–624.
21. Reish O, Ashkenazi S, Naor N, Samra Z, Merlob P. An outbreak of multiresistant *Klebsiella* in a neonatal intensive care unit. *Journal of Hospital Infection* 1993;25:287–291.
22. Rumback MJ, Cancio MR. Significant reduction in methcillin-resistant *Staphylococcus aureus* ventillator-associated pneumonia associated with the institution of a prevention protocol. *Critical Care Medicine* 1995;23:1200–1203.
23. Romance K, Nicolle L, Ross J, Law B. An outbreak of methicillin-resistant *Staphylococcus aureus* in a pediatric hospital—how it got away and how we caught it. *Canadian Journal of Infection Control* 1991(6):11–13.
24. Austin DJ, Bonten MJ, Slaughter S, Weinstein RA, Anderson RM. Vancomycin resistant enterococci (VRE) in intensive care hospital settings: transmission dynamics, persistence and the impact of infection control programs. *Proceedings of the National Academy of Science* 1999;96:6908–6913.
25. Casewell M, Phillips I. Hands as a route of transmission for *Klebsiella* species. *British Medical Journal* 1977;2:1315–1317.
26. Sanchez V, Vazquez JA, Barth-Jones D, Dembry L, Sobel DJ, Zervos MJ. Epidemiology of nosocomial acquisition of *Candida lusitaniae*. *Journal of Clinical Microbiology* 1992;30:3005–3008.
27. Noskin GA, Stosor V, Cooper I, Peterson LR. Recovery of vancomycin-resistant enterococci on fingertips and environmental surfaces. *Infection Control and Hospital Epidemiology* 1995;16:577–581.
28. Bonten MJ, Hayden MK, Nathan C, Van Voortis J, Matushek M, Slaughter S, Rice T, Weinstein RA. Epidemiology of colonization of patients and environment with vancomycin-resistant enterococci. *The Lancet* 1996;348:1615–1619.
29. Anderson RM, May RM. Infectious Diseases of Humans: Dynamics and Control Oxford: Oxford University Press, 1991.
30. Zuckerman et al. *Infection Control and Hospital Epidemiology* 1999;20:686–686.
31. Grundmann H, Kropec A, Hartung D, Berner R, Daschner F. *Pseudomonas aeruginosa* in a neonatal intensive care unit: reservoirs and ecology of the nosocomial pathogen. Journal of Infectious Diseases 1993;168:943–947.
32. Bonten MJ, Bergmans DC, Speijer H, Stobberingh EE. Characteristics of polyclonal endemicity of *Pseudomonas aeruginosa* in intensive care units: implications for infection control. American Journal of Respiratory and Critical Care Medicine 1999;160:1212–1219.
33. Talon D, Mulin B, Rouget C, Bailly P, Thouverez M, Viel JF. Risks and routes for ventilator-associated pneumonia with *Pseudomonas aeruginosa*. American Journal of Respiratory and Critical Care Medicine 1998;157:978–984.

34. Talon D, Capellier G, Boillot A, Michel-Briand Y. Use of pulsed-field gel electrophoresis as an epidemiologic tool during an outbreak of *Pseudomonas aeruginosa* lung infections in an intensive care unit. Intesive Care Medicine 1995;21:996–1002.
35. Flynn DM, Weinstein RA, Nathan C, Gaston M, Kabins SA. Patient's endogenous flora as the source of "nosocomial" Enterobacter in cardiac surgery. Journal of Infectious Diseases 1987;156:263–268.
36. Flanagan PG. Fungal infections in the intensive care unit. Journal of Hospital Infection 1998;38:163–177.
37. Foca M. Jakob K. Whittier S. Della Latta P. Factor S. Rubenstein D. Saiman L. Endemic *Pseudomonas aeruginosa* infection in a neonatal intensive care unit. *New England Journal of Medicine* 2000;343:695–700.
38. Sheretz RJ. Reagan DR. Hampton KD. Robertson KL. Streed SA. Hoen HM. Thomas R. Gwaltney JM Jr. A cloud adult: the Staphylococcus aureus-virus interaction revisited. *Annals of Internal Medicine* 1996;124:539–547.
39. Villers D, Espaze E, Coste-Burel M, et al. Nosocomial *Acinetobacter baumannii* infections: microbiological and clinical epidemiology. Annals of Internal Medicine 1998;129:182–189.
40. Livornese Jr LL, Dias S, Samel C, Romanowski B, Taylor S, May P, Pitsakis P, Woods G, Kaye D, Levison ME, et al. Hospital-acquired infection with vancomycin-resistant *Enterococcus faecium* transmitted by electronic thermometers. Annals of Internal Medicine 1992;117:112–116.
41. VandenBergh MF. Verweij PE. Voss A. Epidemiology of nosocomial fungal infections: invasive aspergillosis and the environment. *Diagnostic Microbiology & Infectious Disease* 1999;34:221–227.
42. Maki DG, Alvarado CJ, Hassemer CA, Zilz MA. Relationship of the inanimate hospital environent to endemic nosocomial infection. *New England Journal of Medicine* 1982;307:1562–1566.
43. Bonten MJ, Bergmans DC, Ambergen AW, et al. Risk factors for pneumonia, and colonization of respiratory tract and stomach in mechanically ventilated ICU patients. *American Journal of Respiratory and Critical Care Medicine* 1996;19:853–855.
44. Talon D, Mulin B, Rouget C, Bailly P, Thouverez M, Viel JF. Risks and routes for ventilator-associated pneumonia with *Pseudomonas aeruginosa*. *American Journal of Respiratory and Critical Care Medicine* 1998;157:978–984.
45. Haley RW, Bregman DA. The role of understaffing and overcrowding in recurrent outbreaks of staphylococcal infection in a neonatal special-care unit. *Journal of Infectious Diseases* 1982;145:875–885.
46. Fridkin SK, Pear SM, Willaimson TH, Galgiani JN, Jarvis WR. The role of understaffing in central venous catheter-associated bloodstream infections. *Infection Control and Hospital Epidemiology* 1996;17:147–149.
47. Badri SM, Sahgal NB, Tenorio AR, et al. Effectiveness of gloves in preventing transmission of vancomycin-resistant enterococcus (VRE) during patient care activities. IDSA'98 1998; Abstract 599.

INDEX

D

E

F